Clinical dental hygiene

Clinical dental hygiene

Shailer Peterson
B.A., M.A., Ph.D., F.A.C.D.(Hon.), F.I.C.D.(Hon.)

Associate Dean and Professor of Dental Education, The University of Texas Dental School at San Antonio, Texas; formerly Dean and Professor of General Dentistry, University of Tennessee College of Dentistry, Memphis, Tenn.; Assistant Secretary for Educational Affairs of the American Dental Association, Secretary of the Council on Dental Education and Council of the National Board of Dental Examiners of the American Dental Association; affiliated with Chicago College of Dental Surgery, University of Chicago, South Dakota State College, University of Minnesota, and University of Oregon

Fourth edition

With 298 illustrations

The C. V. Mosby Company
Saint Louis 1972

Fourth edition

Copyright © 1972 by The C. V. Mosby Company

Previous editions copyrighted 1959, 1963, 1968

Printed in the United States of America

International Standard Book Number 0-8016-3810-0

Library of Congress Catalog Card Number 72-77196

Distributed in Great Britain by Henry Kimpton, London

Contributors

James T. Andrews, B.A., D.D.S., F.A.C.D.

Chairman and Professor of Department of Operative Dentistry and Director of Dental Auxiliary Utilization Program, University of Tennessee College of Dentistry, Memphis, Tennessee

Marilyn Moss Beck, B.S., R.D.H.

Assistant Professor of Dental Hygiene, Marquette University School of Dentistry, Milwaukee, Wisconsin

Harrison M. Berry, Jr., D.D.S., M.Sc., F.A.C.D.

Associate Dean and Professor of Radiology, School of Dental Medicine, University of Pennsylvania, Philadelphia, Pennsylvania

Eugene G. Brunson, D.D.S.

Oral Surgeon, Pensacola, Florida; formerly Associate Professor of Departments of Oral Surgery and Oral Pathology, University of Tennessee College of Dentistry, Memphis, Tennessee

James L. Bugg, Jr., B.A., D.M.D., M.S.

Professor of Department of Preventive Dentistry (Pedodontics), The University of Texas Dental Branch at Houston, Houston, Texas

Michael H. Burns, B.S., D.D.S., M.S.

Associate Professor of Department of Orthodontics, College of Medicine and Dentistry of New Jersey, New Jersey Dental School, Jersey City, New Jersey

Charles O. Cranford, D.D.S., M.P.A.

Graduate of the Lyndon B. Johnson School of Public Affairs, The University of Texas at Austin; formerly Chief, Manpower Development Branch, Division of Dental Health, National Institutes of Health, Department of Health, Education, and Welfare; currently assigned to the Office of the Assistant Secretary for Health and Scientific Affairs

James K. Foster, Jr., D.D.S., F.A.C.D.

Chairman and Professor, Departments of Oral Diagnosis and Roentgenology, The University of Texas Dental Branch at Houston, Houston, Texas

Tillie D. Ginsburg, B.A., R.D.H., M.Ed.

Director and Associate Professor of Dental Hygiene, Marquette University School of Dentistry, Milwaukee, Wisconsin

Kathryn S. Goller, C.D.A., R.D.H.

Clinical Associate, Department of Community Dentistry, Co-director of Dental Therapist Training Program, University of Alabama in Birmingham School of Dentistry, Birmingham, Alabama

Maynard K. Hine,
D.D.S., M.S., D.Sc., F.I.C.D., F.A.C.D.

Chancellor, Indiana University-Purdue University at Indianapolis; Professor, Department of Periodontics, formerly Dean, Indiana University School of Dentistry, Indianapolis, Indiana

Sam W. Hoskins, Jr., D.D.S., M.S.D.

Professor and Chairman, Department of Periodontics, The University of Texas Dental School at San Antonio, San Antonio, Texas

Richard E. Jennings, D.D.S., M.S.D.

Chairman and Professor, Department of Preventive Dentistry (Pedodontics), The University of Texas Dental Branch at Houston, Houston, Texas

Jack C. Miller, B.A., M.S.W.

Professor of Practice Relations, The University of Texas Dental Branch at Houston, Houston, Texas

Sidney L. Miller, B.S., D.D.S., M.P.H., F.A.C.D.

Chairman and Professor, Department of Community Dentistry, The University of Texas Dental School at San Antonio, San Antonio, Texas

James E. Phillips, A.B., D.D.S., M.Sc.

Associate Professor of Radiology, University of Pennsylvania School of Dental Medicine, Philadelphia, Pennsylvania

Ralph W. Phillips, M.S., D.Sc., F.A.C.D.

Assistant Dean for Research, Research Professor of Dental Materials, Indiana University-Purdue University at Indianapolis School of Dentistry, Indianapolis, Indiana

Milton Siskin, B.A., D.D.S., F.A.C.D., F.I.C.D.

Chairman of Endodontics and Professor, Department of Operative Dentistry, University of Tennessee College of Dentistry, Memphis, Tennessee

James F. Smith, B.A., D.D.S., Ph.D., F.A.C.D.

Professor of Oral Pathology, University of Tennessee College of Dentistry, Memphis, Tennessee

James E. Turner, B.A., D.D.S.

Chairman and Associate Professor, Department of Oral Pathology, University of Tennessee College of Dentistry, Memphis, Tennessee

Wade B. Winnett, D.D.S., M.S.D.

Associate Professor of Operative Dentistry, Meharry Medical College School of Dentistry, Nashville, Tennessee; formerly Chairman of Department for Education of Auxiliary Dental Personnel, University of Tennessee College of Dentistry, Memphis, Tennessee

Preface

Since the title for a textbook is often misleading to both the student and instructor, it is fortunate that the publisher requests the author or editor to provide a preface so that the purpose of the book can be fully explained. It is just as important to know what the book does not purport to do as to know its objective and purpose.

Dental hygiene is a young profession, as indicated in the first chapter of this book. The American Dental Association's Council on Dental Education established the first set of educational standards for dental hygiene as recently as 1952. When this was done, there were only twenty-six dental hygiene programs in the United States; practically no books had been written specifically for the dental hygiene student.

I was Executive Secretary of the Council on Dental Education during the time that the educational requirements were being established for dental hygiene, dental assisting, and for the dental laboratory technician. Discussions with officials of The C. V. Mosby Company led to the conclusion that textbooks needed to be developed for these new and special educational programs. Up to this time, dental hygiene students had been using hand-me-down reference books that had been written for dental students, nursing students, and others.

The publisher asked me to be responsible for *Clinical Dental Hygiene,* which would be written by a group of experts whom I would select.

The first edition of *Clinical Dental Hygiene* was published in 1959. Second and third editions followed at 3-year intervals, all leading to this present new fourth edition, which is materially changed. This same commitment to meet the educational needs of dental hygienists led me and my team of contributors to produce *A Comprehensive Review for Dental Hygienists.*

Two major points should be made. First, each of the contributors has had a great deal of experience, not only in the technical field represented by his or her chapter, but also in working with dental hygienists in the classroom or in practice or both. Some of the contributors have written complete textbooks in their special field, and now they have been called upon to write a single chapter for the special needs of the dental hygiene student. Nearly every contributor has played a significant part in changing the history of the dental profession. Without the achievements of these twenty-one persons it is unlikely that dental hygiene could have advanced to the high position it holds today. Without this same dedication to the dental hygiene profession, these textbooks would not have been written.

Second, the reader needs to know the philosophy of this team of writers for this will explain what has been included; it will also explain why it was decided not to include certain other material. The following beliefs or philosophies guided the preparation of these books:

1. A total profession such as dentistry, dental hygiene, or nursing represents too much content and scope for it to be served by a single textbook.

2. Dental hygiene needs a basic textbook that contains chapters and sections prepared specifically for dental hygienists. If suitable textbooks in the needed subject have already been written for the dental hygienist, then the topic probably need not occupy a chapter in this textbook.

3. A dental hygiene textbook or sourcebook should be able to serve as a review book for continuing education classes or as a reference book.

4. A book to be used for a total professional program cannot be written in such a way that a reader will study the chapters for start to finish. Just as a student is enrolled in several different kinds of subjects, so does the dental hygiene student expect to have assignments in two or more chapters of this book at any one time.

5. Dental hygiene students require some of the same courses by title that are included in the dental school curriculum. But dental hygiene students need to have them presented so that they relate to their need for the topic; and also they need to have them taught at a different level of depth and intensity.

6. There should be no attempt to include chapters on the basic sciences. In many cases these courses offered in the dental hygiene curriculum are already established in the institution, so instructors have many suitable textbooks available.

7. There also should be no attempt to include chapters in such subjects as English, speech, economics, and so on for these courses too are usually already established in the institution and are service courses to those majoring in other fields.

8. The topics selected for inclusion represent the clinical and related areas. It is in these areas that there has been the greatest need for new instructional material.

9. Overlapping is to be expected between chapters; there will be some repetition and even some differences of opinion. To remove all duplication and all differences of opinion would be to remove the personality of the author from some of the chapters.

I am greatly indebted to the twenty-one contributors who have assisted me in developing this basic dental hygiene textbook.

Shailer Peterson

Contents

Clinical dental hygiene

part one

PROFESSIONAL BACKGROUND

chapter 1

INTRODUCTION TO THE DENTAL HYGIENE PROFESSION

Shailer Peterson, B.A., M.A., Ph.D.

Dental hygiene is a great and wonderful profession that has earned prestige and dignity. There is a great demand for dental hygienists, and hence the remuneration is greater than it is for many other professions. In spite of all of these benefits, the educational requirements are neither lengthy nor costly. While there are only about 4,196 freshman class positions available each year, it is usually possible for every fully qualified and dedicated applicant to be admitted to a dental hygiene school, since only about 80% of these capacity figures are filled each year.

In the approximately 60 years that dental hygiene has existed, it has been a profession exclusively for young women. In recent years when the courts decreed that educational and career opportunities should be open to all qualified persons regardless of race or sex, men have started to show an interest in entering this field. Even without the intervention of the courts, this interest of men in the field would have followed, for the income from this career is easily sufficient to support a family. Moreover, many dentists would prefer to employ personnel whom they know want to make a real career of the profession and who will stay with them. Nursing also began as a career for young women, but today there is a fair number of men in the field both as technicians and as male nurses. Only fifteen of the 145 dental hygiene programs in the United States stated that they are not equipped to accept males into their programs.

Parents, counselors, and prospective dental hygienists should not be misled by the fact that a profession that is about 60 years of age still has only about 30,000 licensed dental hygienists, of which about two thirds are in full-time or part-time practice. Until about a dozen years ago, there were only about twenty-five dental hygiene programs that graduated about 1,000 students each year; these just about offset the number of dental hygienists retiring from practice each year. The following facts kept the number of dental hygienists relatively small for many years:

1. Few schools and small classes
2. Few applicants
3. Retirement of girls as soon as they married, with very few returning for even part-time work
4. Inadequate salaries in many parts of the nation
5. Lack of dentists' experience in using any auxiliary dental personnel, so no great demand for dental hygienists by dentists in practice

3

6. Relatively few positions for dental hygienists in schools, industry, or public health work
7. Few recommendations from school counselors and advisors on dental hygiene as a career
8. Neglect by dentists to suggest dental hygiene as a career for their patients

In 1970 there were 6,854 students enrolled in dental hygiene programs, and in that same year there were 2,465 dental hygiene graduates. In other words, from 1960 to 1970 the number of graduates had risen from 992 to 2,465, or about a 150% increase. Of the 2,465, 462 received baccalaureate degrees and 2,003 received certificates; 2,044 took positions in private offices.

It is interesting to note that the first time that statistical data were reported on dental hygiene schools by the Council on Dental Education was in 1941, soon after the official requirements had been established by the A.D.A. for an approved 2-year dental hygiene program. At that time, there were only seventeen dental hygiene programs of which thirteen were conducted in dental schools; the other four were in private institutions. The seventeen schools had an enrollment of 504 and 177 (35%) of these were enrolled in the four private, nondental schools. At that same time, there were thirty-nine dental schools in full operation with an enrollment of 8,355.

Between 1941 and the present there has been an increase from seventeen to 121 dental hygiene programs, an increase of 613% in about 30 years. In the same 30 years, there has been a thirteenfold increase in enrollment, from 504 dental hygiene students in 1941 to an enrollment of 6,854 students in 1971.

Although not all those enrolled study dental hygiene in their own state, the five states that are currently producing the greatest number of dental hygiene students are California (544), Illinois (404), Michigan (404), New York (770), and Texas (358).

While dental hygiene has always been a fine and attractive profession, in the last dozen years it has grown very rapidly not only in numbers but also in acceptance by the dental profession and the public, until today there is a demand for dental hygienists that cannot be met even with the increased number of schools. The barriers to the growth of the dental hygiene profession have now either been removed or completely reversed.

1. Many new dental hygiene programs have been started, particularly in junior colleges and community colleges. In 1970-1971 there was a total of 121 programs in the United States with another twenty-five on the drawing board. There were also five in Canada.
2. There is an increasing number of well-qualified applicants, which is the reservoir from which the dental hygiene schools will be filled. Sixty-one of the 121 dental hygiene schools in the United States and all of the five dental hygiene schools in Canada were filled to capacity in 1971. However, applicants were not evenly distributed, with the result that many schools were not filled. A total of 12,329 students made application for the 4,196 freshman openings in the 121 U. S. dental hygiene programs, and 3,265 openings were filled.
3. Girls in dental hygiene still leave their practice to become housewives, but many more of them are indicating their plans to return for at least a part-time position in the dental office after their families are grown.
4. Salaries of dental hygienists in all parts of the nation have increased significantly. However, supply and demand still cause the salaries in some areas to be much higher than in others.
5. For the last dozen years, every dental graduate has been exposed to edu-

cation and experience using a chairside assistant, and most have also been given some information on how to establish a practice by making use of all auxiliary dental personnel. Most of the remaining dentists have taken refresher courses and other continuing education courses on practice management that have made them realize that they need to recruit dental assistants and dental hygienists for their offices. All of this attention has increased the demand for dental hygienists.

6. There has been an increase in the employment of dental hygienists in public school systems and an increase in the number of public health positions for dental hygienists.

7. The increase in the number of school "career days" and the interest shown by civic service clubs in sponsoring job opportunity programs has alerted both students and counselors to the opportunities to be found in dentistry and all of its auxiliary dental personnel fields.

8. It is found now that dentists rank first in recruiting young students to a career in dentistry and its related fields. Fellow students themselves rank second, and parents rank third. Strangely enough, counselors rank far down the list.

Dentistry as a recognized profession is itself very young. The first dental school accepted its first student only 132 years ago (1840), when the Baltimore College of Dental Surgery was started. This contrasts considerably with the history of the medical profession in which the first medical school on record was the University of Pennsylvania, which was started 196 years ago (1776). Nursing also has a longer history than dental hygiene. Its first school was started in 1873, thus making it formally 99 years old as a profession in the United States.

The age of a profession or of a career can be described in several ways. One might think that one should date medicine from the time that the first surgery was performed and dentistry from the time that the first tooth was extracted. This would be possible, but one finds that even the early cavemen found some ways to treat their illness, and some of them apparently found ways to soothe the pain of a toothache. Some would say that the time when the first surgeon started to teach another person to follow his same trade or occupation would be a good time to date the beginning of a profession or a career. This would be possible, but the process that has come to be used is to date the beginning of a profession from the time that the first *formal* education program was established so that students might be enrolled and taught. Therefore, when we say that dentistry is 132 years of age, it means that the first dental school had its official beginning back in 1840, when it took its first class of five students.

For a long time prior to the establishment of the first medical or dental school, there were many self-taught physicians and dentists who in turn would teach their friends and colleagues. Much of this teaching would be done as on-the-job training in which the dentist would bring the prospective dentist into his office and teach him by letting him work with him. This was called the "preceptorship" method. Preceptorships are still being used in some of the trades. Learning on the job and teaching by the employer is also being done for dental assistants, even though schools are gradually replacing these preceptorial and apprenticeship methods. All of the states except Alabama recognize and license only those dental hygienists who have received their education in accredited dental hygiene schools.

Between the time that the first medical and dental schools were started and the present time there was a period when many of these early schools were of the "proprietary" type. This means that they were operated as private businesses for profit. A quarter of a century ago the last of the proprietary schools for dentistry disappeared, and within the last 10 years all of the schools can boast that they are a part of a fully accredited recognized university or college.

It is easy to see that it is not practical for a business organization to operate a college that would produce dentists, physicians, nurses, veterinarians, or dental hygienists. Such educational programs are complicated and expensive. They involve not only lectures and laboratories but also patient treatment, the use of drugs and x-rays, and a host of other things that involve the approval of many other agencies and many controls. It is one thing for a commercial school to teach secretarial work, bookkeeping, office management, and office reception skills. It would be quite another for a business school to try to offer training and experience in scaling a patient's teeth. It is also one thing for a business organization that produces tapes, recordings, slides, film strips, and movies to branch into a program of releasing visual and audio aids that physicians and dentists may use in order to keep themselves up to date on what is being published in their fields, but it would be quite another thing to expect that the total dental curriculum could be taught by the aid of films and tapes.

History dates the origin of the dental hygiene profession from 1913, when Alfred C. Fones organized and sponsored his first course of 6-weeks' training for dental hygienists in order to staff the preventive dental clinic in Bridgeport, Connecticut. In 1916 the first dental hygiene school was established at Hunter College with prescribed admissions requirements. Other courses were soon offered at Rochester Dental Dispensary in Rochester, New York, and at Forsyth Dental Infirmary for Children in Boston, Massachusetts. Dental hygienists were first licensed in Connecticut in 1917. By 1955 all states had made provision for licensing dental hygienists.

Actually the credit for suggesting dental hygiene as a separate career dates before the first course, because as early as 1844 N. W. Kingsley had advocated the employment of women to assist the dentist. In 1902 C. M. Wright proposed a subspecialty of dentistry, namely the polishing of teeth and the care of the mouth, and he went further to suggest that this be practiced by women. He even had the foresight to suggest the content of the training program, its length, the giving of a certificate, and the legal control of this practice.

The dental hygienist should recognize the relative youth of her profession, because this will enable her to understand better the fact that there are still a number of dentists who have never had an opportunity to employ a dental hygienist. Also, there are many patients who never have had a dental hygienist give them an oral prophylaxis.

The dental profession recognizes the need for the dental hygienist as a specially educated person who is primarily concerned with the prevention of oral diseases. The hygienist assists the dentist in this preventive program by giving oral prophylaxis, by discussing dental health problems with patients, and by applying fluorides topically to the teeth of children. The whole field of dentistry today is placing special emphasis on preventive methods, and hence it is easy to understand that the hygienist is engaged in a challenging profession—one that is destined to expand as the science of dentistry continues to develop.

The members of any profession must know more than just the technical and scientific facts that make them expert and skillful in their clinical work. They must be aware of the many problems that affect the growth and development of their profession. The efficient dental hygienist must recognize the important role she is expected to play as a member of the dental health team. She must be able to adjust to the varying situations and needs that arise within the different dental offices, and she must be ready and willing to adjust to these different situations. Her willingness and ability to adjust to the needs of the office in which she works and her ability to demonstrate to her dentist the skill she possesses and the service she can render will contribute tremendously to the increased recognition of the dental hygiene profession by both the dental profession and the public. Since each dentist looks to his own hygienist as one who represents the dental hygiene profession, the usefulness of hygienists and the importance of their profession are influenced by what each individual dentist sees in the work of his own hygienist.

DENTISTRY—A YOUNG PROFESSION

Mention already has been made that dental hygiene is a relatively new pro-

fession. Actually dentistry itself is newer than many persons realize. The term *dentistry* did not appear in the literature until the time of Fauchard in 1728, and the first dental school in the world was not established until 1840, when the Baltimore College of Dental Surgery was started in Baltimore, Maryland. In the 132 years that have followed, about 200,000 dentists have been graduated, and these 121,000 are still alive today, although not all of them are still in active practice. About 102,000 dentists are actively practicing at the chairside, while nearly 3,000 are engaged in research and in full-time teaching, in public health, and in administrative positions.

The educational requirements for dentists increased rapidly, and by 1935 all dental students were required to have had a minimum of 2 years of college prior to starting their 4 years of professional school study. More than half of the dentists now in practice are graduates of this present educational program, and an increasingly high percentage of them have had more than 2 years of preprofessional study be-

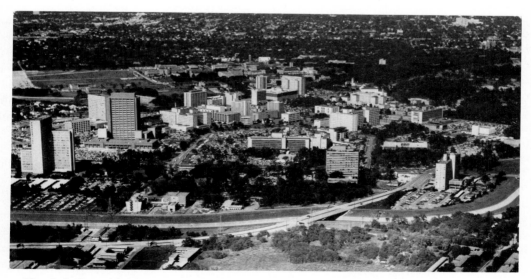

Fig. 1-1. Dental hygiene programs are often located on huge health unit campuses where dental hygienists can learn to work with members of all health professions. (Courtesy Texas Medical Center, Houston, Tex.)

fore being admitted to dental school. At the present time 94% of the freshmen have had more than 2 years of study, and 66.4% possessed college degrees before entering dental school.

All of the fifty states, the District of Columbia, and the Commonwealth of Puerto Rico require the dentist to be licensed to practice in his respective state or locality. The dental practice acts specify the operations and treatments that the dentist can perform, just as the medical practice acts describe the professional duties of the physician and as the dental practice acts describe the work of the dental hygienist. By specifying the operations that the dentist may perform, these acts also indicate what operations cannot be performed by those who are not licensed as dentists.

The dental hygiene profession, like the dental profession, must be concerned with the problems of supplying dental care to the public and meeting the demands of the public for dental care. There are insufficient dentists to care for all the existing dental needs of the public, although there are almost enough dentists and dental hygienists in most areas to meet the demands of the public for dental care. However, the demands are increasing rapidly as the public becomes more conscious of its dental needs and the close relationship between dental disease and diseases in other parts of the body. Further reference to the need for dental care from the dental health *team* is given in other chapters throughout this textbook.

There are now fifty dental schools in the United States and in Puerto Rico, all of which are graduating dental students, and there are nine dental schools in Canada. The schools in the United States and Puerto Rico enroll about 16,008 undergraduate students, and the Canadian schools enroll about 1,580.

In addition to the fifty dental schools that are now graduating students, there are two dental schools, the University of Texas Dental School at San Antonio and the School of Dentistry at the Medical College of Georgia, that are in full operation with classes but not with all 4 years in full operation. In addition, there are also five other dental schools that have been authorized to take classes in the future. These include the School of Dentistry at the University of Colorado, the College of Dentistry at the University of Florida, the School of Dental Medicine at the State University of New York at Stony Brook, the School of Dental Medicine at Southern Illinois University, and the School of Dentistry at the University of Oklahoma. The first four of these have announced that they will admit a freshman class in September of 1972; and the last has announced that its first class will be in 1973.

Dental hygiene

There are currently 121 dental hygiene programs in the United States and five programs in Canada. Thirty-one of the United States' programs and all of the Canadian programs are conducted in dental schools. There is a total of about 6,854 dental hygiene students in United States' programs and about 270 in the Canadian programs. About 2,465 dental hygienists are graduated each year from United States' schools and about 110 from the Canadian schools. There are currently plans for the establishment of about fifteen new dental hygiene programs in the United States.

The dental hygienist deserves to be proud of her profession, and she should strive to learn as much about it and about the dental profession as she can. She must understand what it is about her profession that has made it grow in prestige, because then she can be in a position for helping herself and her colleagues give the proper *image* of the profession to all of her patients as well as to the public.

The dental hygienist must realize that

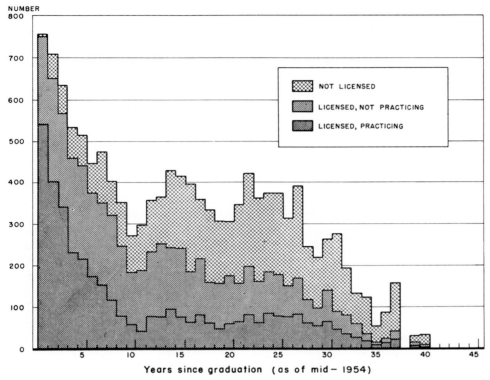

Fig. 1-2. Number of dental hygienists according to years in active practice since graduation. (From Pelton, W. J., Pennell, E. H., and Vavra, H. M.: Dental hygienists, Health Manpower Source Book, Pub. No. 263, Section 8, Washington, D. C., 1957, U. S. Government Printing Office.)

hers is a fairly young but growing profession. The demand for dental hygienists will be increasing rapidly in the future, and there will be a demand for adding new jobs, new functions, and new responsibilities to the work of the dental hygienist.

The reader must study Chapter 10, which explains that the dental hygienist is already being given many more responsibilities. Within a few years both she and the dental assistant will be expected to take over many more of the responsibilities in the dental office. As the only other licensed member of the dental health team, the dentist will expect the dental hygienist to take the responsibility for many important dental services.

The dental hygienist must remember that while licensure gives status and prominence, this carries with it a great deal of responsibility, which in turn is based upon her education, her experience, her competences, and most of all her judgment and discretion. It has only been since 1947, 25 years ago, that the minimum educational requirements at the college level have been increased to 2 academic years. However, many girls in dental hygiene today have had much more than the minimum of 2 years, many have college degrees, and some have graduate degrees. The prestige of a profession grows as the education of its members grow. A profession also grows as those who practice the art and science of the profession become active members of their own association—the American Dental Hygienists' Association.

The opportunities for dental hygiene are tremendous, and dental hygienists are finding important roles to play in hospitals and in various clinics and schools.

Perhaps the greatest limiting factor in the growth of dental hygiene has been that such a high percentage of its members stay in dental hygiene practice for only a few years. It is true that many are returning after they have raised their families, but the short average length of service keeps reducing the effective number of dental hygienists who can serve the public and the dentists. A profession that is growing in prestige and recognition is one that should attract its members back to it, even though they may interrupt their practice for one reason or another. New licensure laws and a greater use of the National Board Examinations, as indicated in Chapter 10, will make it easier for a dental hygienist to move her residence and her practice from one state to another.

There are few professions for women that have as many advantages as does the profession of dental hygiene. This is being recognized, as it is observed that there are four or five times as many girls now applying for admission to dental hygiene programs as there are places for them in the classes. Those who have been successful in becoming dental hygienists represent a choice few, and they should value highly the fine opportunity that has been given to them.

THE DENTAL HEALTH TEAM

In the area of sports everyone knows the significance of a team: a football or baseball game depends upon a "team approach." The eleven men on a football squad are essential for the playing of the game and everyone on the squad or on the team has a certain specific job to perform.

In the professions, and particularly in the health professions, the team approach has developed as the professions themselves have grown and developed and as the need for specialization is created. It was not so many years ago that the family doctor was the one who called on his patients; he was the walking encyclopedia for medical knowledge and the "know-how" at the time; he delivered the babies in the bedroom without the aid of nurses, anesthesiologists, and a host of other personnel who now constitute the medical team in a modern hospital.

Dentistry is a young profession, and only a few years ago no one had heard about a dental hygienist who could assist the dentist and be a member of the *dental health team*. While dentistry is a much younger profession than is medicine, dentistry too is becoming more mature and more sophisticated. The kinds and types of treatment are becoming so many that dentistry now has eight dental specialties, which means that the general practitioner has eight different kinds of dentists with specialized training and experience to whom he can refer patients or refer the problems of dentistry.

The need and demand for dental care has grown much more rapidly than has the number of dentists, so it has been necessary for the dental profession to develop auxiliary members of the dental profession to add their skills, take over specific responsibilities, and lend a helping hand. Actually these extra persons add more than helping hands, for they add their ideas, their suggestions, and their judgments. These extra members of the dental health team are not robots but intelligent, highly skilled persons.

The dental health team today consists of (1) the dentist, (2) the dental hygienist, (3) the dental assistant, (4) the dental laboratory technician (or the commercial dental laboratory), as well as other persons who help make the profession operate at its optimum efficiency, (5) the representative of the dental supply company or representative of the dental manufacturer, and (6) the dental wife. These will be discussed further in Chapter 2.

While the dentist is the key person on the dental health team, just as the physician is the key person on the medical health team, he cannot function to his optimum efficiency unless he makes full use of all his auxiliary dental personnel.

Can anyone imagine a modern physician today doing all of the work that is necessary in connection with the treatment of a patient? Would the physician be making good use of his time if he did the following?

1. Repaired and serviced his equipment
2. Prepared his own pills and capsules
3. Typed his own statements
4. Gave the patient his injections
5. Took blood samples from his patients
6. Did the laboratory work-up on blood and urine
7. Took and developed all of his own x-ray films
8. Gave anesthetics to his patients
9. Performed surgery in every field

Of course one cannot imagine the physician doing all these things. While he has been trained to do many of them, it would be wasteful of his time and talents to elect to do the things that his auxiliary personnel and team members can do for him. As a matter of fact some of these auxiliary personnel can do the work even more expertly than the physician because they specialize in these procedures and practice them to such an extent that they become much more expert than anyone can be who does them only as a small part of his job.

This is also true of the dental hygienist. She devotes most of her time to oral prophylaxis and practices this art much more than her dentist. While he is compe-

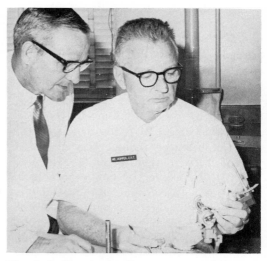

Fig. 1-3. The dentist discusses a set of dentures with his dental laboratory technician. (Courtesy University of Tennessee College of Dentistry, Memphis, Tenn.)

tent to render this service, she often can do it much more expertly and rapidly than he can, for this is her major responsibility.

The same thing is true of the dental laboratory technician. While the dentist has had a great deal of experience in fabricating dentures, crowns, and bridges and knows what to expect and require in terms of quality and excellence, he would rather devote his time to determining the needs of the patient, stipulating through a work authorization and prescription what he wants from the dental laboratory technician and the commercial dental laboratory, than take the time to do all of the laboratory work himself. The dental laboratory technician who spends all of his time doing these procedures also can do a very fine job and usually do it more quickly than a dentist who would be doing this only a small part of his time.

The wise and efficient use of the auxiliary dental personnel by the dentist is a sign of efficient delegation of responsibility and a sign of a well-organized and well-planned office procedure. The use and the value of the team approach is *not* merely the employment of more people or the use of more hands in the dental office. The *dentist* is always responsible for the health, the life, and the welfare of the patient regardless of the other persons to whom he delegates some of the work and responsibility. It is the dentist who is responsible if the patient becomes ill or dies or if the patient becomes disfigured. The persons whom the dentist selects for members of his team must be talented and skilled, but they also must be cooperative and useful in working as parts of a team that functions effectively.

Therefore the *dentist* must select carefully the persons who are to be members of his *team.* He cannot select just any dental hygienist, or any dental assistant, or any commercial dental laboratory to do his work. Also he cannot trade with just any dental dealer or any dental manufacturer. He must select *only* those trained auxiliaries who will work with him as members of the team in which he is both the team coach and playing member. As the chief professional and as the leader of the team the dentist must be constantly watchful of the manner with which each of his team members performs his assignments and the way that each one works effectively with others, and he must be prepared to replace any one of them quickly. One poor team member can almost completely ruin the effectiveness of a fine dental practice. One poor team member also could cause the death of a patient, the loss of the dentist's license, and the ruin of the dentist as a professional man.

While individual members of a team receive some individual praise and credit for their own role and part in a job that has been well done, the perfect team works as a unit without regard to special and individual praise and credit. The mark of a true team is when the individuals forget about the personal praise and, instead, work only for the credit and the accomplishment of the whole team, realizing that they are all important cogs in the machinery but that every wheel must turn and function properly or the job will not get done.

A dental hygienist who has been a member of a large family, who always has been interested in what the whole family does, and who has joined the others in being happy about the success of any member of this family team knows what it means to be able to take pride in what a team has accomplished. A dental hygienist who has learned the expression that "We have done this" instead of always wanting to say "I have done this" has learned to know and understand the meaning of a *team approach.*

Not everyone is a natural-born team member. Many can learn to become team members, but perhaps there are a few to whom this diminution of personal acclaim and constant personal attention might make team membership difficult or even impossible to attain. In any team there is plenty of opportunity for some personal praise and some personal attention, but a team job is surely not intended for the person who always wants to be the center of attention or who feels a need to take all of the credit for everything that turns out well. If you are one of those persons who has never been the member of a team, or if you find that you are one who does not enjoy giving your friends and colleagues credit for helping to get a job done, you had better take another look at whether or not you want to be a dental hygienist. A dental hygienist *must* be willing and even anxious to be a team member and to accept her part of the credit with all the other members of the team.

Certain aspects of "teamwork" have been included in this first chapter because it is an important concept to recognize as part of an introduction to the profession of dental hygiene. However, in order to be an effective team member, there is much more to be said about the dental health team and the role that the dental hygienist must expect to play in it. Therefore, this subject of teamwork is continued and expanded in Chapter 2.

chapter 2

THE DENTAL HYGIENIST AND HER ASSOCIATES

Shailer Peterson, B.A., M.A., Ph.D.

DENTAL HYGIENIST

The modern dental hygienist is a four-faceted person. No one's life is wrapped up in one container and with one purpose; everyone has at least two personalities. For example, a man can be office personality, husband, and father.

The modern dental hygienist has at least the following four interests and challenges:
1. Her personal life
2. Her personal function in the dental office
3. Her function as a member of the office team
4. Her function as a member of her dental hygiene society and associations

As a career woman, all four of these are intertwined and related to each other; only to a degree can they be kept independent or separate. For example, her personal duties and functions in the office are listed as separate from her function as a member of the dental office team, and yet as she works in the office it is difficult to keep them entirely separated. Being a professional person, it is even difficult for her to leave all of her problems about patients and her plans for her appointments at the office. This involvement is one characteristic of those who choose a health profession for a career instead of a clerical position.

When the dental hygienist and her dentist originally chose their professions, they pledged that they would devote time and energy to the improvement and the elevation of the health professions. While they can do this in part by the changes and improvements that they bring into their office practice, there are many local, state, regional, and national questions that arise from time to time that require their attention and their consideration. For example, right now there are people, groups, and agencies that are trying to figure out ways and methods of delivering health care to the public. Some of these people have the interests and the concern of the dentists and the dental hygienists in mind as they formulate their plans. There are others who do not seem to be interested in having the physicians, the dentists, and the other health personnel retain their professional status.

One must remember that the right and the privilege for a physician, a dentist, and a dental hygienist to practice as they do is regulated by state practice acts. These acts and these rules are approved or changed by members of the legislature. While these legislators listen to the professional people when seeking information before they take a vote, they also listen to other nonprofessional persons.

PROFESSIONAL ASSOCIATIONS

Medicine has its American Medical Association and dentistry has its American Dental Association. While the A.D.A. also concerns itself with dental hygiene, the dental hygienists also have their own association, the American Dental Hygienists' Association.

Associations and societies are the organized groups of people who collectively study problems and take action about them. An individual dental hygienist or an individual dentist who asked for an opportunity to take the time of a legislative committee might never be given the opportunity to state his case. However, when the A.D.A. wants to be sure that a legislative committee in Washington understands a problem correctly, it has no difficulty getting a "hearing." Similarly, when new state laws affecting dental hygienists and dentists are proposed, the state dental association has a legislative committee that can easily obtain an opportunity to explain its needs and its wants to the members of the state legislature.

The dentist and the dental hygienist can make many rules within their own office, but they are constantly aware of the fact that their licenses to practice are awarded to them by a state licensing board. If the rules and the laws regulating dental practice were unwisely changed, this could mean a backward step to the practice of dentistry and in the delivery of dental health care. Even though many dentists and their dental hygienists may not want to be bothered with discussions about the dental practice acts and may not be too interested in who is elected to state office, no professional person can afford to be disinterested.

Every dentist and every dental hygienist need their own professional associations and societies. In turn these associations and these societies are only as strong as the persons in them. For the associations to be able to speak for dentistry and for dental hygiene, their spokesmen must be able to say truthfully that they really represent all the members of their profession.

Chapter 10 discusses the very important problem of "expanding the duties" and increasing the responsibilities of dental hygienists and dental assistants. This is a timely subject, since the dental practice acts are going to be changed. As a matter of fact some have already been changed. These changes will affect every dental hygienist who is now in practice, and yet very few dental hygienists have taken an active interest in the hearings held about changing these laws.

Associations and societies prove that there is more strength in numbers than there is in the pleas and the requests of a few individuals. Also, when the members of an association reach agreement on some problem or proposal, their collective opinions when expressed through their association are much more valuable and productive than when an association admits that its own members are confused and cannot make up their minds—or do not care.

Every dental hygienist should be an active member of her local dental hygiene society, of her state dental hygiene association, and her national association, the American Dental Hygienists' Association. Membership in these is combined, for one cannot have membership in one without having membership in the other. This is the same pattern that exists for the A.M.A. and for the A.D.A. and for most other large professional organizations.

As students, every dental hygienist also needs to belong to the Student American Dental Hygienists' Association. This membership becomes good experience for the future.

Just as the dentist, the dental hygienist, and the other auxiliary personnel work together as a team, so do the dental professional associations work closely together. There is strength in teamwork. As you become active in the community in which

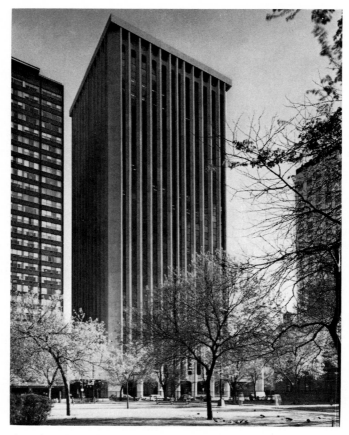

Fig. 2-1. The American Dental Hygienists' Association has offices in the new building of the American Dental Association in Chicago. (Courtesy American Dental Association, Chicago, Ill.)

you practice you will find that you will become a member of other teams. You may become one of the many members of a church team, a choir team, a girls' club team, a knife-and-fork club team, a golfing club team, and many other organizations.

Nothing will be quite as important, however, in all of your teamwork activities as your *dental office team*. This is the place of your chosen profession and chosen career, and this is the place where you can make contributions that only you can make. This is where your membership in the team can be most appreciated and where you will help to render a service that may mean the difference between the life or death of a patient. This is the place where you can hold your head high because the team of which you are a very significant and important part is making a very special contribution to the dental health of the whole community. This is the place where your own team coach, your dentist, is a leader in his community, and this is the very special man whom you help to make successful. When you do a good job, you look good, and you also make him and his office look good.

These things are the ingredients for tremendously happy and successful work.

Few other people have it as good as you can have it—if you become a good team worker and member.

On p. 10 the dental health team was described as having six members. Because the dental hygienist will be working with all of them, it is well that she have a good understanding of who they are, what they do, and what special training they have received.

DENTIST

The dentist is the primary member of the dental team. The more you know about his work, the better you can enjoy and appreciate what he is doing and realize how you and the other team members help him to render service to and for his patients.

The dentist has had 2 or more years of predental education at the university level with prescribed courses. This has been followed by a 4-year program at a recognized dental school. Dentists who are specialists are now required to have completed a minimum of 2 years of formal training at the graduate or postgraduate level. Many dentists have had internships and residencies in hospitals, and many also have had experience in dental public health work at the state or national level. A dentist, like the dental hygienist, must be licensed to practice dentistry in the state in which he practices.

There were 120,916 licensed dentists in 1970, 102,000 of whom were active in their profession of dentistry. Of these, about 8,000 were in federal dental service, more than 1,400 were in dental education, and about 524 were in state dental public health work. There are currently fifty dental schools that graduate about 3,600 dentists every year. There are two new schools that have had no graduates as yet, and there are plans for another five schools to be started in the next few years. See Chapter 1, p. 6.

Dentistry has perhaps the highest per-centage of its professionals as members of its official organization, the American Dental Association. In 1970, 98,240 of them were members.

DENTAL HYGIENIST

The dental hygienist as a team member has many duties that are outlined by her dentist, by the licensure laws of her state, and by the customs and interpretations of these laws by the state licensing board. It is common to find that the duties of a dental hygienist are those of oral prophylaxis and dental health education. While this is true, she also may have many other duties, which include such items as charting the mouth, exposing x-ray films, and a host of other things. The extent to which she specializes, in the sense that she devotes most of her time to oral prophylaxis, depends largely upon the structure of the office in which she works and the assignment of duties by her dentist to other members of the dental health team.

Many states, many schools, and many dentists are now giving a great deal of attention to new and special functions that may in the future be given to the dental hygienist. Every dental hygienist should be aware of the changes that are occurring every year in an effort to make it possible for her to render the best service to the patient and to her dentist as a member of the dental health team. Nearly every chapter in this book alludes to various functions and responsibilities of the dental hygienist, to her professional responsibility to keep herself knowledgeable concerning the advances that are being made in dental hygiene practice, and to the need for high ethical standards in its practice. Refer to Chapter 10, which discusses the expanded functions of all auxiliary dental personnel.

All dental hygienists have had a minimum of a high school education before entering dental hygiene school, which has a 2-year curriculum. Most dental hygiene

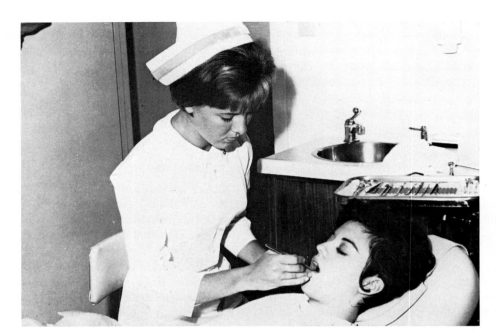

Fig. 2-2. A dental hygienist usually works today without a dental assistant to help her. (Courtesy University of Tennessee College of Dentistry, Memphis, Tenn.)

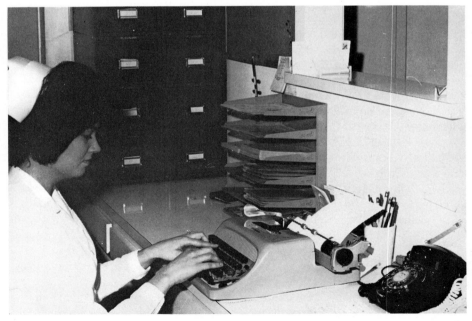

Fig. 2-3. One of the team members is the secretary-receptionist in the dental office. (Courtesy University of Tennessee College of Dentistry, Memphis, Tenn.)

graduates at the present time have had more than the minimum of education, and an increasing number of them have baccalaureate degrees; many have advanced and graduate degrees.

There were in 1968 a total of 30,000 licensed dental hygienists, 23,500 of whom were in active professional practice. There are currently 121 dental hygiene schools graduating students at the rate of 2,500 each year. There are plans for about fifteen new dental hygiene programs to be started in the next few years. There were 9,900 members of the American Dental Hygienists' Association in 1971.

DENTAL ASSISTANT

The dental assistant, as the name implies, may have a large number of duties in the dental office as a member of the dental health team. She assists the dentist and actually assists the entire office in which her team operates. She follows the directive of the dentist, who is both coach and playing member of the team.

In an office in which the dentist has only one or two auxiliary persons, the dental assistant will have many different duties, whereas in an office in which there is a dental hygienist, several dental assistants, and a dental laboratory technician, the dental assistant will be much more specialized in her duties and responsibilities. In an office that has one dental assistant and one dental hygienist it is likely that the dental hygienist may render some of the same assisting services that a dental assistant might be called upon to do in a larger office. The complicated dental office has many jobs to be performed, and obviously these must be delegated between the personnel who are there to make up the team, whether it be small or large.

The responsibilities in the modern dental office are becoming so numerous and so complicated that dental assistants may

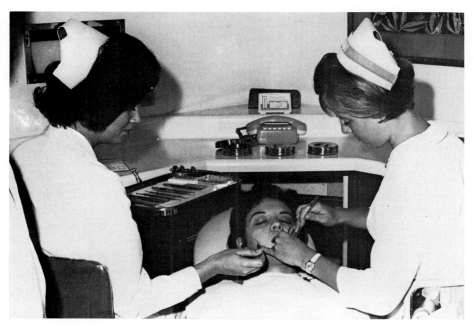

Fig. 2-4. A dental hygienist can use the extra hands of the dental assistant to improve her efficiency. (Courtesy University of Tennessee College of Dentistry, Memphis, Tenn.)

have to become specialists. These specialties may be described as (1) office receptionist, (2) office secretary, (3) office bookkeeper, (4) chairside assistant, (5) roving assistant, (6) laboratory assistant, and (7) housekeeping assistant.

The dental assistant may be any one of the foregoing or may be all seven of them. The dental hygienist in a small office also may have any or several of these same duties delegated to her to perform as a member of the team. In any event the dentist will expect his dental hygienist to know enough about the operation of the entire office, and also about the specific work of every auxiliary, so that she, the dental hygienist, can act as a substitute in emergencies so that the office operation does not fall apart just because one person is absent for a day or a few days.

The important factor in any team approach is that no one is so entrenched in his own usual duties that he cannot or is unwilling to perform almost any of the duties of any other members of the team. For example, it would not be unusual for the dental hygienist, in the absence of the receptionist, to perform the duties of receiving and welcoming the patients and handling the duty of making appointments and the like. Obviously the dental assistant, in the absence of the dental hygienist, cannot take over her responsibility of giving prophylaxis, but she ought to know enough about talking to patients concerning dental health care to be of help.

There were in 1968 about 145,000 dental assistants, of whom approximately 31,000 were secretaries and receptionists. Within recent years formal dental assistant educational programs have been established, and they require high school graduation, plus at least 1 academic year of college or university level instruction. Many programs are 2 years long and lead to an Associate of Arts degree. There are currently 165 accredited dental assistant programs, about thirty-four with provisional or pending approval, and about forty planned to begin within the next few years.

There has been a tremendous growth in the number of dental assisting programs and also in the number of new dental assistants. The number of programs has grown from forty-five in 1968 to 165 in 1971. There were 1,419 dental assistants enrolled in programs in 1962 and 5,812 enrolled in 1970. There were 658 graduates from the schools in 1962 and 2,955 in 1970.

In 1970, 74% of the schools gave a certificate after 1 year of education. The remaining 26% offered an Associate of Arts (A.A.) degree. It is also interesting to note that 40% of the schools reported that they had accepted male students into the class. Of the 5,812 students enrolled in dental assisting programs, it is interesting to note that 4,841 were first-year students and the remaining 971 were second-year students. Therefore, many more become certified after the 1-year program than after the 2-year program for the A.A. degree.

Dental hygienists may need to advise persons who are interested in following dental assisting programs. It is reported that while the costs vary widely from one program to another, the average cost is $414 for residents.

While the dental assistant is not licensed, there is a Dental Assistant Certification Program, which is recognized by both the American Dental Association and the American Dental Assistants Association. Certification depends upon graduation from an accredited dental assisting program, passing a qualification examination, and having had experience in a dental office for a specified number of years.

The American Dental Assistants Association had 18,900 members in 1971.

DENTAL LABORATORY TECHNICIAN

The dental laboratory technician has the responsibility for fabricating various kinds of oral appliances according to the direc-

Table 2-1. Auxiliary dental office personnel*

| Type of auxiliary | Number of auxiliary personnel | | Percentage of dentists using auxiliary personnel† | | |
	Full-time	Part-time	One full-time	More than one full-time	Some part-time
Dental hygienist	11,500	12,000	11.6%	0.7%	12.2%
Dental laboratory technician (employed in office; does not include those employed in commerical dental laboratory)	4,400	1,800	3.6%	0.6%	1.9%
Dental assistant (excluding the office receptionist and secretary)	95,300	18,600	61.6%	21.8%	17.5%
Secretary and receptionist	25,200	5,400	25.0%	1.4%	5.6%
Totals	136,400	37,800			
Grand total	174,200				

*Data compiled from 1968 Survey of Dental Practice, Chicago, American Dental Association (produced by the Bureau of Economic Research and Statistics of the American Dental Association).
†In 1968 7.6% of practicing dentists reported that they did not have any employees.

tions and specifications of the dentist. The dental laboratory technician is not permitted to serve the patients directly. The dentist studies and evaluates the needs of a patient, takes the impressions for a denture, and writes a prescription and work authorization for the dental laboratory technician. The technician fabricates the appliance and returns it to the dentist, who in turn checks first to see whether the appliance meets his specifications and then fits the patient with the appliance. Dental laboratory technicians may be employed by a commercial dental laboratory, they may be self-employed in a one-man dental laboratory, or they may be employed by a dentist or a group of dentists. There was in 1966 a total of 31,300 dental laboratory technicians, of whom about 6,000 were directly employed by dentists; the remainder were employed in about 8,200 commercial dental laboratories.

Most dental laboratory technicians have been trained by the apprenticeship method in the dental laboratories. There is now a recognized 2-year program of education that requires high school graduation as minimum preparation. There are ten accredited schools for training dental laboratory technicians. There is a certification program for dental laboratory technicians that is approved by the A.D.A. and by the national association representing dental laboratory owners. There is also a national program for inspecting and accrediting the dental laboratories themselves, and this is recognized by the A.D.A.

There are now twenty-six schools for the education of dental laboratory technicians. It was only a dozen years ago that there were only four such schools. The undergraduate enrollment went from 295 in 1962 to 1,113 in 1970. In 1962 there were only 95 graduates, but in 1970 there were 359. It is interesting to note that according to the report* of the American Dental Association's Council on Dental Education,

*Annual Report on Dental Auxiliary Education 1970/71, Division of Educational Measurements, Council on Dental Education, American Dental Association, Chicago.

these 1970 graduates took the following types of positions:

Private dental office	46
Commercial dental laboratory	173
Own dental laboratory	12
Dental school laboratory	11
Civil Service	5
Armed services dental laboratory	73
Other	39

Dental laboratory technicians are licensed in only ten states, and some other states are giving licensure consideration.

REPRESENTATIVE OF THE DENTAL INDUSTRY

The representatives of dental manufacturing companies and of dental dealers have become a new type of auxiliary to the dental profession. These are the persons who discuss the problems of dental equipment, dental instruments, and dental supplies with the dentist and other team members at the national and state meetings. They call at the office to acquaint the dentist with old and new instruments and medicaments that are needed. They keep alert to help to supply the needs of the modern-day dental office and modern practice methods, producing the items of equipment and supplies that the dental hygienist and the other members of the dental health team will require to provide the needed service. The dental representatives will help to modernize the dental office and produce the timesaving gadgetry and kinds of equipment that will make dental practice less tiring and more comfortable to perform.

The representative who may have been interested in sales in the past will find in the future that his responsibility as a member of the dental health team is one of service and efficiency. It will be a new concept to many that these "detail men" can be considered members of the auxiliary dental health team, but when their true function is analyzed carefully, it will be obvious that they can serve a needed function of this closely knit team.

While the dental dealer, the service man, and the dental manufacturer all play an important part in keeping the dental hygienist and her employer up to date, it is equally important that the dentist and all of the auxiliary dental personnel continuously let the dealer and the manufacturer know their office needs. As is mentioned in Chapter 9, the manufacturers try to meet the demands and the needs of the dentists and the dental hygienists. For many years, manufacturers made very few changes in their chairs and in their units, thinking that the profession was entirely satisfied with the barber-like chairs and the units that resembled gasoline pumps. With the advent of four-handed dentistry into the curriculum about a dozen years ago, all of the manufacturers began to seek the best ideas from their clients. They also began to perform time and motion studies and to take time-lapse movies to help them improve the product.

It is the dentist and the dental hygienist who use the equipment all day and every day who can point out many of the ways by which the equipment can be improved and ways by which its operation can be handled with more comfort and less fatigue. The members of the dental profession cannot expect the manufacturers to improve on their products unless the operators express themselves and point out their needs.

DENTAL WIFE

The dental wife really should be recognized as part of the dental health team, even though she is not strictly speaking a member of the office team. It is true that there are some who would advocate that dental wives be trained so that they can act as office members of the team. The reason that the dental wife is included here as a member of the team is because she is expected to be a member of the dentist-wife team in the community. It is expected that she will understand about the need for the clinical team and also understand the role that she must play as the wife of a professional man in the community, in the local and state and national dental associations, and in her household operation.

Some dental schools are giving elaborate programs for the education of the dental student's wife or girl friend, with the expectation that she will be better prepared to act as a member of this team in the community.

There are some who advocate that the dental wife should be taught enough about being a dental assistant so that she can work in the dental office either on a part-time basis or in emergencies. Most persons believe that the dentist-wife team functions best as a team for community responsibilities rather than for office responsibilities. It would be useful if the dental wife were knowledgeable and could fill in as a receptionist or a secretary in an emergency, but the work of the dental office team will be most effective with full-time personnel who can be specifically trained and experienced for their teamwork functions and with the minimum of any outside part-time personnel.

NEED FOR THE TEAM

There are many factors that influence and predict the amount of dental service that will have to be performed in the future and hence the demands that will be placed upon the dentist and his dental health team. One must realize that there is a difference between the *need* that exists for dental care and the *demand* that there is for it. A group of persons may have serious oral health problems that should be attended to by a dentist, and yet these persons may not choose to take care of their diseased condition and, hence, will not seek dental care. For example, there are estimated to be 204 million persons living in the United States in 1972, excluding the personnel in the Armed Forces overseas. The need and the demand that these millions of persons have for dental care helps to explain the kind and amount of service that the dental profession will be called upon to produce. Most of these persons need dental care, and certainly all except the very young should have oral examinations to determine whether their dentures are fitting properly and whether sores and irritations have developed.

One sees publicity about the groups of school children who have fewer cavities as a result of using different types of dentifrices. One also knows that the children living in cities in which the water is fluoridated have fewer cavities. It is also a fact that people have a longer life expectancy today than formerly, which means that there are many more years during which every person will require dental service.

It is true that at the present time in the United States only about 40% of all persons seek dental care except on an emergency treatment basis. For example, 50% of the children today have never seen a dentist even once. However, everyone is becoming aware of the importance of dental care, and many more persons than ever before are seeking dental care. This is because they have learned to take pride in their appearance, and they believe that the appearance of their teeth has much to do with their physical attractiveness. Therefore the population is becoming more conscious of the need for dental care on the one hand, and on the other hand the efforts of the dental researcher are reducing the occurrence of decay, which in turn decreases some of the need for restorative dentistry. It must be understood also that the reduction in caries does not eliminate all other oral diseases or the need for regular oral examinations, and therefore the need for dental care continues to rise in spite of research.

Many charts and graphs have been

drawn to trace the increase in the nation's population and to compare it with the number of dentists, physicians, and other health personnel. However, it must be recognized that there is no magic formula or equation that will tell a community how many dentists or dental hygienists it should have, nor will any formula predict how much of a financial success a dentist will be in any given community if he employs one hygienist and two dental assistants and uses a commercial dental laboratory. The charts and the graphs have served their purpose by jarring the dental profession out of its complacency a few years ago through explaining that there were not enough dentists to take on the treatment and care of the entire population if even a goodly portion of them should decide to demand it. As is explained and discussed in other parts of this book, the dental profession has encouraged a number of things such as the following:

1. The building of new dental schools
2. Acceptance of more students by existing dental schools
3. Greater use of all auxiliary dental personnel by dentists
4. Education of all auxiliary dental personnel
5. Experimentation in shortening the dental curriculum
6. Experimentation in the use of auxiliary dental personnel
7. Expansion of the duties and responsibilities of auxiliary dental personnel
8. Financial aid to students
9. Financial aid to schools training health personnel
10. Various methods of prevention such as the fluoridation of communal water supplies
11. Creation of numerous programs to increase the public's awareness of dental health problems

These and many other items demonstrate vividly that the dental profession through organized dentistry, the American Dental Association, has made a tremendous contribution in two specific ways.

1. The Association has encouraged the development of various methods that would help to *prevent* or retard dental disease.
2. The Association has encouraged all sorts of methods to help provide the personnel required to take care of the dental health of those who demand it.

While prevention on one hand tends to remove the need for dental treatment, there are more persons becoming conscious of their dental needs. Some of the various kinds of changes that are taking place are shown below. It is items or changes such as these that will affect the availability of dental care in a community, the income of the dentists in that community, and the demand that will exist for dental hygienists.

1. Dentifrice advertisements and nutrition information are making more persons conscious of their appearance and of their dental needs.
2. The unequal distribution of dentists makes it easier for some persons to obtain dental care than other persons.
3. Rising costs in general cause low-income families to neglect their dental problems.
4. Increase in graduates from dental assisting and dental hygiene schools provide the dentist with more "extra hands" to increase and improve his productivity.
5. Improved teamwork in the dental office increases the amount of dental service that can be rendered in that office.
6. Improved dental instruments, dental furniture, and dental gadgets make it easier and faster for the dental health team to render service.
7. Increase in the number of persons

drinking fluoridated water reduces the incidence of caries.

8. Reduction in caries and in the necessity to extract teeth keeps teeth in the mouth longer.

9. Increase in the diseases of the soft tissue provides added need for dental care.

10. The fact that dental hygienists and dental assistants can perform duties that only the dentist himself was permitted to do a few years ago saves the dentist time and allows the office to serve more persons and more families.

11. Improvements in filling materials and in other dental materials used in dental treatment reduces the frequency of repair of restorative materials or appliances.

All of these factors and many more may have an effect upon the practice of any dentist and his dental hygienist. Good sound business practices coupled with a good realization of the factors that are involved in providing a good, professional dental service are important. One dental team may succeed in a place and a situation where another team failed miserably for any one of a number of reasons. The dental teams whose members hold membership in their professional associations and societies are the ones that invariably succeed and prosper.

chapter 3

THE DENTAL HYGIENIST AND HER SUPERVISING DENTIST

Wade B. Winnett, D.D.S., M.S.D.
Shailer Peterson, B.A., M.A., Ph.D.

Some persons will say that it is always important that there be a good relationship between the employer and the employee in every office. This is true whether it be an attorney and his secretary in a law office, the cashier and her employer in a grocery store, or the teacher and her principal in a school system. In a dental office, in a hospital, in a physician's office, and in all health-related offices it is even more important that the rapport and congenial atmosphere be at a very high level. The life and the safety of a patient depend upon the fine working relationship that must exist between the employer and every member of his health team. When the life or death of a patient is at stake, there is no time for questions, bickering, or dissention. Even when the life of the patient is not at stake, the attention to the patient and to his welfare still demands that every member of the dental health team respect the judgment and decision of the dentist.

Almost everyone who has been a patient in a hospital, in a dental office, or in a physician's office has probably observed that the nurses, technicians, assistants, dental hygienists, and all others demonstrate a high degree of loyalty and allegiance to their chiefs or employers. Most of these conditions of loyalty and allegiance come from respect and admiration, for it is only natural that the dedication that a professional man has for his career and his responsibilities must impress all of those who work with him and for him. There are some men who are thoughtless at times and even inconsiderate on occasion, but in nearly all instances their employees come to accept the fact that, while these are not pleasant traits, these employers must receive the respect and loyalty of their employees.

Regardless of what profession or business an employer represents, he is bound to have his peculiarities, his admirable qualities, and his unfavorable traits. He is bound to have days when he displays more worry and lack of understanding than at other times. A dental hygienist is going to have to do some adjusting to the supervisor she has. The employer also has to contend with the inconsistencies and the peculiar personalities of his employees, so the mutual cooperation and the mutual admiration is not a "one-way" proposition.

Every employee realizes that she must study her boss and determine whether she can be comfortable and happy working in his dental office. She must realize that as a dental hygienist the decision about being comfortable in her working situation is even more important than if she were to be a clerk in a bank. In banks and in grocery stores, the patrons are of concern to both the employer and the employee, but this is much less personal and less involved than in the dental office where the patient must be the focal point of attention and concern. In other words, it is very important that the dental hygienist be able to enjoy her working relations. Employees in many offices and stores have little conversation and contact with their fellow employees and with their employers. However, in a health profession where the close working relationship and teamwork are so vitally important, compatibility is essential.

AN OBLIGATION TO BE EFFICIENT

Finding an office where the dental hygienist can comfortably and efficiently continue in her career in the health professions is not just for her own convenience and comfort; it is basically her obligation to the profession. When the dental hygienist chose dental hygiene as a profession and when a school admitted her for her education, she obligated herself to put her time, skills, and education to work in a profitable fashion. Anything less than an efficiently conducted practice is less than she agreed to perform when she accepted her position in a dental hygiene class. So it is easy to understand that the dental hygienist not only has a right to be selective in choosing the office in which she will work, but it is for her own comfort and for her obligation to the dental hygiene and dental profession that she must find an office environment and an employer with whom she can work at her optimum efficiency.

The fact that one dental hygienist cannot work efficiently in a dentist's office does not mean that his office tactics are

difficult. There are frequently clashes of personality, and there are times when the circumstances are such that a different dental hygienist could function in a certain dental team more easily and more comfortably than the former dental hygienist could. Finding the proper niche and office is extremely important. No dental hygienist can ever expect to find an office that meets every one of her expectations. One might categorize the kinds of problems that one finds as she seeks a position as a dental hygienist in a modern dental office. These are:

1. Undesirable office from standpoint of location, distance from home, personality of employer, outdated equipment, salary, fringe benefits, and so on
2. Apparently desirable office that apparently requires no change in procedures and expects no added duties
3. Apparently desirable office that does not require learning any new procedures or technics at this time. However, the dentist says that he may be adding new, expanded duties in the future that will require some continuing education courses and some study.
4. Apparently desirable office that employs now (or anticipates utilization of) certain expanded duties that would demand additional study and the acquisition of new skills

The question is often asked as to what a dental hygienist should do if her dentist were to request that she perform some operatory function that only a dentist is permitted to do according to the state's dental practice act. This could be a double-barreled question. The dentist-employer may be testing her to see if she is even aware of the dental practice act, or he could be testing her in regard to some of the new trends in liberalizing the dental practice acts. Probably the best answer to this question is for the dental hygienist to explain the following to her new employer:

1. According to her educational program and her study of the dental practice acts, she did not believe that she was permitted to perform this particular task.
2. She realizes that the dentist-employer always takes full responsibility for what is done in the dental office. However, as his employee, she would always want to share in this responsibility. If this service involves some act or treatment not specifically permitted in the dental practice act, she should suggest that the dentist-employer discuss this item with the board of dental examiners to learn whether the state board will permit this service or treatment to be given either routinely or under some experimental arrangement. She could also add that such a situation was discussed at the school where she received her education and that this procedure was suggested by the faculty.
3. She realizes that the A.D.A. and the state dental licensing boards are liberalizing what the dental hygienist is permitted to do, and hence she is not sure whether her dentist-employer really wants her to perform this task or whether he is just checking on her knowledge of the current dental practice act.

There is also the problem of the dental hygienist who is asked by her new employer to perform certain tasks and functions for which she does not feel competent. In this case, she could also use some of the items suggested above and also explain:

1. I was not given sufficient education and experience in this operation and function when I took my training at —————— University, and I have not taken a short course in this subject.
2. My previous employer did not want me to perform this type of function in his office. I feel very inexperienced and would need some refresher training and experience before I would feel that I should attempt it.
3. I admit that I do not feel competent to perform this function, but if you wish me to become expert in this, I shall be glad to follow your recommendations and suggestions.

There may be dental hygienists who do not wish to perform the new functions or even to learn how to perform them. In this event there are two possibilities for the dental hygienist in an office in which her dentist-employer has requested that she "expand her duties." She has the following choices:

1. Find another position.
2. Ask her employer to assign her only to operations and functions that she does enjoy and feels competent to perform.

The foregoing paragraphs have indicated that the assigned duties in a dental office can sometimes become a problem. Some of this depends upon the degree to which the dentist-employer is changing or enlarging the duties of his dental assistant and his dental hygienist. This point is discussed at some length in Chapter 10 and should be studied thoroughly.

It is very important for every dental hygienist as well as her dentist-employer to keep well informed on the changes that are made periodically in both the dental practice act and the interpretation of the state licensing board regarding the functions permitted for all of the auxiliary dental personnel. If one has an opportunity, it is also a good idea to keep in touch with the dental school or school for dental hygienists in the area, because these institutions are always a good index of what functions the practicing dentist will be expecting from his dental hygienist and his dental assistant.

The dental hygienist must realize that she has a professional responsibility to her dentist-employer to let him know if:

1. She encounters a patient problem that she does not feel competent to handle.
2. She is asked to use a piece of equipment that she does not feel that she is experienced in using or manipulating.
3. She does not feel competent to employ a certain new technic on a patient that the dentist has requested.

For example, some states do not permit the use of topical applications of fluorides. While schools in those states still teach the technic, they may not provide the students with as much experience in it as in other technics. Also, patients available to some school clinics may not provide examples of extremely heavy calculus deposits, and a dental hygienist from such a school may not feel competent to treat such a patient without some help or without very close supervision. Without this kind of an explanation she may be called upon to render a treatment that she is unqualified to perform and may actually cause damage and harm to the patient. Also, without this precaution, she could also cause her employer to be taken into court because of the damage that could be caused by her treatment. The employee-employer relationship in a professional office should be such that problems of competency and expertise can be discussed honestly in private. The employee should be able to expect an interested and considerate listener.

Similarly, the dental hygienist should feel free to talk to her dentist-employer about her accomplishments. If she has taken a refresher course and has learned about some new technics, her dentist will be interested in learning of this. If she goes to an exhibit of dental equipment and sees some new equipment that she thinks will be of interest to her employer, she should want to tell him about this. If a special course is being given to help dental hygienists learn how to use a new piece of equipment, she will want to talk to her employer and see whether he wants her to enroll in this course.

Every employer deserves an allegiance and loyalty from every employee during the time that she is accepting salary checks for her services. As a matter of fact, while it is inexcusable to criticize one's employer while working for him, it is also not professionally ethical or proper to criticize or slander a previous employer, no matter how unhappy one might have been in that office. As a rule, one praises and compliments the employers who have been fine persons to work for; when one has no compliments to offer about a previous position, this is enough of an indictment of that office without becoming unethical in trying to elaborate upon this fact. Every dental hygienist should also keep in mind that a prospective employer does not want to employ any person who makes a point of criticizing her former employers. He knows that she would not be changing positions if she did not have some reasons, but he will respect her more if she refuses to criticize her former employers.

THE BEST STUDENT DOES NOT ALWAYS MAKE THE BEST EMPLOYEE

The best grades do not always guarantee success in the dental office. Grades are very important, but it takes much more than good grades to make one a success in a dental office. This is also true of the dentist himself. There are many fine dentists who are very skillful and talented, and yet if they do not know how to get along with their patients or with people in general, then they are usually failures. This is true also of the employees in a dental office. The *super* dental assistant and the *unusual* dental hygienist may both find that they are misfits in an office in spite of the fact that they have passed all of their school courses with high grades. When one listens to many employers talk about their office problems, it becomes evident that nearly all of them have had the unfortunate experience of having to fire an employee who was actually outstanding in every way except one—the art of getting along with other people.

A certain percentage of those who are reading this chapter will have the unfortunate characteristic of irritating other people from time to time or doing something that will distract tremendously from her true ability and talent. This inability to be able to get along with other people takes many different forms. Some of the various kinds of traits are as follows:

1. Trouble-makers in the office—those who constantly try to make everyone suspicious of everyone else
2. So-called perfectionists who constantly brag about their skills and belittle their colleagues' abilities
3. Interfering persons who are never content to attend to their own assignment but who always have to inject themselves in other people's business
4. Persons who can never work with anyone else on a project without trying to make the other person feel insecure and inferior
5. Persons who consistently break office rules and flaunt the fact that they can get by with it
6. Persons who can never follow an outlined procedure but who always insist upon doing it in a different way just to be different and contrary
7. Persons who will never take advice or follow suggestions of their superiors but who instead always try to criticize other people
8. Persons who try to see only the bad side to things and are ever mindful of telling everyone about these bad omens

There are, of course, many, many more examples of people who have one or two qualities and characteristics that are so self-destructive that these people can never hold a job for very long. They only end up by making even themselves very unhappy. It is not easy to help these people because most of them refuse to recognize that they have any personal problems. Those who feel that a problem exists usually feel that they are blameless and that their problems are caused by the other people around them.

In this chapter, it has been emphasized that every employee should try to have an excellent working relationship with her dentist-employer. If this is a good relationship, then the dentist-employer will probably feel free to give advice, and he can help his employees to correct their faults. However, there are still some who have these peculiar faults so firmly ingrained in them that they will not be helped.

There is no single formula for success in a dental office, just as there is no single kind of person who is the troublemaker for the office. It is unfortunate that the willing and able employee is not permitted to exert all of his energy and his skill in doing a good job for the office. However, in every office every good employee has to spend a goodly portion of time helping to make the teamwork system operate. When one finds that she is working in an office in which there is harmony and respect among most of the employees, then she can feel very fortunate, and she can also take a measure of credit for this situation for she is a part of this team.

There is no simple formula for knowing how to get along with the boss or for knowing how to let the boss know that there are unscrupulous employees who are "robbing him blind." There are no simple, unfailing methods of being able to work efficiently in a complex situation in which the wrong people seem to have all of the power and get all of the attention. The fact that there are many successful and highly professional offices proves that some persons have found some workable formula for getting along well with their colleagues. This means that there is a large number of very fine employees who operate successful offices in spite of any failings and shortcomings that they may have.

Dental hygienists are cognizant that in most offices there is a definite, clearcut distinction between the various members of the dental health team. Dental assistants are usually aware that a type of "caste system" exists in most dental offices. Everyone abhors any kind of "caste system" unless it is perhaps the person who is at the top of the "caste." It will aid employees as well as employers to have a sound philosophical understanding of what is meant by a dental health team and what the advantages and disadvantages of a "caste system" can be.

It is difficult to think of any group of persons or any organization in which there isn't some sort of rank order given consciously or subconsciously to its members. In a school, it may be the Board of Regents, the President, the various vice-presidents, the deans, the department chairmen, the individual teachers, the assistants, and so on. In the military, there is the President, who is the Commander-in-Chief of all of the military divisions, the cabinet officers for the different armed services, the generals, the other officers, the noncommissioned personnel, and so on. Even in the family household there are sequences of authority and responsibility. There are some households in which the responsibilities are as well defined and as carefully followed as in the military or in a school system.

In the dental hygiene department of any school, there is a sequence of authority and a sequence of responsibility. Normally, those at the top of the listing who have the responsibility for the program have had the most training and experience. This is not always true, for sometimes some of the instructors have had even more experience and education than their supervisors, but they are occupying positions that do not require them to make the same kinds of

decisions. There are many retired persons who have come back into educational programs who have education, training, and experience that far surpasses that of those in charge of the total program. However, one should always realize and recognize that when a director or supervisor of dental hygiene has been selected, that person not only has the authority to do some things that an ordinary faculty member cannot do but he also has chosen to take on a multitude of responsibilities for which he will be held responsible. One should not forget this parallelism between authority and responsibility. If the program is found to be failing, it is not the assistant, the instructor, or even the assistant supervisor who is called to task for this failure. The failure is blamed on the top administrative officer of the program. Deans and departmental chairmen and dental hygiene supervisors can be fired from their prestigious positions if their programs fail, but it is interesting to note that the instructor is rarely affected by matters of this importance.

The dental office is no exception to this general rule. If a patient dies in the office, it will be the dentist who will be called upon to explain the situation, for he is the one who is responsible for everything that takes place in that office by the whole "dental team." Similarly, if something about the prophylaxis treatment given by the dental hygienist is questioned, it is she who will be questioned by her employer and by those who are in turn bringing legal action. The dental assistant, the dental laboratory technician, the bookkeeper, and the receptionist are not the ones who will worry about this incident.

There are many unhappy persons today who want added prestige and jobs that offer the ultimate in importance and authority. But such persons should realize that they must justify the preparation and ability to hold such a responsible position. They must realize that with added prestige and added authority also comes added responsibility and the likelihood for blame when things go wrong. The employee who is interested first of all in how well she can do the job for which she was hired and how well she can please her employer so that she can be worthy of advancement or even a good recommendation for another position is the employee who invariably makes a success of herself.

The best employee is the one who is a bit humble—humble enough at least to let herself know that she is still learning and that success and advancement will come when she proves that she deserves it.

The successful employee is the one who does the following, among others:

1. Tries to select for an employer a person whom she admires greatly
2. Tries to select the boss to whom she can be loyal
3. Tries to make the best of difficult situations as they occur
4. Tries to work cooperatively with every other employee
5. Tries to overlook the faults of other employees
6. Tries to overlook the bad features of the "caste system" and accept the fact that the higher the authority, the greater the responsibility
7. Tries to seek help from her employer in attaining the education and experience that will make her eligible for the advancements
8. Tries to overlook the petty jealousies and gossip of the average office
9. Refrains from criticizing her boss to his colleagues or to any others
10. Tries to improve herself in her present job

These ten items merely scratch the surface of a list of the kinds of things that could be helpful to a career woman who wants to be a success.

Some employees listen to and depend upon the advice of their fellow workers. This is not always a good plan. No one but the employer can tell an employee exactly what it is that he expects of her and her work. What he expects of someone else may be different. Also, the translation of what he wants may sound quite different by the time that it is told to her. In other words, no employee should depend upon getting her directives from anyone but her supervisor or her boss. One should never be satisfied with secondhand information, for it is usually wrong or slanted.

Even though one wants to trust her office friends, there may be a few colleagues and fellow workers who would much rather see themselves succeed than to help anyone else be successful. If this selfishness is strong enough, then it is conceivable that there might be some workers who would devote some attention to discouraging the new employee, giving the new employee slightly warped information on what she is expected to do, and completely misrepresenting many things.

In Chapter 11 of this book, attention is given to the importance of studying the patient's background, fears, problems, apprehensions, and so on. It is important to understand the patient if the dental hygienist and her doctor are going to be successful in serving and treating that patient.

If it is important for the dental hygienist to understand the patient with whom she comes in contact a few hours during a lifetime, then it is even more important that she understand her employer and her colleagues. Not everything can be taken for granted and not everything can be taken for "face value." If the dental hygienist likes her job and wants to succeed, then she should be willing to devote a good many hours to studying her job, her employer, her colleagues, her surroundings, and the total office picture. Every student knows that if she wants to learn and if she wants to earn good grades on examinations, she must study her professors as much as she studies her textbooks. A new dental hygienist in an office should study her employer and her fellow workers in depth, for her career and her future depend upon these persons. (This suggestion seems so logical and so sensible, and yet it is rather surprising that very few classroom discussions are devoted to this practical approach to "success in the professions.") This is also good advice for the dental hygiene supervisor and dental hygiene instructor. They must also study the philosophies of their supervisors, namely, the dean and the directors of instruction for whom they work, if they are going to succeed and receive promotions.

The dental hygienist who reads this chapter and who studies this textbook has already decided that she wants to make a success of dental hygiene as her career. She has chosen not only an important health profession, but she has chosen a career in which her success depends upon how well she can treat patients and one in which her productiveness, her efficiency, and her future depend upon how well she can work as a member of a "team" of persons. This means that she must concentrate on such things as the following:

1. Improving her knowledge
2. Improving her skill and competence
3. Learning to understand her patients
4. Learning to understand her dentist-employer and interpreting how best she can serve in this office as a dental hygienist
5. Learning to understand her role as a member of the office's "dental health team" and to improve her efficiency as a team member

As one can see from the preceding summary list, knowledge, skill, and work are only a few of the items that will influence the dental hygienist's success and future. Equally as important, and probably more important, is the dental hygienist's ability to discover her role in the dental office and learn how to work successfully with all of the people with whom she comes in contact. Success will come to those who follow this kind of advice.

part two

THE PRACTICE OF DENTAL HYGIENE

chapter 4

CASE HISTORIES, CHARTING, AND DIAGNOSIS

James Foster, Jr., D.D.S.

One of the most vital areas in the operation of a dental office is that of keeping accurate patient records. It is an area of shared responsibility in most private offices today and in the near future may well be a task primarily delegated to the nondentist office team member.

In dental record keeping, tooth designation by number has varied somewhat over the past 20 years, and the method most often used was that with which the dentist became familiar during his student experience. Recently, a standardized method of tooth designation for both primary and permanent teeth has been proposed by the Fédération Dentaire Internationale. It is a two-digit numbering system that offers simple and fast identification of tooth location, indicates whether it is primary or permanent dentition, and is compatible with computerization of records when such methods of record keeping are used. This approach is particularly helpful in research projects where large numbers of entries are made. Specifically, the proposed international tooth numbering method is a step toward simplification in the sharing of information in the field of dentistry and foreseeably will lead toward a better understanding of the incidence, frequency, and management of dento-oral disease. It can be assumed that the acceptance of this system will be widespread in universities, hospitals, and very likely, in time, by federal health agencies (Fig. 4-1).

In many physicians' offices today, the medical history is taken and recorded by an office member other than the doctor himself. With a greater appreciation of the role of systemic disease as it relates to oral health, wound healing, and the like, the dentist today needs to know a great deal more about his patient other than just his current dental complaint. The task of taking and recording a definitive past medical history and past dental history may well become a routine duty of the dental hygienist.

Many commercially produced forms for this purpose are available, most of which are very adequate. Most are a "check sheet" type questionnaire designed to review past medical experiences, diseases, operations, or conditions that might have a bearing on the selection of dental treatment or medication for the individual patient.

At the University of Texas Dental Branch at Houston, a health questionnaire (Fig. 4-2) form was developed using the checklist approach. It is a composite reflection of the basic information requirements of all clinical departments. This health questionnaire is included in each patient's chart and is completed on each patient to be

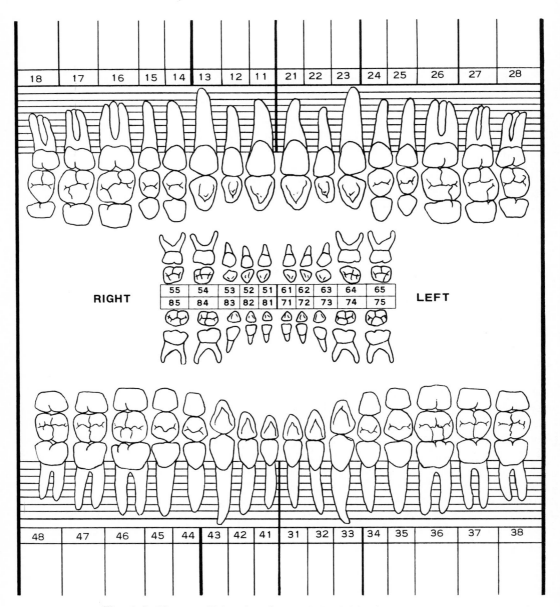

Fig. 4-1. (Courtesy University of Texas Dental Branch, Houston, Tex.)

U.T.D.B. HEALTH QUESTIONNAIRE

SPECIAL CASE NOTES

NAME _____ DATE OF BIRTH _____ SEX ___ _____

WEIGHT _____ HEIGHT _____ MARRIED _____ _____

NAME OF FAMILY PHYSICIAN OR PEDIATRICIAN _____ _____

ADDRESS _____ PHONE _____ _____

WHAT IS YOUR CHIEF COMPLAINT ABOUT YOUR MOUTH OR TEETH? _____ _____

_____ _____

DATE OF LAST PHYSICAL EXAMINATION _____ _____

HAVE YOU EVER HAD OR SUSPECTED?	YES	NO
CANCER		
RHEUMATIC FEVER		
HEART TROUBLE		
ABNORMAL BLOOD PRESSURE		
CHEST PAIN		
SHORTNESS OF BREATH		
ASTHMA OR HAY FEVER		
SINUS TROUBLE		
TUBERCULOSIS		
DIABETES		
FREQUENT THIRST		
KIDNEY OR BLADDER TROUBLE		
BLOOD DISEASE		
HEPATITIS OR JAUNDICE		
PROLONGED BLEEDING		
SEVERE HEADACHES		
TREATED BY RADIATION (X-RAY)		
ANY DIFFICULTY IN THE PAST ASSOCIATED WITH DENTAL TREATMENT		
HAVE YOU HAD?	YES	NO
FAINTING TENDENCY		
ANY RECENT MEDICAL TREATMENT		
YOUR TONSILS REMOVED		
ANY OTHER OPERATIONS		
ARE YOU TAKING OR HAVE YOU EVER TAKEN THE FOLLOWING DRUGS?	YES	NO
CORTISONE DRUGS, STEROIDS, ACTH OR ANTI REJECTION DRUGS		
ANTICOAGULANTS OR BLOOD THINNERS		
TRANQUILIZERS OR SEDATIVES		
ANY OTHER MEDICINES OR DRUGS		
ALLERGIES	YES	NO
ARE YOU ALLERGIC TO PENICILLIN		
ARE YOU SENSITIVE OR ALLERGIC TO ANY OTHER MEDICINE OR FOOD		
HAVE YOU EVER HAD NOVOCAINE OR SIMILAR LOCAL ANESTHETIC		
HAVE YOU EVER HAD A GENERAL ANESTHETIC		
HAVE YOU HAD ANY UNDESIRABLE EFFECTS FROM ANY ANESTHETIC		
TO BE COMPLETED ON ALL PATIENTS UNDER 14 YEARS OF AGE		
DO YOU CONSIDER YOUR CHILD TO BE	YES	NO
ADVANCED IN THE LEARNING PROCESS		
PROGRESSING NORMALLY IN THE LEARNING PROCESS		
A SLOW LEARNER		
HAS THE CHILD EXPERIENCED ANY UNFAVORABLE REACTION FROM ANY PREVIOUS DENTAL OR MEDICAL CARE?		
WOMEN ONLY	YES	NO
ARE YOU PREGNANT		
DO YOU HAVE ANY PROBLEMS ASSOCIATED WITH YOUR MENSTRUAL PERIOD		
ARE YOU PRESENTLY TAKING ANY MEDICINE OF ANY KIND ROUTINELY (BIRTH CONTROL, THYROID, ETC.)		

SIGNATURE OF PATIENT, PARENT, OR LEGAL GUARDIAN   SIGNATURE OF FACULTY ADVISOR

Fig. 4-2. Health questionnaire. (Courtesy University of Texas Dental Branch, Houston, Tex.)

PRELIMINARY EXAMINATION   Date _____

Chief Complaint: _____
        History of Complaint: _____

Past Medical History: _____
_____
_____
_____
_____
_____

General Health: Excellent □   Good □   Average □   Fair □   Poor □
        Current Medical Treatment: _____
_____

        Drugs Being Taken: _____

        Nutritional Status/Diet: _____
_____

        Age _____ Sex _____ Weight _____ Height _____ Blood Pressure _____ Pulse _____
        Temperature _____ Respiratory Rate _____

Past Dental History: _____
_____
_____
_____

Hygiene Index: _____
_____
_____

Past Personal History (Birthplace, Residences, Occupation): _____
_____
_____

Special Medical or Dental Considerations: _____
_____
_____

Referral Consultations: _____
_____

    Student _____ Faculty Advisor _____

Review of above findings for change which might alter further treatment:

DATE OF REVIEW	CHANGES IN GENERAL HEALTH OR MEDICATION	INITIALS

Fig. 4-3. Preliminary examination. (Courtesy University of Texas Dental Branch, Houston, Tex.)

treated by dental students and by students in the School of Dental Hygiene.

The hygienist must have a basic level of understanding in interpreting such information to properly care for her patients and to be able to alert the dentist of possible medical conditions that warrant further inquiry prior to treatment of any kind.

The dentist's background, training, and experience enable him to follow up his investigations in those medical areas of concern noted in the health questionnaire and to project a treatment plan that will best care for the patient's dental needs. Often medical consultations between the physician and the dentist are required.

To enable our students to understand *first* why each question is included in the health questionnaire and *second* the significance of the patient's response, a copy of the "Student Guide to the Interpretation of the Health Questionnaire" is distributed to each dental and hygiene student during their training. The contents of this guide are given in the accompanying box.

The explanations are brief but serve to offer to the student an insight in areas of patient management where an understanding of the patient's general health, disease, current medications, and past complications associated with treatment guide and direct treatment choice.

There is little doubt that in the future dental practice will be a team effort. This will come as a response to the challenge of a growing population interested in oral health through better education, ability to afford comprehensive dental care, or assurance of treatment payment through third-party payment.

With team effort in the private office, it becomes readily apparent that a sharing of responsibilities would extend primarily to the best-qualified member of the office team, the hygienist. Such an expansion of responsibilities will, no doubt, include preliminary examination and provisional

diagnosis. Included are two of the proposed forms prepared by the Chart Revision Committee at the University of Texas Dental Branch. These deal with the recording of examination findings. The items included in the forms will be discussed individually to clarify the type of entries to be made (Figs. 4-3 and 4-4).

PRELIMINARY EXAMINATION

Chief complaint. This should be stated in the patient's own words and should concern itself with the problem that caused the patient to seek dental treatment.

History of complaint. Document the onset, frequency, severity, and type of discomfort the patient has experienced.

Past medical history. Include a recording of all past experiences of surgical or medical nature. Note whether the patient has had radiation therapy and to what area of the body. Include any past traumatic experiences to the jaw or face.

General health. This should reflect basically the patient's own feeling concerning his general health status. If it differs from the clinical impressions of the examiner, further interrogation is indicated.

Current medical treatment. Include any medical treatment that the patient has received within the past year.

Drugs being taken. Include any medication that the patient has had prescribed or self-administered during the past year. Of particular interest are those patients who are taking or have received cortisone or anti-coagulant drugs during the preceding year. Record the type and daily dosage of all drugs received by the patient. Patients under therapy for diabetes must be under control and current status verified.

Nutritional status/diet. Give a brief summation of the patient's dietary status indicating relative adequacy, predominance of protein or carbohydrate ingestion, habitual skipping of meals, or special diets, prescribed or otherwise. Note dietary analysis requirements as indicated.

EXAMINATION FINDINGS

(Description of findings)

SOFT TISSUE EXAM:

Lips _____

Tongue _____

Cheeks _____

Floor of mouth _____

Palate _____

Throat _____

Ridge Form _____

Mucosa _____

Saliva _____

ROENTGENOGRAPHIC FINDINGS:

Apical lesions _____

Trabecular Pattern _____

Pulp Cavity calcifications _____

Periodontal ligament space _____

Bone height-alv. crest _____

Defects _____

Dental caries _____

Root tips (residual) _____

Foreign bodies _____

Other _____

EXAMINATION OF HEAD AND NECK:

Regional nodes _____

Skin _____

Face Form _____ Arch Form _____

OCCLUSION:

Classification _____

Freeway Space _____

Prematurities _____

Missing Teeth _____

Specific abnormalities _____

PERIODONTAL CHARTING:

Diagnosis _____

Etiology _____

Prognosis _____

Tissue reaction after scaling _____

Fig. 4-4. Examination findings. (Courtesy University of Texas Dental Branch, Houston, Tex.)

STUDENT GUIDE
For the interpretation of the UTDB health questionnaire

This questionnaire, despite brevity, offers a fairly wide scope of general information to guide your treatment selection in patient management.

Affirmative answers do not necessarily preclude patient acceptance but in all instances should stimulate further questioning to achieve a better understanding of the patient's health status.

Where medical clearance by the patient's physician is determined advisable by the student's Faculty Advisor, this should be noted in the "Special Case Notes" section in the upper right corner of the Questionnaire Form. All such requests are processed through the Office of the Clinical Coordinator (Rm. 223).

Each area of the questionnaire is considered in sequence with brief discussion of possible implication of affirmative answers.

U.T.D.B. HEALTH QUESTIONNAIRE

SPECIAL CASE NOTES

NAME_____ DATE OF BIRTH_____ SEX____ _____

WEIGHT_____ HEIGHT_____ MARRIED_____ _____

NAME OF FAMILY PHYSICIAN OR PEDIATRICIAN_____ _____

ADDRESS_____ PHONE_____ _____

WHAT IS YOUR CHIEF COMPLAINT ABOUT YOUR MOUTH OR TEETH? _____

DATE OF LAST PHYSICAL EXAMINATION _____ _____

Vital statistics—Self explanatory.

Special case notes—Includes any comments of conditions, past treatment, or medication that would affect treatment choice, such as cardiac disease, allergies, rheumatic fever, radiation to jaws, anticoagulant medication. Enter in this section request for medical clearance when indicated.

Chief complaint—Enter in the "patient's own words."

Date of last physical examination—Unless this date is within the past year, its value is questionable, and medical clearance for dental treatment by the patient's physician will probably not be given without a current examination.

HAVE YOU EVER HAD OR SUSPECTED?	YES	NO
Cancer		
Rheumatic fever		
Heart trouble		
Abnormal blood pressure		
Chest pain		
Shortness of breath		
Asthma or hay fever		
Sinus trouble		
Tuberculosis		
Diabetes		
Frequent thirst		
Kidney or bladder trouble		
Blood disease		
Hepatitis or jaundice		
Prolonged bleeding		
Severe headaches		
Treated by radiation (x-ray)		
Any difficulty in the past associated with dental treatment		

Continued.

Cancer—Current therapy includes surgery, radiation, chemotherapy, or combinations thereof. When the treated lesion was located in the head and neck area, special precautions are required when *radiation* to the jaws has occurred. The resulting reduction in vascularity may eventuate an osteoradionecrosis following dental surgery. *Cytotoxic* drugs used in cancer chemotherapy are often used in the management of chronic leukemia. These drugs produce oral ulcerations as a side effect. Such patients' resistance to dental infection is lowered. *Surgical treatment* of oral malignancy often results in loss or reduced function of the jaws and tongue complicating dental prosthetic consideration.

Rheumatic fever—Patients with RF history often have damaged heart valves. Prophylactic antibiotics should be given prior to any dental procedure that involves the oral soft tissues (including periodontal examination). Such patients are susceptible to subacute bacterial endocarditis. See recommendations of American Heart Association—A.D.R. *(Accepted Dental Remedies).*

Heart trouble

Abnormal blood pressure—Blood pressure to be taken and recorded on patient's first visit. Medical clearance is advisable on any patient with history of hypertension or cardiac disease.

Chest pain—On exertion may be indicative of angina pectoris.

Shortness of breath—May be associated with valvular heart disease with associated atherosclerotic changes, or may be a reflection of pulmonary disease.

Asthma or hay fever—Often reported in patients with multiple allergies. Past episodes of asthmatic crisis should be recorded. Specific allergies should be noted.

Sinus trouble—Due to the proximity of the inferior convolutions of the maxillary antra to the apices of maxillary bicuspids and molars, pain from an acute sinusitis is often described by the patient as dental pain. In chronic sinus disease, a thickening of the sinus membranes is apparent on dental x-ray films. When fluid accumulation is present, the sinus appears cloudy on x-ray films and will not transilluminate.

Tuberculosis—In affirmative response to this question, the operator should wear protective mask and gloves during treatment. Instruments and towels used should be autoclaved. Granulomatous oral lesions of tuberculosis are rarely seen.

Diabetes

Frequent thirst, frequent urination, and dry mouth often are suggestive of diabetes mellitus. The controlled diabetic offers no difficulty in dental treatment except for a reduced resistance to infection. Antibiotic coverage during surgical procedures is advisable. The uncontrolled diabetic should not be considered for elective dental care. Verification of control level in known diabetics is mandatory.

Kidney or bladder trouble—Oral sepsis is often associated with glomerulonephritis. Dental surgery should not be done on patients with acute kidney disease. If emergency extractions are necessary, antibiotics should be given prophylactically.

Blood disease—While this question is primarily concerned with hemorrhagic diathesis, patient response to this question may vary. "Bad blood" is a colloquialism describing syphilis. Anemia is often a self-diagnosed state that will require verification.

Hepatitis or jaundice—The student should wear gloves, mask, and eye glasses while treating patients giving a positive history. All instruments used should be autoclaved.

In patients with severe liver disease, bleeding problems may be present due to their inability to absorb and utilize vitamin K, as well as to reduced prothrombin production.

Severe headaches—Rarely associated with dental disease except in patients with acute pulpitis or TMJ pain dysfunction syndrome. May be related to hypertension, sinus disease, migraine, or disease or lesion of CNS or of psychogenic basis.

Treated by radiation (x-ray)—To include all types of treatment by ionizing radiation. Of particular interest are patients who have had radiation to the jaws—no extractions should be done in areas receiving tumoricidal doses of radiation due to the possibility of a subsequent osteoradionecrosis.

Any difficulty associated with past dental treatment—When answered in the affirmative, determine date, degree, and type of problem, as well as how often problems have been associated with dental treatment. Being forewarned of possible complications of treatment allows the operator to prevent repeating past errors.

HAVE YOU HAD?		
Fainting tendency		
Any recent medical treatment		
Your tonsils removed		
Any other operations		

Have you had?

Fainting tendency—A history of repeated episodes of fainting or blackouts may be associated with epilepsy. If such is the case, special care and sedation may prevent precipitating a seizure during the course of dental care. Unexplained, repeated episodes of syncope should be referred to the patient's physician for evaluation and treatment.

Any recent medical treatment—Most patients under current care by a physician are taking one or more varieties of medication. Knowing what a patient is being treated for and what medications he is receiving reduces the possibility of the dentist prescribing drugs, diet, or therapy that would conflict with medical treatment in progress. For example, a patient on a salt-free diet should not be advised to use saline irrigation. The diabetic should not be instructed to drink several large glasses of orange juice daily. Great care must be taken in prescribing sedatives for patients on antihypertensive drugs because of their potentiating capabilities, which can produce severe hypotension.

Your tonsils removed

Any other operations—Often a patient's only reportable experience with local or general anesthetics will be associated with a T & A. Bleeding tendencies may be associated with such procedures. Patients giving a history of being treated for an oral neoplasm should be examined carefully for recurrence.

ARE YOU TAKING OR HAVE YOU EVER TAKEN THE FOLLOWING DRUGS?		
Cortisone drugs, steroids, ACTH, or anti-rejection drugs		
Anticoagulants or blood thinners		
Tranquilizers or sedatives		
Any other medicines or drugs		

Cortisone drugs, steroids, ACTH, or antirejection drugs—These drugs depress inflammatory response and can shield the clinical appearance of oral infection. In addition, their administration depresses the function of the adrenal cortex. The inherent problem is in the patient's inability to compensate for stress. Dental surgery may precipitate adrenal insufficiency in patients on long-term steroid therapy.

Continued.

Anticoagulants and blood thinners—Usually patients on such drugs are being treated for coronary occlusion, CVA's, or clots. Elective surgery is not to be done because of the bleeding problems that can be anticipated. When emergency dental surgery is required, cooperative effort with the attending physician is a must.

Tranquilizers and sedatives—Many of your patients will be receiving routine daily medication with one or more of the above. Care must be taken in prescribing for such patients as the action of barbiturates are potentiated by tranquilizers with resultant severe hypotension as a possibility. General anesthetics given to patients on tranquilizers have the same inherent danger.

Any other medication or drugs—The dentist should be aware of all medication the patient is taking. Many women carry their medication in their purses and the identification of drugs (not labeled) is often possible using the product identification section of the P.D.R. This is available in the oral surgery office, the examination clinic, and the clinical coordinator's office.

ALLERGIES		
Are you allergic to penicillin		
Are you sensitive or allergic to any other medicine or food		
Have you ever had Novocaine or similar local anesthetic		
Have you ever had a general anesthetic		
Have you had any undesirable effects from any anesthetic		

Allergy to penicillin—When acknowledged by the patient, note in RED in the special care note section *and* on the front cover of the dental chart.

Sensitivity to other medicine or food—Known allergies should be recorded. Of specific interest are those drugs and medications in common dental usage.

Have you ever had undersirable effects from Novocaine or similar local anesthetics

Have you ever had a general anesthetic

Have you had any undesirable effects from any anesthetic

Most patients will report having received local anesthesia without ill effects. Syncope associated with the injection of a local anesthetic is, in most instances, of psychogenic basis today. There is an extremely low incidence of allergy to the local anesthetics (Lidocaine, Carbocaine) in common usage. The use of an aspirating syringe reduces the possibility of inadvertent intravascular injection. All anesthetics should be injected slowly so that should an adverse reaction occur, the injection can be stopped immediately.

Where past ill effects following dental anesthesia are reported by the patient, care should be taken in the selection and use of a suitable alternate anesthetic agent.

TO BE COMPLETED ON ALL PATIENTS UNDER 14 YRS. OF AGE

DO YOU CONSIDER YOUR CHILD TO BE		
Advanced in the learning process		
Progressing normally in the learning process		
A slow learner		
Has the child experienced any unfavorable reaction from previous dental or medical care		

In child growth and in development of the dentition, the chronological and biological ages do not always coincide. The child classified as a slow learner may reflect an overall picture of delayed physiological development including the dentition. Conversely, there are child patients who present a state of dental development that may be 1 year or more ahead of that considered average for their actual age.

Unfavorable past dental experience should be determined at the time of initial interview to guide the operator in future patient management.

WOMEN ONLY

Are you pregnant		
Do you have any problems associated with your menstrual period		
Are you presently taking any medicine of any kind routinely (birth control, thyroid, etc.)		

Signature of patient, parent, or legal guardian

Signature of faculty advisor

Are you pregnant—Elective dental treatment is best accomplished during the second trimester of pregnancy. Should spontaneous abortion occur, it most often is during the first trimester. Nausea, when present, is primarily during this early period. During the last 2 months of pregnancy, routine care is best deferred.

Whenever pregnant patients are to have dental x-rays made, a lead apron shield should be used to protect the developing fetus from stray radiation.

Do you have any problems with your menstrual cycle—Many patients show evidence of gingival change during menstrual cycle due to alterations of hormonal balances. In women who report excessive menstrual flow, elective endodontic or surgical procedures should be deferred during the period.

Are you presently taking medicine of any kind—(birth control pills, thyroid) The effects of birth control medication on oral tissues is unproved but suspected in many instances of nonspecific gingivitis and in apparent altered healing processes.

Patients receiving 3 or more grains of thyroid daily should have medical clearance prior to dental treatment.

Age, sex, weight, height, blood pressure, pulse, temperature, and respiratory rate. A patient's age in most instances is accurately given; however, in middle-aged female patients this answer may become more of an estimate than a fact. The examiner should be alerted to the possibility of potential medical problems whenever the chronological age reported by the patient is not compatible with the physiological aging in the appearance of the patient. For example, premature graying seen in a young person may be indicative of pernicious anemia. The blood pressure, pulse, temperature, and respiratory rate should be recorded at the patient's first visit. This establishes a baseline of normal physiological functions that is most valuable in the event that the patient becomes ill or requires emergency treatment during a dental visit. The greatest accuracy in judging respiratory rate can be achieved if the evaluation of the patient's breathing is done at the time the pulse is being recorded for invariably if the patient is aware of one's counting his number of respirations, he will alter his breathing pattern.

Past dental history. Past dental treatment should be recorded along with the reasons for any extractions that may have been done in the past. When a tooth is missing in the arch, the patient should always be asked when and why it was extracted. If the patient has no recollection of an extraction in the area, it is advisable to take additional dental x-rays of approximating areas of the jaw to determine whether the tooth is congenitally missing or impacted. Patients who wear prostheses should be asked how long they have been wearing them. The frequency of oral prophylaxis should be recorded along with the number of times a day the patient brushes his teeth, the type of brush used, and whether or not any auxiliary aids to oral hygiene are used (for example, dental floss, toothpicks, Stimu-dents, interdental stimulators, or water irrigation devices). Any difficulty associated with past dental treatment should be noted.

Hygiene index. Plaque indices are best recorded on the patient's first office visit. This gives a basis for comparison at a later date of the effectiveness of the oral hygiene instruction.

Past personal history. The birthplace, residences, and occupation often give an insight into deviation from norm, particularly with regard to calcified dental structures. An example would be mottled enamel associated with the patient's having lived in areas with an unusually high fluoride ion concentration in the water supply during the period of tooth development. Certain other changes are associated with the individual's occupation. Pastry chefs, employees of candy factories, and bakers in general, because of their breathing sugar fumes, show a very high caries activity index, particularly in gingival areas. Operators of heavy equipment such as bulldozers, farmers who drive tractors, and operators of pneumatic hammers will inevitably demonstrate a loss of tooth structure on occlusal surfaces as a result of the jiggling together of teeth by vibration while the individual is breathing in abrasive dusts. Abnormal wear facets associated with bruxism are often present on the chewing surfaces of the teeth of individuals who are subjected to high levels of stress. Airplane pilots, race drivers, policemen, firemen, and young mothers are included in that group.

Special medical or dental considerations. List any factors such as current medications, medical conditions, past radiation therapy, sensitivities, or special diets that might alter or cause modification of a projected dental plan.

Referral consultations. Any patient whose past history or preliminary examination indicates the presence or direct suspicion toward systemic disease should have a medical consultation prior to the initiation of any dental procedure. Special dental consultation will be determined following the comprehensive dental-oral examination by the attending dentist.

Review of findings. Whenever an interruption has occurred in the sequence of treatment or upon routine recall for dental maintenance appointments, the preceding material should be reviewed for changes in the health status or medications.

EXAMINATION FINDINGS
Soft tissue examination

Lips. Examination of the lips should include bidigital palpation of the upper and lower lips along with a careful visual examination of the dried vermilion as well as mucosal portions. Any abnormalities are to be described in detail.

Tongue. The tongue should be dried with cotton sponges and carefully examined. The base of the tongue can best be seen by pulling the tongue slightly forward and lateral. This makes it possible to examine both its dorsal and ventral surfaces.

The lateral borders of the tongue should be palpated between the thumb and fore-finger and any discrepancy noted.

Cheeks. The cheeks, including the accessible zones over the parotid gland and duct, are to be examined by direct visualization as well as by manual palpation for the presence of swelling or masses.

Floor of mouth. The floor of the mouth is best visually examined by deflecting the tongue laterally using a mouth mirror as a retractor. Palpation of the floor of the mouth for masses is most simply accomplished by having the patient lean his head slightly forward. Place the first finger of the left hand medial to the inferior border to the mandible while exerting a slight upward pressure, then palpate the floor of the mouth with the first finger of the right hand.

Palate. Both the soft and hard palate should be dried with cotton sponges and examined visually and by palpation. Abnormalities should be noted.

Throat. The examination of the throat is best accomplished with the patient sitting vertically under adequate illumination. The tongue is depressed with either a wooden tongue blade placed well back on the dorsum of the tongue or with a mouth mirror. Particular attention should be paid the tonsillar areas.

Ridge form. Note the form of the alveolar process after the teeth have been removed.

1. Maxillary ridge
   a. Class 1: square, gently curved, or ovoid
   b. Class 2: tapering or V-shaped
   c. Class 3: flat
2. Mandibular ridge
   a. Class 1: inverted U; parallel walled, broad crested
   b. Class 2: flat, inverted, U-shaped
   c. Class 3: U shaped; inverted V; parallel walled, thin ridge; undercut ridge
3. Soft tissue of ridge
   a. Class 1: normal uniform density of the soft tissue approximately 1 mm. over the supporting area; tissue firm but not tense
   b. Class 2: tissue thin and highly susceptible to irritation; mucoperiosteum approximately twice normal thickness
   c. Class 3: tissue excessively thick and flabby or alternately thick and thin, making equalization of pressure difficult
4. Border tissue and frenum attachments
   a. In the maxilla
      (1) High—over 12 mm.
      (2) Medium—8 to 12 mm.
      (3) Low—under 8 mm.
   b. In the mandible
      (1) Low—over 12 mm.
      (2) Medium—8 to 12 mm.
      (3) High—under 8 mm.
5. Ridge relation
   a. Class 1: normal—upper ridge crest directly above the lower ridge
   b. Class 2: prognathic or crossbite—all or a portion of the mandibular ridge crest lying outside the crest of the maxillary ridge
   c. Class 3: retrognathic—the mandibular ridge is lingual to the maxillary ridge
6. Ridge parallelism
   a. Class 1: ridges parallel to occlusal plane
   b. Class 2: mandibular ridge divergent anteriorly
   c. Class 3: maxillary ridge divergent anteriorly
   d. Class 4: both ridges divergent anteriorly

Mucosa. All of the alveolar mucosa should be carefully examined. A pallor of the mucosal surfaces is a common finding in anemia and the leukemias. Abnormal pigmentation or localized tissue changes should be recorded in detail and serve as a baseline for further investigation.

Saliva. Note whether the saliva is normal, thick, or reduced.

Roentgenographic findings

Apical lesions. When present, describe the size, appearance, and location.

Trabecular pattern. Describe the variations from normal and identify the area.

Pulp cavity calcifications. Specify whether of linear or nodular type, by tooth number, and specify canals involved in posterior teeth.

Periodontal ligament space. Locate and describe any abnormalities of width or appearance.

Bone height—alveolar crest. Describe horizontal bone loss in millimeters using the cementoenamel junction as the reference point.

Defects. Include vertical bone loss adjacent to the teeth, postsurgical and developmental defects, or others apparent in the calcified structures.

Dental caries. Record by tooth number and surface of apparent involvement and include root caries.

Root tips (residual). Describe and locate any root tips or fragments.

Foreign bodies. List size, shape, and location.

Other. Enter any abnormality noted in the roentgenograms not included in the preceding sections.

Examination of head and neck

Regional nodes. Any regional enlargement of lymph nodes should be entered along with the number palpable, size, tenderness, and duration, if known by the patient.

Skin. Describe the general texture and color and list any defects—for example, scars, lesions, dermatological disease, skin changes from radiation therapy.

Face form. Face form is the outline of the face from an anterior view. In nature the most pleasing objects are those that blend in harmony with their immediate surrounding environment. Square teeth for a patient with an ovoid or tapering face present a disharmony that is usually not esthetically pleasing. The general outline of the teeth should harmonize with the form of the face. The basic geometrical forms—square, tapering, ovoid, and combinations of the same—provide a baseline for selecting tooth form. Therefore, the basic classifications of the face forms are:

1. Square—temple, condyle, and angle of mandible fall in straight line as viewed on frontal plane
2. Round—condylar area lateral to temple and mandibular angle areas as viewed on frontal plane
3. Tapering—mandibular angle area medial to temple and mandibular angle as viewed on frontal plane

Face profile. Face profile is the outline form of the face from a lateral view. It may be classified as:

1. Straight—forehead, base of nose, and point of chin on straight line as viewed on sagittal plane
2. Curved (prognathic or retrognathic) —point of chin forward or backward of line joining forehead and base of nose

Arch form. Note the shape of the dental arch.

1. Physical size of the jaws
   a. Class 1: large upper and lower jaws offer the greatest possibility for retention and stability
   b. Class 2: medium size upper and lower arches
   c. Class 3: small size upper and lower arches
   d. Class 4: small lower and large upper jaws, worst prognosis for prosthesis
2. Physical form of arch and vault
   a. Class 1: square or U shape; gently curved or ovoid
   b. Class 2: tapering or V shape
   c. Class 3: flat vault

The general classification of the arches

is square, tapering, or ovoid. Many mouths present combination type arches. The presence of an upper arch of one class and the lower arch of another class can present many problems.

Occlusion

Classification. Use Angle's classification.

Freeway space (interocclusal distance). Note the distance between the occluding surfaces of the maxillary and mandibular teeth when the mandible is in its physiological rest position.

1. Class 1: just sufficient interarch distance to accommodate artificial teeth
2. Class 2: excessive interarch distance
3. Class 3: insufficient or limited distance to accommodate artificial teeth

Prematurities. Record the presence and location of premature contacts, centric closure slip, and locate, if possible, central relation (RC) to centric occlusion (IC) interferences when present.

Missing teeth. List by number. In edentulous patients, list by arch.

Specific abnormalities. Malpositions (including drifting and rotation) along with supernumerary teeth should be described and located.

Periodontal charting

Diagnosis

Gingivitis. Describe type, whether it is acute or chronic, and specify whether it is generalized or localized.

Periodontitis. Note whether the condition is acute or chronic, localized or generalized, and mild, moderate, or severe.

Periodontosis. Describe areas and degree of involvement.

Etiology. Try to determine all local factors that may have contributed to the initiation or perpetuation of the periodontal problems (examples: calculus, plaque, defective restoration margins, food impaction, uneven marginal contacts, inadequate home care). Include any known systemic condition that may contribute to the etio-

logical complex—for example, diabetes, hormonal imbalances, or drug therapy.

Prognosis. Give an estimate of ultimate results of the therapy (good—fair—poor—guarded). The prognosis may require qualification. For example, "The periodontal prognosis with therapy is good providing the patient will maintain an adequate level of home care" or "Periodontal prognosis with therapy is good with the exception of the maxillary molars, which is poor."

Tissue reaction after scaling. Describe the observed clinical changes following initial scaling. Examples would be reduced swelling of the gingiva or gingival bleeding previously reported by the patient has stopped following scaling.

As the duties of the dental hygienist may be expanded into areas involving diagnosis as well as delegated treatment that was previously solely in the domain of the dentist, so does the requirement for professional competence. The need for a fuller appreciation of normal as well as pathological physiology becomes apparent.

Dentistry in the United States today can only meet the challenge that it faces in delivering dental health care to all of those who need it by the fullest utilization of all of the members of the dental health team. The sharing of this task will encompass not only patient education, examination, and diagnostic evaluation, but will involve therapy as well. The most qualified ancillary member of this team today is the dental hygienist.

SUGGESTED READINGS

American Dental Association, Council on Dental Therapeutics: Accepted dental therapeutics, ed. 33, Chicago, 1969-1970, The Association.

Bhaskar, S. N.: Roentgenographic interpretation for the dentist, St. Louis, 1970, The C. V. Mosby Co.

Burket, L. W.: Oral medicine, ed. 5, Philadelphia, 1965, J. B. Lippincott Co.

Ellinger, C., and others: A synopsis of complete dentures, Philadelphia, 1971, Lea & Febiger.

Goldman, H. M., and Cohen, D. W.: Periodontal

therapy, ed. 4, St. Louis, 1968, The C. V. Mosby Co.

Heartwell, C. M., Jr.: Syllabus of complete dentures, Philadelphia, 1968, Lea & Febiger.

Kerr, D. A., Ash, M. M., Jr., and Millard, H. D.: Oral diagnosis, ed. 3, St. Louis, 1970, The C. V. Mosby Co.

Ramfjord, S. P., and Ash, M. M., Jr.: Occlusion, ed. 2, Philadelphia, 1971, W. B. Saunders Co.

Shafer, W. G., Hine, M. K., and Levy, B. M.: Oral pathology, ed. 2, Philadelphia, 1963, W. B. Saunders Co.

Sharry, J. J.: Complete denture prosthodontics, ed. 2, New York, 1968, McGraw-Hill Book Company.

Stafne, E. C.: Oral roentgenographic diagnosis, ed. 2, Philadelphia, 1963, W. B. Saunders Co.

chapter 5

RECOGNIZING NORMAL CONDITIONS IN THE ORAL CAVITY

Michael H. Burns, B.S., D.D.S., M.S.

It is the responsibility of the dental hygienist, as she inspects the tissues of the mouth, to inform the dentist of any deviations from the normal that she may observe. The tissues of the oral cavity are sensitive indicators of the general health of the patient. These structures undergo changes that may be symptomatic of dental disease or may indicate a subclinical disease process elsewhere in the body. Therefore it is imperative that the dental hygienist have an adequate knowledge of the normal appearance of the oral and dental tissues as well as an understanding of the basic anatomy of their supporting structures.

BONES OF THE ORAL CAVITY
Maxillae

The upper jaw consists of two bones, a right maxilla and a left maxilla, joined together at the median line at a suture. The maxillae give general shape to the face, form the palate and a portion of the orbit and nasal cavity, and support the upper (maxillary) teeth (Figs. 5-1 to 5-3).

Each maxilla is an irregularly shaped bone and consists of a central body and four processes: (1) the zygomatic process, directly superior to the maxillary first molar tooth and connecting to the zygomatic bone (this process may extend laterally along the roots of the molar teeth, making examination of these teeth somewhat difficult); (2) the nasal process, extending toward the nose and connecting with the nasal and frontal bone; (3) the palatine process, uniting with the process from the other maxilla at the intermaxillary suture to form the major anterior portion of the skeleton of the hard palate; and (4) the alveolar process, which forms the sockets for the maxillary teeth.

A large cavity inside the body of each maxilla, the maxillary sinus, extends from the apical portions of the molar and premolar teeth superiorly toward the floor of the orbit. This air space communicates with the nose through a small opening. Infections sometimes develop in the sinuses that may produce symptoms that the patient may frequently confuse with those involving the maxillary teeth.

Each maxilla contains holes called *foramina*. Through four of these foramina pass nerves and blood vessels of important dental significance: (1) the incisive foramen, located in the palate just lingual to the central incisor teeth; (2) the greater palatine foramen, located in the palate just lingual to the last molar teeth; (3) the

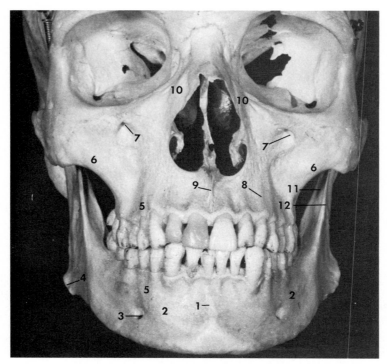

Fig. 5-1. Anterior view of the skull. *1*, Symphysis; *2*, body of mandible; *3*, mental foramen; *4*, angle of mandible; *5*, alveolar process; *6*, zygomatic process; *7*, infraorbital foramen; *8*, canine eminence; *9*, median suture; *10*, nasal process; *11*, internal oblique ridge; *12*, external oblique ridge.

posterior superior alveolar foramen, located on the posterolateral surface of the maxillary body just above the last tooth; and (4) the infraorbital foramen, located just below the orbit on the anterior side of the maxilla.

Mandible

In form the mandible resembles a horseshoe. It is the strongest and heaviest bone and the only movable bone of the skull. It gives shape to the lower face, forms the skeletal support for the floor of the mouth, and supports the lower (mandibular) teeth (Fig. 5-4). On either side the mandible is hinged to the skull at the temporomandibular joint.

The mandible consists of a body, two rami, and five processes. The rami are the two vertical portions of the mandible. Along the superior border of each ramus are found two processes. The posterior process, the condyloid process, articulates with the skull. The anterior process is the coronoid process. These processes are separated by the sigmoid notch. The alveolar process supports the teeth and is located along the superior portion of the body of the mandible.

The four foramina of the mandible transmit blood vessels and nerves to the lower teeth, alveolar bone, and gingivae. Each of the two mandibular foramina is located on the lingual surface of the ramus. There are two mental foramina, each located on the outer surface of the body of the

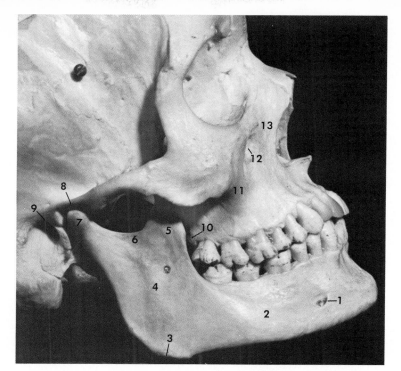

Fig. 5-2. Lateral view of skull. *1,* Mental foramen; *2,* body of mandible; *3,* angle of mandible; *4,* ramus of mandible; *5,* coronoid process; *6,* sigmoid notch; *7,* condyloid process; *8,* temporomandibular joint; *9,* external auditory canal; *10,* maxillary tuberosity; *11,* zygomatic process; *12,* infraorbital foramen; *13,* nasal process.

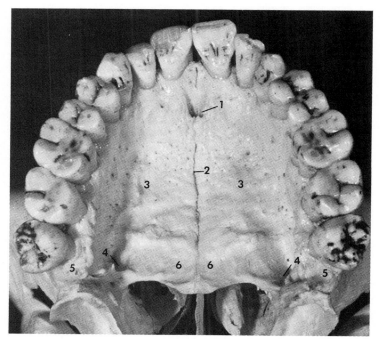

Fig. 5-3. The palatal aspect of the maxilla. *1,* Incisive foramen; *2,* intermaxillary suture; *3,* palatal process; *4,* greater palatine foramen; *5,* maxillary tuberosity; *6,* palatine bone.

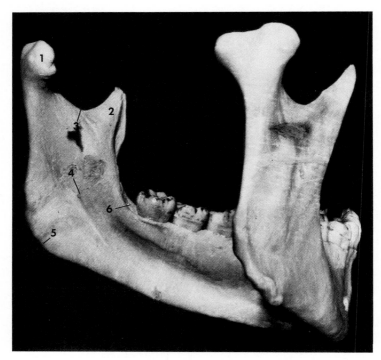

Fig. 5-4. Lingual view of the mandible. *1*, Condyloid process; *2*, coronoid process; *3*, sigmoid notch; *4*, mandibular foramen; *5*, angle of the mandible; *6*, retromandibular triangle.

mandible approximately between the root portions of the first and second premolar teeth.

TEMPOROMANDIBULAR JOINT

The proper function of the mandible depends upon the normal relationships of the various structures comprising the articular mechanism of the temporomandibular joint. Each temporal bone presents a depression anterior to the auditory canal called the mandibular fossa. Each fossa receives one of the knob-like mandibular condyles.

Interposed between the condyle and the mandibular fossa is the articular disk, sometimes referred to as the meniscus. This movable cartilaginous disk permits the mandible to function in a variety of movements. These movements are protru-

sion, retrusion, lateral excursion, and vertical or hinge.

The temporomandibular joint is covered by a fibrous capsule. This capsule contains a small amount of synovial fluid that fills the lower cavity between the articular disk and the condyle and the upper cavity between the articular disk and the mandibular fossa.

MUSCLES OF MASTICATION

The movements of the mandible are primarily effected by the action of the following mucles: masseter, temporal, internal (medial) pterygoid, and external (lateral) pterygoid. Each of these muscles is paired, controlling the movements of the mandible from either side of the jaw.

The masseter, temporal, and internal pterygoid muscles act to effect closure of

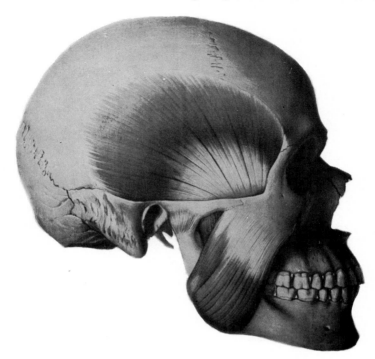

Fig. 5-5. Masseter and temporal muscles. (From Sicher, H., and DuBrul, E. L.: Oral anatomy, ed. 5, St. Louis, 1970, The C. V. Mosby Co.)

the jaws, while the small lateral pterygoid muscle acts to open the jaws. The force exerted in closing the teeth is considerable and has been measured up to 300 pounds per square inch.

Masseter

When the fingertips are placed on the face along along the lower border of the zygomatic bone and the mouth is opened or closed, the masseter muscle can be palpated during function. It is considered one of the most powerful muscles in the body and functions to close the jaws (Fig. 5-5).

The masseter muscle originates from the zygomatic arch and inserts principally on the broad lateral side of the ramus of the mandible, including the angle of the mandible.

Temporal

The fan-shaped temporal muscle is the largest of the muscles of mastication. During the process of mastication, the bulging of this muscle can often be observed. It is easily palpable above the zygomatic arch as the teeth are clenched. The muscle originates from the broad external surface of the temporal bone and inserts on the coronoid process and the anterior border of the ramus of the mandible (Fig. 5-5).

The functions of the temporal muscle are to close the jaws and to retract the mandible from a protruded position.

Internal pterygoid

The internal pterygoid muscle is located on the opposite, or medial, side of the ramus of the mandible from the masseter. Together they form a type of sling that

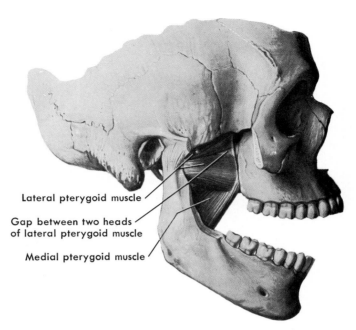

Lateral pterygoid muscle

Gap between two heads
of lateral pterygoid muscle

Medial pterygoid muscle

Fig. 5-6. Lateral and medial (external and internal) pterygoid muscles, lateral aspect, after removal of zygomatic arch and coronoid process. (From Sicher, H., and DuBrul, E. L.: Oral anatomy, ed. 5, St. Louis, 1970, The C. V. Mosby Co.)

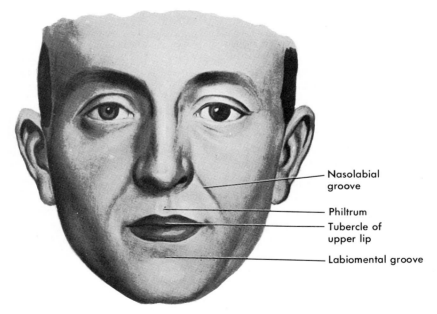

Nasolabial groove

Philtrum

Tubercle of upper lip

Labiomental groove

Fig. 5-7. Semidiagrammatic drawing of the face of an adult. (From Sicher, H., and DuBrul, E. L.: Oral anatomy, ed. 5, St. Louis, 1970, The C. V. Mosby Co.)

cradles the mandible, and their collective action produces an extremely strong closure of the jaws (Fig. 5-6).

The origin of the internal pterygoid is the pterygoid fossa of the sphenoid bone. It inserts on the medial surface of the ramus of the mandible near the angle.

In addition to the function of jaw closure the internal pterygoid also acts to effect lateral movements of the mandible.

External pterygoid

The external pterygoid muscle has dual origins from the sphenoid bone, one in the infratemporal fossa and also an area just external to the origin of the internal pterygoid muscle. The fibers are directed posterolaterally to insert near the condyle of the mandible and into the articular capsule and anterior border of the articular disk (Fig. 5-6).

This muscle functions to open the jaw and in protrusion of the jaw.

SALIVARY GLANDS

The saliva of the mouth is produced by a vast number of glands. Some small glands are located just beneath the mucosal lining, while some glands are large, densely packed, and further removed from the inner lining of the oral cavity. The latter group is connected to the mouth by ducts. Their secretions are controlled by stimuli such as smell, sight, or thought of food, as well as by physically touching the oral mucosa.

Saliva functions in the following ways: (1) it is a lubricating agent for the mouth and food, thus facilitating the act of swallowing; (2) it is a cleansing agent for food particles that may adhere to the teeth; and (3) it aids in digestion by secreting the enzymes ptyalin and erepsin.

The glands are classified according to their secretions and may be divided into serous, mucous, and mixed glands. Anatomically they may be designated as major and minor glands. The minor salivary glands are named according to their location and are the labial, buccal, palatine, and lingual glands. The major salivary glands are the parotid, submandibular, and sublingual glands (Fig. 5-8).

Parotid gland

The parotids are the largest of the salivary glands and one is located on each side of the face, in front of and beneath the ear. A number of important vessels and nerves passes through this gland.

The parotid duct (Stenson's duct) penetrates the mucous membrane of the oral cavity just opposite the buccal surface of the maxillary second molar teeth. The duct opening may be identified in the oral cavity by the presence of a small flap of tissue, the parotid papilla.

The secretion of the parotid gland is serous, giving it a thin and watery consistency.

Submandibular gland

The submandibular glands are two in number, each located below the floor of the mouth in the region of the premolar and molar teeth. These are the second largest of the salivary glands, about the size of a walnut.

The submandibular ducts (Wharton's ducts) transmit the secretions of glands to an opening located on either side of the frenulum of the tongue. Each opening is marked by an elevation, the lingual caruncle. Occasionally the duct may be blocked by calcareous deposits that result in a swelling of the floor of the mouth.

This gland is considered a mixed salivary gland, since it contains both serous and mucous-secreting cells; however, the serous cells contribute the majority of the secretion.

Sublingual gland

The sublingual glands, one on either side, are located beneath the tongue. The secretions reach the mouth through a number of small sublingual ducts that terminate lingual to the lower anterior teeth. The secretions of this gland are thick and mucous.

ORAL CAVITY

Anteriorly and laterally the oral cavity is bounded by the lips and cheeks, superiorly by the palate, and inferiorly by the muscular floor including the tongue. It is subdivided into an outer smaller portion, the *vestibule,* and an inner larger portion, the *mouth cavity proper.* The vestibule is the space bounded by an outer wall of lips and cheeks and by an inner wall of teeth and alveolar processes. The mouth proper is located within the confines of the dental arches. The oral cavity communicates with the outside through the opening between the lips, the *oral fissure,* and with the pharynx through the *fauces.*

LIPS

The lips are two muscular and highly vascular folds covered by skin externally and mucous membrane internally. The upper lip extends up to the nose and laterally to the *nasolabial groove.* This groove is almost nonexistent in the young but increases in depth with age. In the central portion of the upper lip is a shallow depression, the *philtrum.* A thin fold, the *labial commissure,* connects the upper lip with the lower lip. The lower lip is separated from the chin by a depression, the *labiomental groove.*

Between the skin and mucous membrane of the lips is the *red, or vermilion, border.* The skin of this area is thin and transmits the color of the blood in the underlying vessels. It is nonglandular and is richly supplied with sensory nerves and blood vessels. Immediately below the philtrum on the vermilion border is a prominence, the *tubercle* of the upper lip. It rests in a slight indentation in the lower lip (Fig. 5-7).

The inner surface of each lip is connected at the midline to the gingiva of that arch by a fold of mucous membrane, the *frenulum.*

CHEEKS

The cheeks form the sides of the face, being continuous with the lips. They are composed externally of skin and internally of mucous membrane. Between the two layers is a muscular stratum composed of the masseter, one of the muscles of mastication, and the buccinator, one of the associated muscles of mastication. Parts of the largest salivary gland, the parotid, its duct, and its duct opening are also structures comprising the cheek. The parotid duct opens into the oral vestibule opposite the second maxillary molar. It is usually marked by an eminence of the mucous membrane, the parotid papilla (Fig. 5-8).

The cheek also contains a generous amount of fat tissue, a collection of which is sometimes called the buccal fat pad. In the newborn and older infant the fat pad is relatively large and is thought to be of aid in the sucking movement. The sinking inward of the cheeks in thin or emaciated individuals is caused by the loss of an appreciable portion of the buccal fat.

As seen from the oral cavity, the cheek terminates in the reflection of the mucous membrane onto the alveolar process, forming the fornix of the vestibule. In the posterior part of the mouth the cheek terminates in a linear fold, which joins the maxillary and mandibular alveolar processes. This fold is formed by a tendinous strip, the *pterygomandibular fold,* which passes from the pterygoid hamulus of the palatine bone to the retromolar triangle just behind the last molar tooth.

ORAL VESTIBULE

From the base of the lips and cheeks the mucous membrane is reflected onto the corresponding alveolar process, forming a furrow, the fornix of the oral vestibule. The tissue beneath the mucous membrane is

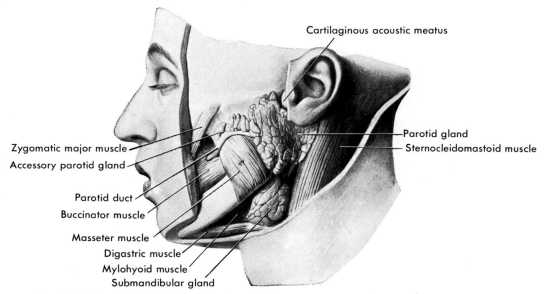

Fig. 5-8. Parotid and submandibular glands. (From Sicher, H., and DuBrul, E. L.: Oral anatomy, ed. 5, St. Louis, 1970, The C. V. Mosby Co.)

loose, permitting flexibility of the lips and cheeks. The reflected mucosa onto the alveolar process is interrupted by a sharp, distinct line that parallels the free margin of the gingiva. Thus the wall of the oral vestibule formed by the alveolar process is divided into two zones, the mucosa of the alveolar process and the gingiva, or gum tissue. The alveolar mucosa is considerably thinner than the gingiva, has a more delicate texture, is more mobile, and is dark red in color. The gingiva, because of its thickness, bulges beyond the mucosa and is pinker in color with a smoother texture.

HARD AND SOFT PALATE

The palate forms the roof of the mouth and extends posteriorly to an incomplete posterior wall and laterally and anteriorly into the alveolar process of the maxilla. It is divided into the bony hard palate and a movable portion, the soft palate. The skeleton of the hard palate consists of the palatine process of the maxilla and the horizontal plates of the palatine bone.

When seen from a dry skull, the palate is more flattened than that of the living individual. This is because of the thick layer of soft tissue covering the bony skeleton, giving the palate its more oval contour. In the anterior part of the hard palate, immediately behind the contacts of the maxillary central incisor teeth, is an oval, smooth prominence, the *incisive papilla* (Fig. 5-9). This papilla contains important nerves and blood vessels to the anterior portion of the hard palate. From the papilla a narrow ridge, the palatine raphe, extends over the entire length of the hard palate. Ridges of dense connective tissue extend laterally, radiating from the incisal papilla and the palatine raphe. These are called *palatine rugae*. The hard palate contains an abundance of fat tissue and mucous glands. These provide a resilient cushion for the palatine mucosa. At approximately the level of the maxillary second or third molars on either side the palatine foramen transmits the nerves and

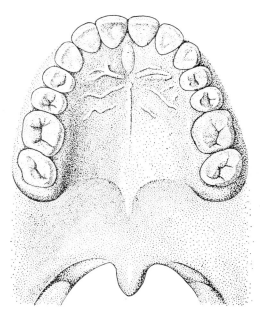

Fig. 5-9. Hard and soft palates. (From Sicher, H., and DuBrul, E. L.: Oral anatomy, ed. 5, St. Louis, 1970, The C. V. Mosby Co.)

blood vessels that supply the posterior portion of the hard palate.

The mucosa of the soft palate is thinner than that of the hard palate and, unlike the hard palate, is not hornified. It is densely supplied with mucous glands. Intraorally the soft palate is readily differentiated from the hard palate. The mucosa of the hard palate is thick and dense, and the thick hornified layer gives it a pale pink color. The soft palate has a thinner mucosa that is more loosely textured and, because of its rich blood supply, appears more darkly red. A definite boundary is readily apparent between the two zones that duplicates in contour the posterior boundary of the skeleton of the hard palate but is slightly anterior to it.

Frequently a small depression is seen on either side of the midline just behind the boundary between the hard and soft palates. Into these *palatine fovea* empty some of the ducts of the palatine glands.

In the lateral area of the root of the soft palate, just medial and posterior to the posterior end of the alveolar process, a small prominence elevated by the hamulus of the pterygoid process can be felt. With the mouth wide open this elevation may be readily apparent. Also seen with the mouth open is a linear elevation extending from the pterygoid process to the retromolar pad at the posterior end of the mandibular process. This is called the pterygomandibular fold, and it marks the posterior boundary of the cheek (Fig. 5-10).

The free border of the soft palate is doubly concave and extends in the midline as the *palatine uvula*. Along this free border the oral mucosa changes character and continues as the nasal mucosa.

On either side the free border of the soft palate splits into two folds. The most anterior of these passes downward from the uvula and into the lateral surfaces of the posterior root of the tongue. This is the *palatoglossal arch*. Posterior and medial to the palatoglossal arch is the *palatopharyngeal arch*. It passes from the soft palate to the lateral wall of the pharynx, where it gradually flattens out. Between the palatoglossal arch and the palatopharyngeal arch lies the *palatine tonsil*.

FLOOR OF THE MOUTH

The mucosa of the floor of the mouth reflects onto the alveolar process from the lingual or tongue surface, as does the mucosa of the vestibule from the buccal or cheek surface. A horseshoe-shaped sulcus is formed in the floor of the mouth with an outer wall of mandibular alveolar process and an inner wall formed by the lateral sides of the base of the tongue. The mucous membrane of the mouth floor folds at the midline to form the *frenulum of the tongue* (Fig. 5-11). Only rarely does this fold attach to the mandibular alveolar process. In some instances it may be overdeveloped in such a way as to restrict the movement of the tongue, resulting in a

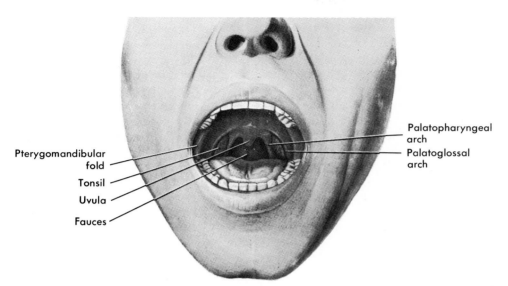

Pterygomandibular fold

Tonsil

Uvula

Fauces

Palatopharyngeal arch

Palatoglossal arch

Fig. 5-10. Soft palate, palatine pillars, and tonsils. (From Sicher, H., and DuBrul, E. L.: Oral anatomy, ed. 5, St. Louis, 1970, The C. V. Mosby Co.)

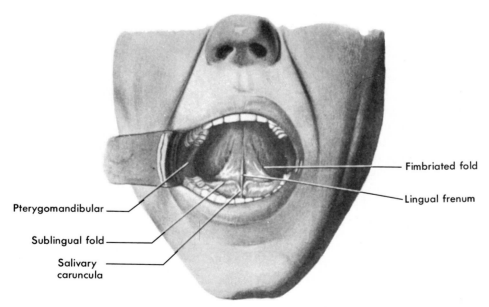

Pterygomandibular

Sublingual fold

Salivary caruncula

Fimbriated fold

Lingual frenum

Fig. 5-11. Sublingual region. (From Sicher, H., and DuBrul, E. L.: Oral anatomy, ed. 5, St. Louis, 1970, The C. V. Mosby Co.)

so-called "tongue tie." On either side of the frenulum is a rounded elevation of the mucous membrane of the floor of the mouth, formed by the sublingual salivary glands.

Each of these glands has ten to fifteen small ducts that open along the base of the tongue. Across the surface of the sublingual glands the submandibular duct forms a tortuous linear elevation in the floor of the mouth that terminates on either side of the frenulum of the tongue in a small papilla. From an opening in this papilla the mucous and serous secretions of the submandibular gland empty into the oral cavity. Upon stimulation the gland may secrete so strongly that the saliva may spurt completely out of the mouth.

An examination of the floor of the mouth may reveal rounded bony elevations on the inner surfaces of the mandible called *mandibular tori.*

TONGUE

The tongue is a very muscular organ composed of many muscle fibers that cross each other at various angles, enabling the structure to readily change contour, shape, and position. It functions not only to position the food but also to provide the sense of touch and taste.

The dorsum of the tongue is divided into two separate, distinctly different surface areas. The anterior two thirds of the tongue turns upward; the posterior third faces backward. The two regions are separated by a V-shaped groove, the *sulcus terminalis,* with the angle of the V pointing backward.

Four types of papillae cover the dorsum of the tongue. The *filiform papillae* are by far the most numerous and cover the dorsum almost in its entirety. All the filiform papillae are inclined anteroposteriorly, which gives the tongue a smooth, velvety appearance. These papillae also account for the tongue's grayish pink color.

Irregularly distributed between the fili-

form papillae are the *fungiform papillae.* They are small mushroom elevations with a deep red color. On their slopes are found taste buds.

The *foliate papillae* are few in number, usually being situated along the lateral margins of the tongue. They contain many taste buds and, although being well developed in animals, may be absent in man.

Just in front of the sulcus terminalis is a row of quite large papillae, the *vallate papillae.* These are shaped like a mushroom with a flattened superior surface surrounded by a deep groove that contains serous glands and taste buds.

Behind the sulcus terminalis is a rough surface with many mounds of tissue, the *lingual tonsillar tissue.*

GINGIVA

Of particular interest to the dental hygienist is the appearance of the normal gingival tissue. In order to be aware of unhealthy conditions she must have a thorough understanding of healthy gingival tissue.

The gingiva is that part of the oral mucosa that is attached to the teeth and alveolar process of the jaws, both maxilla and mandible (Fig. 5-12).

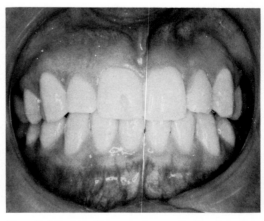

Fig. 5-12. Maxillary and mandibular frenulum of the oral vestibule. (Courtesy University of Tennessee College of Dentistry, Memphis, Tenn.)

The gingiva may be divided into two distinct areas, *free gingiva* and *attached gingiva*. The attached gingiva is demarcated from the loosely attached and movable alveolar mucosa by a scalloped line that is the mucogingival junction. This line of demarcation between the gingiva and the alveolar mucosa occurs on the vestibular surface of the alveolar process and also on the inner surface of the mandible between the mucosa and the floor of the mouth. Since the palatal mucosa has such a firm attachment, no clear dividing line is evident.

The free gingiva is the sleeve-like coronal portion of the gingiva that encircles the tooth with a knife-edged margin to form the gingival sulcus. This sulcus is the space between the unattached free gingiva and the tooth, and it is approximately 2 mm. in depth. A jet of air will blow the free gingiva away from the tooth surface, but it will settle back into place quickly. At the bottom of the sulcus is the epithelial attachment of the gingiva to the tooth. Frequently the depth of the gingival sulcus is marked on the outer surface by a fine groove running parallel to the gingival margin. This is called the free gingival groove, which is the dividing line between the free gingiva and the firmly adhering, attached gingiva.

The surface of the attached gingiva is characterized by an "orange peel" appearance called stippling. The degree of stippling varies. It is finer in females than in males, and it is absent in children.

The gingival tissue continues between the teeth and fills each interproximal space to the contact area, thus forming the *interdental papillae*. In the normal dentition papillae are pyramidal in shape and end in a crest of free gingiva. In cases of diastema between teeth there is no crest, but rather, the interproximal gingiva is blunt or sometimes is a concave surface.

The color of the normal gingiva varies, depending upon ethnic background, from pale pink to black. In the adult the tissue is dense, firm to the touch, and does not bleed easily.

Age has a pronounced effect on the appearance of the normal gingiva. In children no stippling is seen, and the gingiva appears redder and more delicate. With increasing age the papillae and other part of the gingiva may atrophy. A blunted contour in older individuals must be considered normal also. With increased age the gingival attachment to the tooth moves from the enamel to the surface of the cementum. Thus in aged persons the clinical crown of the teeth undergoes a continuing exposure.

TEETH

During an individual's lifetime two different sets of teeth erupt into the mouth, the deciduous or primary dentition and the permanent or secondary dentition (Fig. 5-13).

Deciduous teeth

At birth the individual has no functioning teeth in the mouth. However, the infant's jaws have many teeth in various stages of formation. Eruption of the primary or deciduous teeth usually begins at the age of 6 months, and by the age of 2 years it is complete.

Although there is some variation in the eruption dates of the teeth, Table 5-1 will serve as a guide to the normal eruption pattern.

The terms *baby* or *temporary* should not be used when referring to the deciduous teeth, since they imply that these teeth will be needed for only a short period of time. It cannot be overemphasized that these teeth are most important for the child's welfare and comfort, so premature loss should be avoided.

As the terms *deciduous* or *primary* imply, these teeth are shed. This process of exfoliation occurs between the seventh and twelfth years of age. After the primary

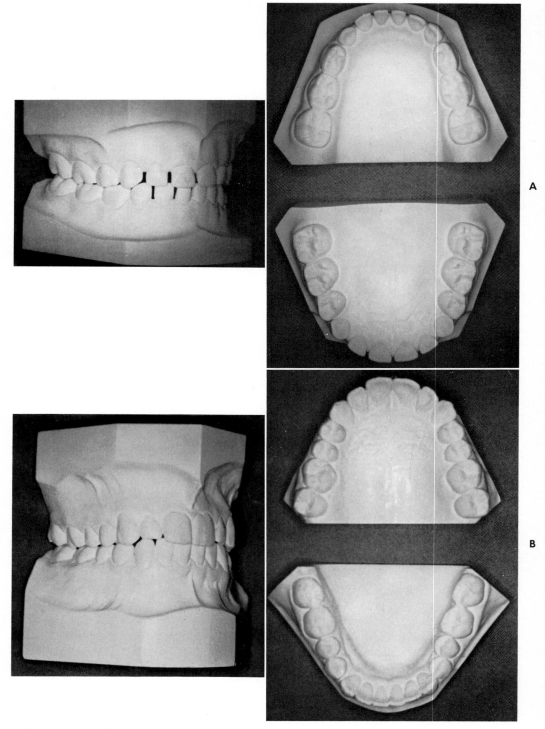

Fig. 5-13. A, Plaster casts of deciduous or primary dentition, including the first permanent molars. **B,** Casts of permanent dentition. (Courtesy University of Tennessee College of Dentistry, Memphis, Tenn.)

Table 5-1. Eruption chart of human dentition

			Months
Deciduous teeth	Maxillary	Central incisor	7 ½
		Lateral incisor	9
		Canine	18
		First molar	14
		Second molar	24
	Mandibular	Central incisor	6
		Lateral incisor	7
		Canine	16
		First molar	12
		Second molar	20
			Years
Permanent teeth	Maxillary	Central incisor	7- 8
		Lateral incisor	8- 9
		Canine (cuspid)	11-12
		First premolar (bicuspid)	10-12
		Second premolar (bicuspid)	10-12
		First molar	6- 7
		Second molar	12-13
		Third molar	17-21
	Mandibular	Central incisor	6- 7
		Lateral incisor	8- 9
		Canine (cuspid)	9-11
		First premolar (bicuspid)	10-12
		Second premolar (bicuspid)	10-12
		First molar	6- 7
		Second molar	11-13
		Third molar	17-21

tooth has erupted and its root is completely formed, a process of resorption occurs until the crown is lost because of insufficient root support.

There are twenty deciduous teeth, ten in each jaw. These ten include four incisors, two canines, and four molars. Beginning at the midline they are named as follows: central incisor, lateral incisor, canine, first molar, and second molar. These teeth are replaced by the following permanent succedaneous teeth: central incisor, lateral incisor, canine, first premolar, and second premolar.

The deciduous molars are replaced by permanent premolars. There are no deciduous premolars, and there are no teeth in the deciduous dentition that resemble the permanent premolar. The maxillary primary molars have three roots like those of the maxillary permanent molars. The deciduous mandibular first molar has a crown form unlike any permanent tooth. It and the second primary molar have two well-developed roots like those of the permanent molars.

The following essential differences between permanent and deciduous teeth can be noted:

1. The primary teeth are usually lighter in color than are the permanent teeth.
2. The crowns of deciduous anterior teeth are usually wider mesiodistally in relation to crown length.

3. The roots of deciduous teeth are usually longer in comparison to crown length and are narrow.
4. There is a distinct constriction at the neck of the deciduous teeth.
5. The buccal and lingual surfaces of deciduous molars are usually flatter and more occlusally converged, thereby narrowing the occlusal surfaces.
6. The cervical ridge of enamel buccally and lingually is more pronounced on deciduous teeth.

The deciduous teeth should be erupted and in normal alignment and occlusion at about 2 years of age. The roots should be fully formed about a year later. After the teeth have erupted and assumed their position in the arch the rapid development of the jaws causes a space, or *diastema,* to occur between the anterior teeth.

Permanent teeth

These permanent teeth are sometimes called the secondary teeth. At approximately 6 years of age the child's jaws have grown enough to accommodate some of the permanent dentition. These teeth must function throughout the individual's life since they have no successors except those prosthetic substitutes provided by the dentist.

The first of the permanent teeth to erupt are the maxillary and mandibular first molars, which take their place just posterior to the deciduous second molars. A natural process of resorption of the roots of the deciduous teeth allows the eruption of those permanent teeth that replace the primary ones, called *succedaneous teeth.* In addition to these the maxillary and mandibular first, second, and third molars erupt, completing the permanent dentition of thirty-two teeth, which are:

Sixteen maxillary teeth (eight right and eight left)
    Central incisors
    Lateral incisors
    Cuspids
    First premolars or bicuspids
    Second premolars or bicuspids
    First molars
    Second molars
    Third molars (called wisdom teeth)

Sixteen mandibular teeth (eight right and eight left)
    Central incisors
    Lateral incisors
    Cuspids
    First premolars or bicuspids
    Second premolars or bicuspids
    First molars
    Second molars
    Third molars

Supporting structures of the teeth

The supporting structures of the teeth, both deciduous and permanent, are the alveolar process and the periodontal ligament (Fig. 5-14).

Alveolar process. The alveolar process is that portion of the maxilla and mandible that invests the roots of the teeth. It consists of a thin layer of dense bone surrounding the root of each tooth and provides attachment for the fibers of the periodontal ligament.

Periodontal ligament. The periodontal ligament is a thin but very dense and tough layer of tissue found interposed between the root (cementum) of the tooth and the alveolar bone. It provides attachment and retention for the tooth in the bony socket. The fibers of the periodontal ligament are directed in such a manner as to cushion the forces of mastication.

Anatomy of the teeth

The teeth can be compared to instruments that do a specific job. Thus the functions of the teeth require a specific design in order to give the maximum efficiency during mastication. The incisors are used for the incision of food. The canines have a pointed cusp and are used for the tearing or prehension of food, whereas the

val tissue, but as age increases there may be gingival recession and bone loss, which exposes the cementum to the oral cavity. When this condition occurs, that portion of the root exposed to the oral cavity becomes a part of the clinical crown.

To understand the design of the instruments of mastication and the dental apparatus as a complete unit one must know and fully understand the specialized form of each individual tooth and the relationship that each tooth bears to its adjacent tooth, its opposing tooth, and its surrounding and supporting structures.

At eruption the crowns of incisors and canines present four surfaces and one ridge; after wear they present five surfaces. At eruption the crowns of premolars and molars present five surfaces. These surfaces are named according to their position and use. The *labial* are those surfaces of the incisors and canines that face the lips. The *buccal* are those surfaces of premolars and molars that face the cheeks. The *facial* are the labial and buccal surfaces when they are used collectively. The *lingual* are those surfaces of all the teeth that face toward the tongue. The *occlusal* are those surfaces of premolars and molars that come in contact during the action of closure or occlusion. The *incisal* are those surfaces found on incisors and canines formed after wear that come in contact during the act of incising, or biting. Those surfaces of the teeth that face adjacent teeth in the same arch are called *proximal* surfaces. They may be called *mesial* if they face toward the midline or *distal* if they face away from the midline.

The midline, or median line, is a line or plane drawn through the center of the face passing between the central incisors, both maxillary and mandibular, at their area of contact. There are four teeth with contacting mesial surfaces. These are the maxillary and mandibular central incisors.

The place where the surfaces of adjacent teeth in the same arch contact is called a *contact area*. Those points where teeth of opposing arches meet or touch during the process of closure, or occlusion, are called *contact points*.

When the maxillary and mandibular teeth come together in a functional relationship, they are said to be in *occlusion*. The teeth are in equal contact, and in a central relationship of one arch to the other they are said to be in *centric occlusion*.

On the buccal surfaces, in normal relationship, the cusps of the maxillary premolars and molars overlap the cusps of the mandibular teeth. The maxillary central and lateral incisors overjet and overbite the mandibular central and lateral incisors. The *overbite* is the vertical distance from the incisal edge of the maxillary incisors to the incisal edge of the mandibular incisors. The *overjet* is the horizontal dimension between the labial surfaces of the mandibular incisors and the lingual surfaces of the maxillary incisors. There is usually about 2 mm. of normal overbite and overjet.

When the occlusion between the maxillary and mandibular teeth is abnormal, the teeth are said to be in *malocclusion*.

Maxillary permanent central incisor

The eruption time of the maxillary permanent central incisor is approximately 7 to 8 years of age. It is the most prominent tooth in the mouth and is the first tooth from the midline in the maxillary arch.

Its distal surface contacts the mesial surface of the lateral incisor. This contact area, which is at the junction of the incisal and middle third of the crown in the central, forms an *embrasure*. An embrasure is a triangular space radiating from the contact area in incisal, gingival, labial, and lingual directions. The gingival tissue normally fills the gingival embrasure (Fig. 5-16).

The contact of the mesial surface is near the mesioincisal angle, which approximates a right angle. The distoincisal angle is rounded.

The labial surface is broad and is less

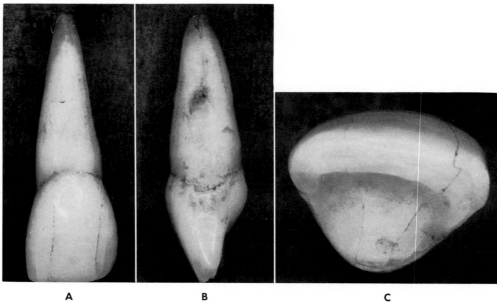

Fig. 5-16. Labial **(A)**, proximal **(B)**, and incisal **(C)** views of an extracted maxillary permanent central incisor. (Courtesy University of Tennessee College of Dentistry, Memphis, Tenn.)

convex than that of the maxillary lateral or cuspid, thus giving a more squared or rectangular appearance.

Upon eruption the incisal ridge presents three rounded elevations. These elevations are called *mamelons* and represent the three lobes of development of the labial surface. As wear of the tooth occurs, these elevations flatten into a smooth incisal edge.

The lingual surface presents a concavity with varying depths, the *lingual fossa*. Gingival to this fossa is a rounded elevation in the gingival third of the crown, the *cingulum*. It represents the fourth lobe of formation. Elevations of enamel bordering the lingual fossa on the mesial and distal surfaces are the *marginal ridges*. The mesiodistal measurements of the tooth from the lingual are much smaller than those of the labial. This is caused by the convergence of the tooth from labial to lingual.

The mesial and distal surfaces have a "shovel appearance" typical of all incisor teeth. The labial and lingual crests of curvature are in the gingival third of the crown and protect the gingiva. These crests of curvature give the crown its greatest labiolingual measurement. The labial outline is slightly convex, while the lingual outline is quite convex in the cervical third and becomes concave in the middle and incisal thirds. The cervical line shows its greatest curvature on the long axis and is greater on the mesial than on the distal.

From the incisal view the tooth appears triangular with a broad, flat labial surface, the rounded cingulum comprising the lingual surface.

Although the maxillary centrals present square, ovoid, and tapering crown forms in different individuals, there are only rare occasions when this tooth presents an anomaly.

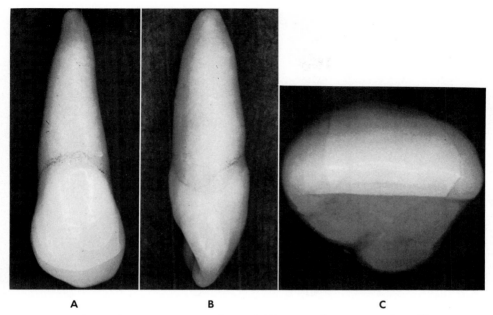

A   **B**   **C**

Fig. 5-17. Labial **(A)**, proximal **(B)**, and incisal **(C)** views of an extracted maxillary permanent lateral incisor. (Courtesy University of Tennessee College of Dentistry, Memphis, Tenn.)

Maxillary permanent lateral incisor

The eruption time of the maxillary lateral incisor is approximately 8 to 9 years of age. It is the second tooth from the midline in the maxillary arch and supplements the central incisor in function and closely resembles it in form. With the exception of the third molars it varies more in its development than any other tooth (Fig. 5-17).

The mesial contact area approximates the distal surface of the maxillary central incisor. The distal contact area is in contact with the mesial surface of the canine.

Because of the close resemblance in shape and form to the maxillary central, direct comparisons between the two will be made. The crown is proportionately smaller than the central, although the root is as long or longer. The labial surface of the crown has more curvature, with an incisal edge being more convex. The mesioincisal edge is rounder than the central but not as round as the distoincisal edge.

The entire incisal edge has a distal slope of approximately 1 mm. The distal outline is rounded, with the height of contour in the middle of the middle third of the crown. The height of contour on the mesial outline is somewhat higher, being at the junction of the middle and incisal thirds.

The lingual surface greatly resembles that of the central incisor. The marginal ridges and cingulum are more prominent because of a more concave lingual fossa. There may be a deep lingual pit in the lingual fossa that is conducive to decay. Removal of such decay may be a hazard in young teeth because of the proximity to the pulp. The mesial and distal surfaces converge to the lingual as they do in the central incisor.

From the mesial and distal aspects the tooth appears as a small central incisor with a long root. The labial and lingual surfaces appear gently convex, with the crest of curvature being in the gingival third.

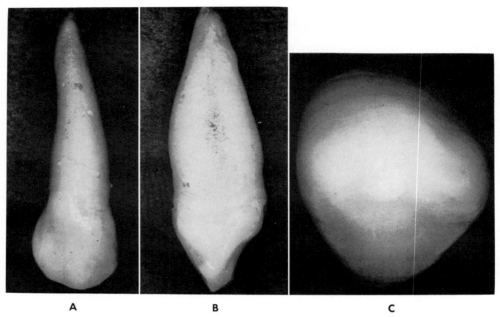

Fig. 5-18. Labial **(A)**, proximal **(B)**, and incisal **(C)** views of an extracted maxillary permanent canine. (Courtesy University of Tennessee College of Dentistry, Memphis, Tenn.)

The resemblance of the maxillary central and lateral incisor is again evident from the incisal view. The labial surface is more convex than the central, as seen from this surface.

This tooth is occasionally congenitally missing; that is, no tooth bud was ever present for its development. Also the mesial and distal lobes may be underdeveloped, giving the tooth a pointed appearance. These teeth are called "peg laterals."

Maxillary permanent canine

The eruption time of the maxillary permanent canine is at approximately 11 to 12 years of age. It is located at the corners of the mouth and is the third tooth from the midline. Mesially it contacts the distal surface of the lateral incisor. Distally it contacts the mesial surface of the first premolar (Fig. 5-18).

The maxillary canine is the longest tooth in the mouth. The tooth length together with its labiolingual thickness gives it added anchorage in the alveolar process of the jaws, making it and its mandibular counterpart the most stable teeth in the mouth. The position and form of the tooth, along with the bony ridge over the labial surface of the root, forms the "canine eminence," which has great cosmetic value.

From the labial view the central lobe can be seen as being much more developed than the mesial and distal lobes. This gives the crown a more pointed appearance and results in a very convex labial surface. This shape allows the crown to be self-cleansing, and this is usually the last tooth lost. Mesially the outline is convex with the height of contour or contact area at the junction of the incisal and middle thirds of the crown. Distally the outline is concave between the cervical line and the contact area, which is located in the center of the middle one third. The cusp has a mesial and distal slope, with the mesial

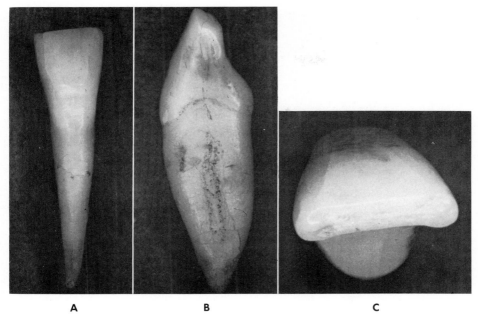

Fig. 5-19. Labial **(A)**, proximal **(B)**, and incisal **(C)** views of an extracted mandibular permanent central incisor. (Courtesy University of Tennessee Colllege of Dentistry, Memphis, Tenn.)

being the shorter, thus placing the tip of the cusp mesial to the long axis of the tooth. The labial surface has a strong *labial ridge* and a developmental depression distal to the ridge.

The general features of the lingual surface greatly resemble those of the maxillary central and lateral, but the surface is distinctive in that the cingulum is always better developed. This tooth also converges more from labial to lingual. There are definite mesial and distal marginal ridges along with a strong lingual ridge. All three blend in with the cingulum. Occasionally small concavities called mesial and distal lingual fossae are present between the lingual ridge and the marginal ridge.

From the mesial and distal views the labial outline appears more convex than that of either the central or lateral incisors, the greatest convexity being located within

the cervical third. The lingual surface is distinctly S shaped, with the deepest concavity within the middle and incisal thirds. The large cingulum, in the cervical third, bulges over the cervical line to create a sharp contrast between crown and root.

Mandibular permanent central incisor

The eruption time of the mandibular permanent central incisor is approximately 6 to 7 years of age. It is the smallest tooth of the dental arch and is located adjacent to the midline (Fig. 5-19).

Its mesial surface contacts the mesial surface of the mandibular central on the other side of the arch. Its distal surface contacts the mesial surface of the mandibular lateral incisor.

The labial surface appears smooth and tapers sharply from the incisal edge in a gingival direction. The contact areas on the mesial and distal are near the incisal

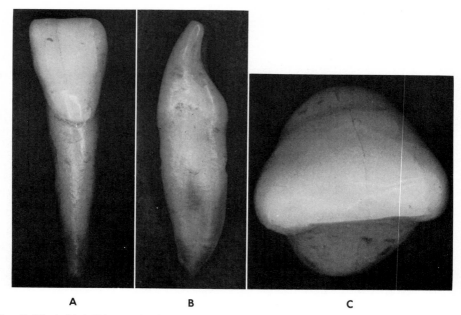

A   B   C

Fig. 5-20. Labial **(A)**, proximal **(B)**, and incisal **(C)** views of an extracted mandibular permanent lateral incisor. (Courtesy University of Tennessee College of Dentistry, Memphis, Tenn.)

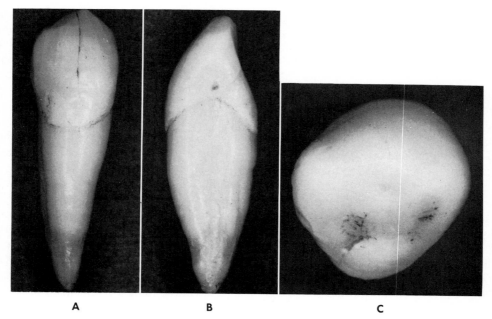

A   B   C

Fig. 5-21. Labial **(A)**, proximal **(B)**, and incisal **(C)** views of an extracted mandibular permanent canine. (Courtesy University of Tennessee College of Dentistry, Memphis, Tenn.)

angle, which is sharp and acute. The incisal edge is almost straight and is at right angles to the long axis of the tooth.

The lingual surface is smooth with a slight concavity in the incisal third, becoming less concave in the middle third and convex in the cervical third. There are usually no marginal ridges present.

From the mesial and distal aspects, this tooth shows a sharp lingual inclination of the incisal edge; that is, the incisal edge is lingual to the long axis of the tooth. Otherwise the contour is similar to that of maxillary incisors.

The incisal view illustrates the bilateral symmetry of the tooth, with the mesial half of the crown almost identical to the distal half. The labiolingual diameter is greater than the mesiodistal diameter. Viewing the tooth from the incisal, one sees more of the labial surface than the lingual.

Mandibular permanent lateral incisor

The eruption time of the mandibular permanent lateral incisor is approximately 7 to 8 years of age. It is the second tooth from the midline and greatly resembles the mandibular central incisor both in form and in function. The mesial contact area, like the distal contact area of the lateral incisor, is near the incisal edge. The distal contact area is next to the mesial contact area of the mandibular canine, located more gingivally in the incisal third than the mesial contact (Fig. 5-20).

The overall measurements are somewhat larger than those of the central incisor, and the incisal edge slopes in a distal direction unlike the central.

The labial, lingual, and proximal surfaces differ from the mandibular central incisor in only minor details.

Unlike the central incisor, however, the crown appears to be slightly twisted on its root. This is apparent from the incisal view. This is necessary, since the tooth is located on the curve of the arch.

Mandibular permanent canine

The eruption time of the mandibular permanent canine is approximately 9 to 11 years of age. It is the third tooth from the midline in the mandibular arch (Fig. 5-21).

The mesial contact area is next to the distal contact area of the mandibular lateral incisor, while its distal surface contacts the mesial surface of the mandibular first premolar.

This tooth resembles its counterpart in the maxillary arch, with several differences. The crown is narrower than the maxillary canine and is as long or longer. The root is usually shorter than that of the maxillary canine.

From the labial view the mesial outline follows an almost vertical course from the cervical line to the mesial contact area, where it curves abruptly to terminate at the pointed cusp tip. The distoincisal angle is rounder, with the distal contact area being in a more cervical direction.

The lingual view shows a cingulum that is well developed but smooth in contour.

From the proximal surface the tip of the cusp is seen to lie lingual to the long axis of the tooth like that of the mandibular incisor. Otherwise there is very little difference from the maxillary canine.

Maxillary permanent first premolar

The eruption time of the maxillary permanent first premolar is approximately 10 to 12 years of age. It is the fourth tooth from the midline in the maxillary arch.

The mesial surface contacts the distal surface of the canine. The distal surface contacts the mesial surface of the second premolar (Fig. 5-22).

The maxillary first premolar has certain characteristics common to posterior teeth and differing from anterior teeth. Posterior teeth have greater buccolingual measurements than mesiodistal measurements. The reverse is true relative to anterior teeth. The contact areas in posterior teeth are broader and at more the same

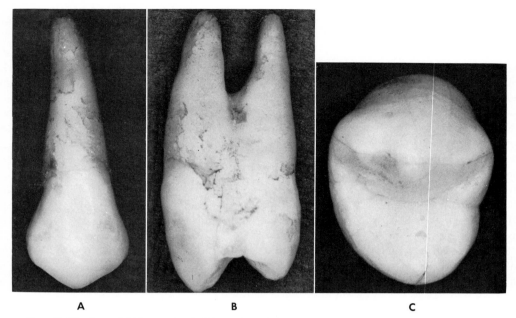

A   B   C

Fig. 5-22. Buccal **(A)**, proximal **(B)**, and occlusal **(C)** views of an extracted maxillary permanent first premolar. (Courtesy University of Tennessee College of Dentistry, Memphis, Tenn.)

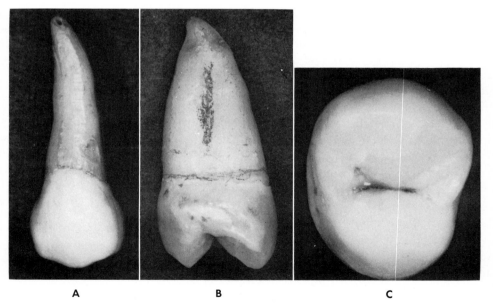

A   B   C

Fig. 5-23. Buccal **(A)**, proximal **(B)**, and occlusal **(C)** views of an extracted maxillary permanent second premolar. (Courtesy University of Tennessee College of Dentistry, Memphis, Tenn.)

level. The crowns are shorter cervico-occlusally, and there is less curvature to the cervical line.

The buccal surface of the maxillary permanent first premolar resembles that of the canine in appearance, with a cusp less pointed. There is a strong buccal ridge but no buccal development grooves. The tip of the buccal cusp lies distal to the long axis.

The lingual surface is smaller, since the tooth has distinct lingual convergence. This allows portions of the buccal section of the tooth to be seen from this view.

From the mesial and distal views the buccal cusp is slightly longer than the lingual cusp. The buccal surface shows a gentle slope from the cervical line to the cusp tip, with the crest of curvature being in the cervical third. In the middle of the mesial surface in the cervical third is a definite concavity. This view exhibits two well-developed roots.

The occlusal surface shows the buccal and lingual cusps between which, passing mesial to distal, is the central developmental groove. At the termination of the groove are the mesial and distal pits. Bordering the occlusal surface are the mesial marginal ridge on the mesial and the distal marginal ridge on the distal.

Maxillary permanent second premolar

The eruption time of the maxillary permanent second premolar is approximately 10 to 12 years of age. It is the fifth tooth from the midline in the maxillary arch.

It contacts the distal surface of the first premolar on the mesial and contacts the mesial surface of the first molar on the distal (Fig. 5-23).

This tooth bears a striking similarity to the maxillary first premolar. The buccal contour is slightly rounder than that of the first premolar. Also the tooth is generally smaller than its first premolar neighbor. The buccal cusp is more blunted.

On the mesial surface no concavity is

found above the cervical line as in the first premolar.

The occlusal surface of this tooth is symmetrical and shows many supplemental grooves and appears wrinkled, or crenated. The pits are closer together than in the first premolar. The occlusal outline is generally less angular and more rounded. The cusp tips are more nearly the same height. The maxillary second premolar usually has only one root.

Maxillary permanent first molar

The eruption time of the maxillary permanent first molar is approximately 6 to 7 years of age. It generally erupts after the mandibular first molar; however, both are called the "6-year molars" (Fig. 5-24).

The mesial contact area proximates the distal surface of the maxillary second premolar, and its distal contact area proximates the mesial surface of the maxillary second molar.

As is true of all maxillary molars, each is firmly anchored in the alveolar process by three well-developed roots. The first molar appears to be a "double premolar." It takes its place distal to the second deciduous molar and therefore is not a succedaneous tooth.

The 6-year molars are usually lost before any other permanent teeth. Three reasons for this are given:

1. They stay in the mouth longer and therefore are exposed to sweets longer.
2. These teeth frequently are not brushed fully because of their position in the arch.
3. Parents may not be aware that these are permanent teeth.

The relationship of the maxillary to the mandibular permanent first molar is very important to the development of a normal relationship between the arches. They are referred to as the "keys to occlusion." Since the jaws do not grow anterior to the teeth once they have erupted, the available

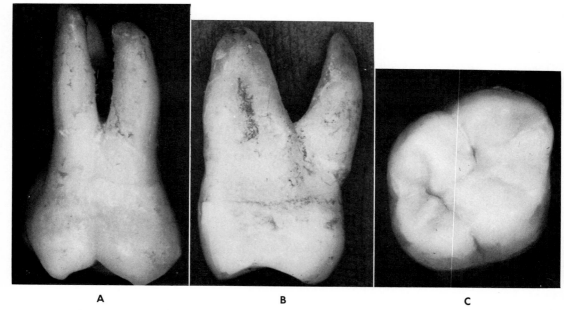

A   B   C

Fig. 5-24. Buccal **(A)**, proximal **(B)**, and occlusal **(C)** views of an extracted maxillary permanent first molar. (Courtesy University of Tennessee College of Dentistry, Memphis, Tenn.)

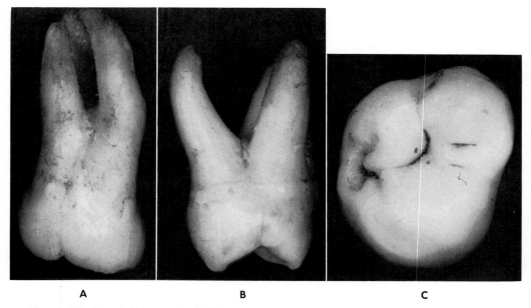

A   B   C

Fig. 5-25. Buccal **(A)**, proximal **(B)**, and occlusal **(C)** views of an extracted maxillary permanent second molar. (Courtesy University of Tennessee College of Dentistry, Memphis, Tenn.)

space in front of them is determined, and any change in the maxillary to mandibular first molar relationship can cause a malocclusion of teeth because of the loss of available space.

The maxillary first molar presents four well-developed cusps: mesiobuccal, mesiolingual, distobuccal, and distolingual. A tubercle sometimes seen on the mesiolingual cusp is called the cusp of Carabelli.

There are two buccal roots and one lingual root. The lingual root is the strongest, and the distobuccal root is smallest and more fragile.

From the buccal view this tooth resembles two fused premolars. At the junction of the two buccal cusps a Y-shaped groove is formed. A pit may appear at the center of the Y, which is the site of occasional decay. The buccal groove passes onto the occlusal surface into the central fossa.

The lingual surface differs from the buccal in that there is no cervical ridge. A lingual groove between the two lingual cusps arises from the distal fossa of the occlusal surface.

Prominent on the occlusal surface is a *transverse ridge,* which passes from the tip of the mesiolingual cusp to the tip of the distobuccal cusp. The central developmental groove begins in the mesial pit, passes into the central fossa and central pit, crosses the transverse ridge, and ends in the distal pit.

Maxillary permanent second and third molars

The maxillary permanent second molar erupts at approximately 12 to 13 years of age and is the seventh tooth from the midline. The maxillary permanent third molar erupts at approximately 17 to 21 years of age and is the eighth tooth from the midline. Both teeth will be considered together since they resemble each other in form and function (Fig. 5-25).

The roots of the maxillary second molar are as long or longer than those of the first molar but not as well developed. They are closer together, more susceptible to breakage, and have a distal curvature.

The crown of the second molar is somewhat smaller than that of the first molar. The distolingual cusp is much less developed on the second molar and even more poorly developed on the third molar. No cusp of Carabelli is seen on either second or third molar.

The maxillary third molar is the last tooth in the dental arch and presents more anomalies than any other tooth. Because of its late formation and crowded jaw position the tooth is "compressed" mesiodistally and wide buccolingually. It is common for this tooth to be impacted, and it is often congenitally missing.

The maxillary third molar may present three types of crown formation. It may have four cusps, three cusps (heart shaped), or two cusps (premolar type).

Mandibular permanent first premolar

The eruption time of the mandibular permanent first premolar is approximately 10 to 12 years of age. It is the fourth tooth from the midline in the mandibular arch (Fig. 5-26).

The mesial contact area meets the distal surface of the mandibular canine, whereas the distal contact area proximates the mesial surface of the mandibular second premolar.

The mandibular first premolars are similar to the maxillary premolars in that they are developed from four lobes, three buccal and one lingual. The first premolar has a large, well-formed buccal cusp, with a small nonfunctioning lingual cusp, sometimes no larger than the cingulum found on the maxillary canines. The mandibular first premolar is characteristically like the canine in that it functions with the canine, and its sharp buccal cusp is the only part of it occluding with maxillary teeth. The first premolar is always the smaller of the

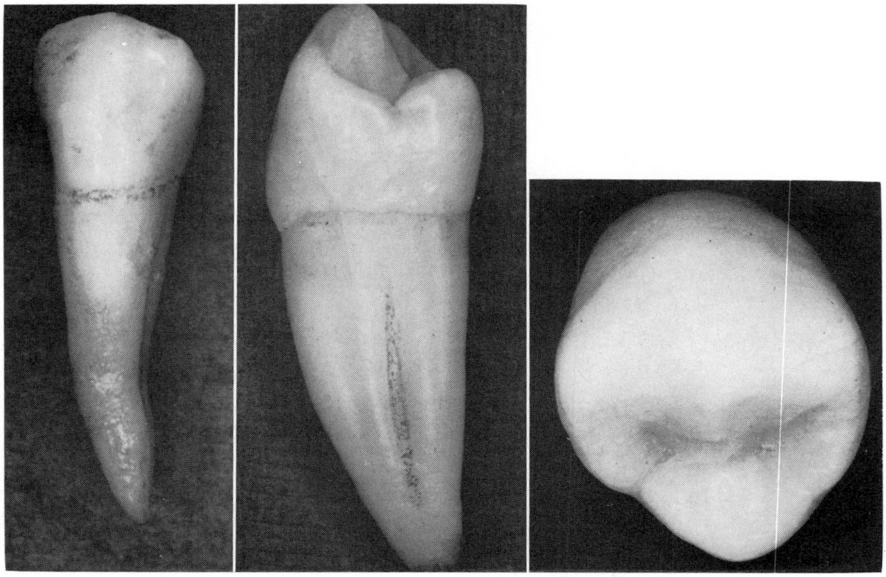

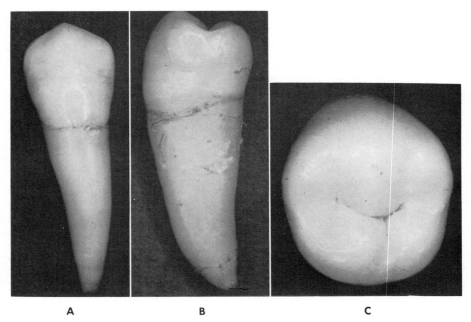

Fig. 5-26. Buccal **(A)**, proximal **(B)**, and occlusal **(C)** views of an extracted mandibular permanent first premolar. (Courtesy University of Tennessee College of Dentistry, Memphis, Tenn.)

A   B   C

Fig. 5-27. Buccal **(A)**, proximal **(B)**, and occlusal **(C)** views of an extracted mandibular permanent second premolar. (Courtesy University of Tennessee College of Dentistry, Memphis, Tenn.)

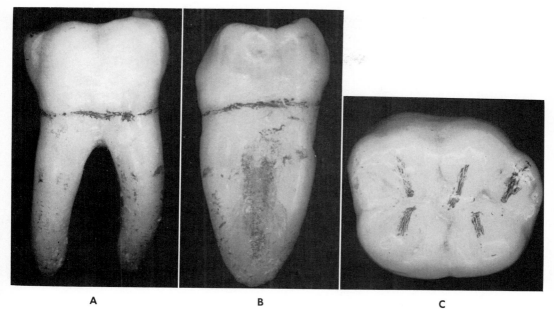

Fig. 5-28. Buccal **(A),** proximal **(B),** and occlusal **(C)** views of an extracted mandibular permanent first molar. (Courtesy University of Tennessee College of Dentistry, Memphis, Tenn.)

two mandibular premolars, whereas the opposite is true, in many cases, of the maxillary premolars.

From the mesial and distal aspects a feature characteristic of mandibular teeth is quite apparent—this is the lingual inclinations of the buccal surface and lingual surfaces. Thus the entire crown appears to be tilted in a lingual direction. This feature is characteristic because of the occlusal angle of the opposing maxillary arch.

This tooth is almost always single rooted with a distal apical curvature.

Mandibular permanent second premolar

The eruption time of the mandibular permanent second premolar is approximately 10 to 12 years of age. It is the fifth tooth from the midline in the mandibular arch (Fig. 5-27).

The mesial contact area meets the distal surface of the mandibular first premolar, whereas the distal contact area proxi-

mates the mesial surface of the mandibular first molar.

This tooth usually has three cusps on the occlusal surface, one well-developed buccal cusp and two less developed lingual cusps.

The buccal view strongly resembles that of the mandibular first premolar. The lingual view, however, differs because of the presence of two lingual cusps. Between these cusps is a groove that passes onto the occlusal surface and terminates in a central pit at the base of the lingual ridge of the buccal cusp.

There may be many variations in the occlusal surface of this tooth. The most common form is that of the Y-shaped central grooves that divide the three cusps. In some cases there may be only two cusps, as in the first premolar.

Like the mandibular first premolar this tooth is usually single rooted with the apex curved in a distal direction.

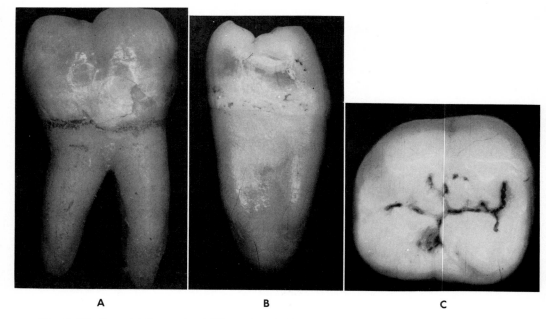

A   B   C

Fig. 5-29. Buccal **(A)**, proximal **(B)**, and occlusal **(C)** views of an extracted mandibular permanent second molar. (Courtesy University of Tennessee College of Dentistry, Memphis, Tenn.)

Mandibular permanent first molar

The eruption time of the mandibular permanent first molar is approximately 6 to 7 years of age. It is the sixth tooth from the midline, is usually the first permanent tooth to erupt, and is of great importance in the formation of the occlusion of the arches (Fig. 5-28).

The mesial contact area touches the distal surface of the second premolar. Its distal contact area proximates the mesial surface of the mandibular second molar.

This is the largest tooth in the mandibular arch and has five true cusps and two well-developed roots.

From the buccal view three buccal cusps may be seen: mesiobuccal, distobuccal, and distal. A buccal groove separates the mesiobuccal from the distobuccal cusp and runs for half the length of the crown. A distal groove separates the distobuccal from the distal cusp and slants in a distal direction.

The lingual surface presents two cusps,

the mesiolingual and the distolingual, which are about the same size and shape. There is a slight lingual groove.

The mesial and distal views show the crown tipped at a slight angle toward the lingual surface. The crest of curvature on the buccal is in the cervical third, while on the lingual it is at the junction of the occlusal and middle third.

There are five distinct cusps on the occlusal surface. The three buccal cusps are arranged so that the mesiobuccal and the distobuccal cusps form the major portion of the occlusal surface, with the small distal cusp crowded into the distobuccal area. The central developmental grooves follow a straight course from the mesial pit through the central pit to the distal pit.

Mandibular permanent second and third molars

The eruption time of the mandibular permanent second molar is approximately 11 to 13 years of age. The eruption time of the mandibular third molar is approximately 17 to 21 years of age. They are respectively the seventh and eighth teeth from the midline (Fig. 5-29).

The mandibular second molar has four cusps on the occlusal surface and two well-developed roots.

The buccal surface presents two buccal cusps that are similar in size and shape. Separating the two buccal cusps is a buccal groove, which is deep and passes down the buccal surface to a buccal pit.

The lingual surface is similar to the buccal surface, with two similar lingual cusps separated by a lingual groove.

The proximal views of this tooth are similar to those of the mandibular first molar; however, there is no distal cusp.

The occlusal surface is symmetrical, with four cusps of almost equal size and a central groove passing mesiodistally. The buccal and lingual grooves cross the central groove in a right angle at the central pit.

The mandibular third molar may present various forms. The four-cusp type resembles the mandibular second molar, whereas the five-cusp type resembles the mandibular first molar. The crown is usually larger than that of the second mandibular molar and is usually crenated on the occlusal surface. The roots may be fused, crooked, and multiple in number.

SUGGESTED READINGS

Goldman, H. M., and Cohen, D. W.: Periodontia, ed. 4, St. Louis, 1969, The C. V. Mosby Co.

Goss, C. M., editor: Gray's anatomy of the human body, ed. 28, Philadelphia, 1966, Lea & Febiger.

Shapiro, H. H.: Maxillofacial anatomy, Philadelphia, 1954, J. B. Lippincott Co.

Sicher, H., and DuBrul, E. L.: Oral anatomy, ed. 5, St. Louis, 1970, The C. V. Mosby Co.

Wheeler, R. C.: Textbook of dental anatomy and physiology, ed. 3, Philadelphia, 1958, W. B. Saunders Co.

Woodburne, R. F.: Essentials of human anatomy, ed. 3, New York, 1965, Oxford University Press.

Young, J.: Outline of oral and dental anatomy, New York, 1964, McGraw-Hill Book Company.

Zeisz, R. C., and Nuckolls, J.: Dental anatomy, ed. 1, St. Louis, 1949, The C. V. Mosby Co.

chapter 6

RECOGNIZING ABNORMAL CONDITIONS IN THE ORAL CAVITY

Eugene G. Brunson, D.D.S.
Maynard K. Hine, D.D.S., M.S., D.Sc.
James E. Turner, B.A., D.D.S.
James F. Smith, B.A., D.D.S., Ph.D.

This is a companion chapter to Chapter 5, in which the dental hygiene student studied what she may expect to see when she looks into the normal mouth. She has learned the proper names that she must use to describe the hard and the soft tissues, and she has learned some of their functions.

In this chapter the dental hygiene student will learn the meaning and significance of the telltale marks that appear in an oral cavity in which something abnormal is taking place. The dental hygienist may be the first trained person to recognize or suspect abnormalities that may be related to the local or general health of the patient.

Admittedly not all of the abnormalities that she sees will have a "life or death" aspect to them. Most of them either will be an index to what she will be doing for the patient or will provide some advance information that her dentist will need to know before he examines the patient further.

In most instances the dental hygienist is privileged to see the "before" in the patient, and she actually can derive great satisfaction in seeing both the "before" and the "after" and in recognizing the tremendous improvements that have taken place as a result of the dental service that the office has provided. It is important for the dental hygienist to realize that when she sees and recognizes abnormal conditions, these are "privileged" bits of information. This may be "classified information" or "personal information." Some of these telltale marks can be disturbing and even exciting, but the dental hygienist must never discuss them with the patient. When and if it is to be discussed, it *must* be the dentist who reveals and discusses it and *not* the dental hygienist.

STAINS AND DEPOSITS

Among the first abnormal conditions that will be observed by the dental hygienist are the stains and deposits on the teeth. Since one of her prime responsibilities is the removal of these stains and deposits, more emphasis will be placed on this than on other abnormal conditions.

Often an attractive person has his appearance marred by unsightly teeth covered with deposits, stains, and cavities and by reddened, swollen gingiva. A primary responsibility of the dental hygienist is to remove all the many stains and accretions that collect on the exposed surfaces of teeth, so that when the person smiles, the teeth appear clean and well polished and the soft tissues normal.

Not only do stains and deposits on teeth interfere with esthetics, but they also contribute to unpleasant breath (halitosis) and in many cases result in irritation to the soft tissues around the teeth. As a result a chronic inflammatory gingivitis occurs, and the mouth may be tender, with red, bleeding gums. Deposits also make it more difficult for the patient to clean the teeth and gums properly, and resistance of gingival tissues is lowered so that a gingivitis (infection of tissues around the teeth) that ordinarily would be of little significance may become quite severe.

The degree of uncleanliness in the mouth varies from patient to patient and from area to area in the same mouth. The amount of debris collecting in a mouth depends upon many factors; some mouths are naturally quite free of accumulations and debris, while others are difficult to keep clean.

The character of the tooth surface is important in determining how much foreign material collects upon it. *Hypoplastic* (poorly formed) enamel makes it easier for stains to collect. The composition and quantity of saliva also aid in controlling the amount of stain and calculus that collects on the teeth. Saliva is usually a thin, watery secretion that keeps the teeth and gingival tissues moist at all times. If, however, it is too viscid or is below normal in quantity, the natural cleansing of the oral cavity is ineffective, and stains and debris tend to collect. It is recognized that complete absence of saliva (*xerostomia*) occurs rarely, and in such cases gingival tissues are irritated and deposits on teeth increase in amount.

The arrangement and contour of teeth and dental restorations will influence the amount of foreign material collecting in the mouth; a study of the normal contours of the teeth and arches indicates that teeth are arranged in the mouth in such a way that they usually protect underlying soft tissues. Deviation from the normal contour will result in a collection of debris, in food impaction, and eventually in chronic gingivitis.

Constant motion of the tongue and cheeks aids in keeping the mouth cleaned. It will be noted, for example, that if the patient refrains from using one side of the mouth because of a toothache or for some other reason, the unused side of the mouth will show many more deposits on the teeth.

Also, the type of food ingested and method of mastication can be a factor in keeping the mouth clean. Individuals who eat many raw vegetables and chew their food thoroughly will usually have a cleaner mouth than those who eat soft foods.

There are many personal dental care measures that the patient may use to aid in keeping the mouth clean, such as toothbrushing and use of dental floss. Frequent visits to the dental office and the excellence of the oral prophylaxis will also have a role in determining the cleanliness of the oral cavity.

In most cases collections of foreign material in the mouth are limited to the teeth themselves, to tissues immediately around or between the teeth, to artificial replacements of teeth, and to the dorsum (central part) of the tongue.

Types of deposits on teeth

The types of deposits that occur in the oral cavity may be classified into two general groups: those that are calcified and those that are not.

Plaque. All exposed enamel surfaces except those that are subjected to friction during mastication are always covered with a thin, usually invisible coating com-

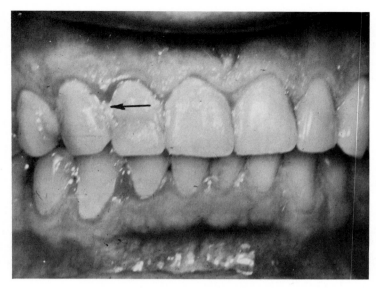

Fig. 6-1. Clinical photograph showing plaque that collected in the mouth of an adult who did not brush his teeth on one side of the mouth (see arrow). Note the chronic inflammatory gingivitis present on the unbrushed side.

posed of bacteria, food debris, and desquamated epithelial cells. In most cases this thin film, or plaque, is not noticeable unless stained by a disclosing solution. These plaques are actually accumulations of bacterial colonies consisting of many types of oral microorganisms. Interspersed between these bacterial growths can be found occasional desquamated epithelial cells and, rarely, minute particles of food (Fig. 6-1).

Disclosing solutions. Disclosing solutions are applied to the teeth and gums to disclose the presence of plaques that are difficult to see with the naked eye. In the past there were three commonly used solutions in the dental office: one in which the Mercurochrome produces the color, one in which Bismarck brown produces the color, and another in which iodine produces the color (see accompanying formulas). All three solutions are effective, but those containing Mercurochrome and iodine produce the heaviest stain.

Formulas for disclosing solutions

1		
Mercurochrome	1.5	gm.
Water q.s. ad	30	ml.

2		
Bismarck brown	3	gm.
Alcohol	10	ml.
Glycerin	120	ml.
Oil of anise	1	minim

3		
Potassium iodide	1.6	gm.
Iodine crystals	1.6	gm.
Water	13.4	ml.
Glycerin q.s. ad	30	ml.

Keep in glass-stoppered bottle.

More recently, disclosing agents containing erythrosin (F.D.C. Red No. 3), as advocated by Arnim,* have become the standard for both office use and for use by the patients in their home mouth care procedures. This disclosing agent can be prepared as a solution for office use or as a

*Arnim, S. S.: Thoughts concerning cause, pathogenesis, treatment and prevention of periodontal disease, J. Periodont. 29:217-223, 1958.

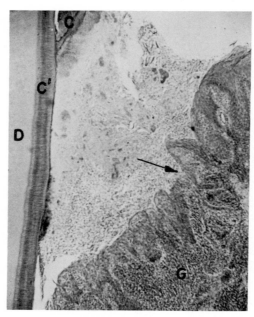

Fig. 6-2. Photomicrograph of a gingival pocket. Note the space between the tissue and the tooth is filled with debris and many microorganisms. The arrow indicates a break in the epithelium which allows the bacteria to enter directly into the gingival tissue, G. C, Calculus; C', cementum; D, dentin. (Modified from Box, H. K.: J. Ontario Dent. Assoc. **31**:204, 1954.)

chewable tablet for home use. In the tablet form, flavoring agents are added that makes its use pleasant and effective. Erythrosin adequately stains the plaque so that its location and extent can be readily determined by the patient, yet it does not permanently stain clothing or bathroom fixtures.

Probably no other single factor has had as much influence upon the development of effective mouth cleaning procedures by patients as the use of the disclosing tablet.

Bacteria of plaque. The types of bacteria growing in plaque vary greatly for reasons not well understood. In most mouths they consist of a heterogeneous collection of cocci, bacilli, spirilla (vibrios), spirochetes, and filamentous organisms. Some of these organisms can break down carbohydrates to produce acids that decalcify the teeth and cause dental caries. Other microorganisms produce toxins and invade oral soft tissues and cause gingivitis (Fig. 6-2).

Noncalcified deposits and stains. Noncalcified deposits and stains include materia alba; green, orange, tobacco, and black stains; brown pellicle; stains from foods and metals; and intrinsic stains.

Materia alba. If the bacterial plaque on a tooth is so thick that it is easily seen without staining, it is often referred to as materia alba. This is a white deposit that accumulates, particularly around necks of teeth and on the free margin of the gingiva, although in mouths poorly cared for it may cover much of the crown of the tooth. It consists of a soft, cheese-like substance that, when examined under the microscope, will be found to consist of the same elements as those of the bacterial plaque (Figs. 6-1 and 6-2).

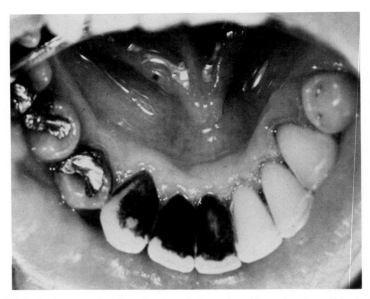

Fig. 6-3. Clinical photograph of teeth of a pipe smoker. Note the dense black stain on the lingual surface of the lower anterior teeth. Stain has been removed on one side.

Green stain. Occasionally the gingival third of the teeth will be covered with a relatively thick, dense, furry type of deposit that is pale green or gray-green in color. This stain usually occurs on the upper anterior teeth of children or young adults and is very difficult to remove. Its etiology is unknown, although it is assumed that the stain is caused by an overgrowth of green pigment–producing microorganisms of some unknown type. Often its removal will reveal an etched enamel surface below the stain. Removal of the stain requires a rather strong abrasive, and frequently two or three treatments are needed. Sometimes painting the stain with an iodine solution, such as dental glycerite, seems to "fix" the plaque and make it a little easier to remove.

Orange stain. Occasionally in children and young adults a diffuse, brick red to orange stain is seen in the gingival third of certain teeth. This stain usually is easily removed by polishing the tooth with a mild abrasive. The stain has no known significance, and its etiology is not understood.

It is supposed that the stain is either from food pigments or from some chromogenic microorganisms, but neither has been identified.

Tobacco stain. The tars and resins from smoking usually cause a diffuse, powdery stain on the surfaces of the teeth. The color ranges from light yellow to almost black. Cigarette smoking produces the least stain, cigar smoking somewhat more, and pipe smoking the most (Fig. 6-3). It is not known why more stains accumulate on the teeth of some smokers than on those of others, but it is known that both the type and amount of smoking are important.

Black stain. Occasionally a dark brown or black stain may be found on teeth of nonsmokers, particularly on the lingual surface and close to the gingival tissues. This stain is believed to be caused by food pigments or a breakdown of hemoglobin or perhaps chromogenic microorganisms, but its etiology is unknown and it has no significance.

Brown pellicle. A thin, brownish deposit,

or pellicle, is occasionally noted on teeth that are poorly cleansed. This type of stain often covers most of the crowns of teeth. It is easily polished away and has no known significance.

Stains from food and metals. Some candies and highly colored foods often will produce pigmentation of bacterial plaques on the teeth and soft tissues of the mouth, particularly the tongue. Recognition of these stains may be made by the bizarre appearance of teeth and oral tissues and the history of ingesting colored foods. Occasionally teeth will be stained by deposit of drugs used in dental treatments (such as silver nitrate) and metals inhaled in industry (such as copper).

Treatment. All the stains and deposits discussed, with the exception of green stain, are quite easy to remove by polishing the teeth, but they may recur within a few hours or days after removal. For this reason the patient must be taught exactly how to brush the teeth, since these stains can be brushed away if the brushing is done effectively and often.

Intrinsic stains. It should be mentioned that the enamel of teeth sometimes becomes stained so that a tooth or many teeth will appear dark because of the stain in the tooth itself. These so-called intrinsic stains are caused by many conditions. For example, if water containing fluorides in a proportion of more than 2 parts per million (p.p.m.) is ingested by an individual at the time his teeth are forming, the teeth may show a collection of white spots (if the fluorosis is mild) or a mottled brown or black appearance (if the fluorosis is severe). This stain is actually deposited between the tiny rods that make up the enamel. It can be removed only with great difficulty and care. One technic for removal includes the use of 30% hydrogen peroxide solution in repeated applications (protecting the gingival tissue carefully) and perhaps polishing away some of the surface of the enamel.

Stains from filling materials may penetrate the enamel and dentin, causing the tooth to be bluish black in color. This is particularly true if a germicidal silver cement is used in a base of the filling or if amalgam is packed carelessly into a cavity.

In many cases breakdown of blood pigmentation after removal of the dental pulp will result in intrinsic black or brown staining of the tooth. The tooth will lose its translucency and assume a color varying from a light yellow to a slate gray, brown, or black. Treatment of such discolored teeth is difficult, and the dentist should use all precautions to prevent stain from forming by removing all hemorrhage from the pulp chamber at the time of pulp removal. If the pulp chamber is then enlarged and several applications of 30% hydrogen peroxide are used, sometimes the tooth can be bleached in a satisfactory manner.

Trauma will occasionally result in hemorrhage in the pulp, which makes the tooth turn pink. In some cases the trauma results in an internal resorption of the tooth so that the tooth assumes a pink color because of the loss of tooth substance and increases the vascular pulp.

In cases of pronounced jaundice, teeth have been known to turn green or yellow-green. The pigment disappears shortly after the jaundice clears up. Occasionally acute exanthematous diseases have resulted in teeth turning pink.

Rarely teeth of children with an Rh-negative factor have turned green or blue-green, probably as the result of hemorrhage into the developing tooth germ.

Calcified deposits. In many young adults and most adults hard, stone-like concretions are often found on teeth (Fig. 6-4) or on other hard substances in the oral cavity (Fig. 6-5). The deposits are called dental calculus. Synonyms are sialolithiasis, odontolithiasis, and the lay term, tartar.

Calculus is light yellow to dark brown in color, depending upon the amount of stain

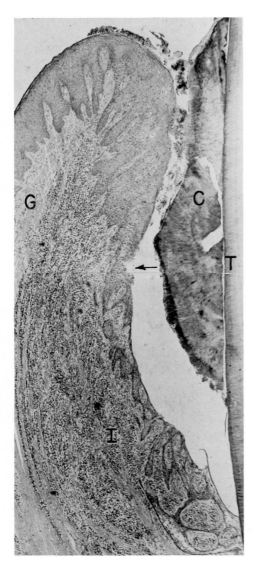

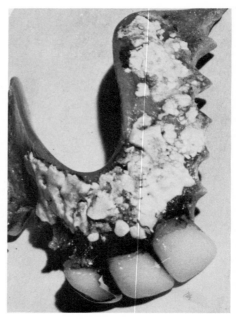

Fig. 6-5. Calcareous deposits on the lingual surface of a poorly fitting maxillary denture.

Fig. 6-4. Photomicrograph showing calculus and gingival tissue. Note the heavy deposit of adherent calculus which has been formed layer upon layer, C. The arrow indicates a break in the epithelium which allows invasion of the gingival tissue by bacteria. Note the low-grade chronic inflammation, I, below the epithelium in the gingival tissue, G. Calculus is adherent to the tooth, T. (Courtesy Weinmann, J. R., and Winn, W. W. From Burnett, G. W., and Scherp, H. W.: Oral microbiology and infectious disease, Baltimore, 1957, The Williams & Wilkins Co.)

and food debris trapped in it. Newly deposited calculus is light yellow and soft and gradually hardens until it is at least as hard as cementum. It must be emphasized that the chemical composition of calculus is quite similar to that of cementum. Therefore it is difficult to remove calculus chemically or physically without also threatening the integrity of the cemental surface of the tooth. The calcareous deposits are quite firmly attached to the teeth and hence often difficult to remove.

Since microorganisms form the framework for deposits of calculus, it is possible that they actually attach themselves directly to the tooth. Sometimes the calcified matrix of the calculus will fit into an irregularity in the cemental surface of the tooth or into areas of cementum that have been previously resorbed. A study of calculus deposits under the microscope also suggests that there actually may be a penetration of microorganisms into the cementum in some cases.

Location of calculus. According to its location, calculus is classified into two general groups: supragingival and subgingival (or submarginal and supramarginal). Supragingival or salivary calculus is commonly found on teeth opposite the salivary ducts (lingual side of the lower anterior teeth and buccal side of the upper molars). Its color is buff to dark brown, and it often assumes an alarmingly large size. Subgingival calculus is located just below the free gingival margin on the enamel or cemental surface of the tooth. This type was formerly called serumal calculus, since it was believed to come from blood serum. It occurs usually as narrow dark brown to black bands, which, when removed, are found to be brittle and almost metallic in hardness. The color of subgingival calculus is probably caused by a breakdown of blood pigments. It is now believed that both types of calculus are formed in the same way and that the difference results because of the location of the calculus. Obviously calculus above the gingival tissue would contain more food debris, while the calculus below the free gingiva would be compressed and hence more dense. Many deposits show both types of calculus together, with one shading into the other so that a division is indistinguishable.

Supragingival calculus is easily located by a visual examination with a good light and a mouth mirror. Location of subgingival calculus, however, is often difficult and requires an instrument, since the calculus is usually covered by gingival tissue. Since subgingival calculus is very dark in color, it will sometimes give the free margin of the gingiva a dark color. Gently blowing the gingiva from the tooth with a blast of air will occasionally bring the calculus into view. Generally, however, subgingival calculus is located by gliding an instrument over the surface of the tooth; a rough, irregular surface indicates the presence of calculus.

Theories of formation of calculus. Many theories have been formulated to explain the deposition of calculus. It was early thought to be merely a result of a decomposition of some elements of saliva. Black believed that calculus was caused by a decomposition of colloidal suspension of calcium combined with a globulin of saliva. Others (Kirk) believed that calcium was deposited when carbon dioxide was lost from the saliva upon excretion—that loss of carbon dioxide resulted in a lessening of the ability of saliva to hold calcium, and so the calcium was deposited as calcium phosphate. Others thought that ammonia from decomposing food resulted in a more alkaline reaction of the saliva and hence caused a deposition of calcium phosphate.

A study of calcareous deposits will show that they are deposited in layers, with the innermost layers being the most heavily calcified. Often a matrix or network of long rods or thread-forming microorganisms *(Leptotrichia)* are found. It is believed by some that these organisms serve as a matrix or nidus for calculus and that they produce a localized alkaline reaction that precipitates calcium from saliva. Another theory is that in some individuals there is present a microorganism producing a phosphatase that accelerates the deposition of calculus.

Careful studies have been made of salivary variations that occur in individuals with and without calculus. It is apparently true that patients with excessive deposits of calculus do have saliva with a slightly higher calcium and phosphate content, a slightly higher alkalinity, and a slightly lower protein content. However, these variations are slight, and many calculus-free individuals have more calcium in their saliva than do those who have calcareous deposits. It is probable that many of the foregoing factors combine to result in deposits of calculus. Fig. 6-6 diagrammatically illustrates the formation of calculus.

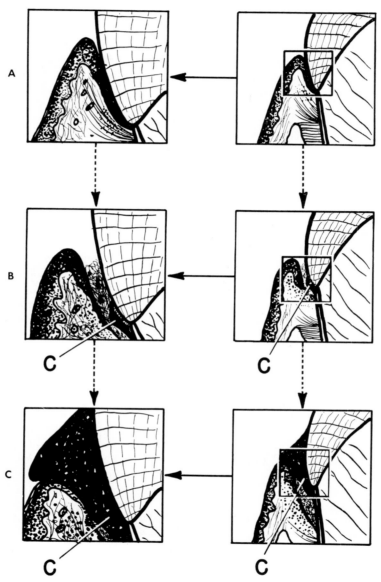

Fig. 6-6. Diagram of the development of calculus, C. **A,** Normal sulcus with "epithelial attachment" closely adapted to enamel surface. **B,** Matrix of motile and nonmotile bacteria, protozoa, leukocytes, and desquamated cells in thick, viscous, serous exudate has formed in the sulcus. Gingiva is displaced from its adaptation to the tooth. Mineralization of the mass to form calculus (C) has begun. **C,** Mineralization continues until mass of both subgingival and supragingival calculus is present. Inflammation of the inner gingival wall and a breakdown of the gingival fibers, resulting in an enlarged and deepened sulcus, has occurred.

Composition of calculus. The composition of calculus varies according to the length of time it has been present. Newly formed calculus is soft and amorphous and contains much more water and organic material than calculus that has begun to harden. At this time it can be brushed away or removed easily; after 36 to 48 hours it begins to harden and becomes firmly attached to the tooth or prosthetic appliance.

In general hardened calculus deposits are composed of approximately 67% calcium phosphate, 20% water and organic material, and 13% calcium carbonate, with traces of potassium, sodium, and iron. Calcium carbonate closely resembles dentin, cementum, and bone in its chemical composition and physical hardness. For this reason it is almost impossible to dissolve calculus with any chemical compound without also injuring the adjoining tooth surface.

Incidence of calculus deposition. Careful clinical observations have indicated that calculus is deposited at irregular intervals. Patients will sometimes demonstrate a rapid deposition for a short time and then have no deposition for days or weeks. It is therefore difficult to give accurate statistics on the incidence of calculus, but it is apparent that there is a great increase in calculus deposition as individuals approach their twentieth year. This increase is even greater in the third decade of life and with advancing age until finally nine out of ten individuals past 50 years of age have calcified deposits on their teeth. Calculus is slightly more common in males than in females. Usually both supragingival calculus and subgingival calculus are found in the same patients; only occasionally will subgingival calculus alone be found.

Removal of calculus. Removal of the calculus before it hardens is relatively easy and usually can be accomplished by the patient who uses a good toothbrushing technic. However, once the calcification has started, the deposits must be removed by a dentist or dental hygienist. Removal is best accomplished by scaling the teeth (using instruments called scalers, Fig. 6-7) in the manner described in Chapter 8. After the removal of calculus with scalers it is necessary that the teeth be polished with a brush or a rubber cup and a porte-polisher, using a very mild flour pumice or tin oxide polishing agent. After scaling and polishing it is advisable to paint the tissues liberally with a mild antiseptic such as a dental glycerite (see accompanying prescription).

The prescription for dental glycerite is as follows:

R̸ Zinc phenosulfonate
　Potassium iodide　　　　　　āā gr. xx
　Iodine crystals　　　　　　　　gr. xxx
　Methol　　　　　　　　　　　　gr. iij
　Thymol　　　　　　　　　　　　gr. ij
　Glycerin　　　　　　　q.s. ad f℥ j
M. Sig:　Apply in teeth and gingival tissue

Many chemical agents have been recommended for the removal of calculus, but these cannot be recommended routinely. For example, solutions containing a weak solution of hydrochloric acid will soften calculus but also injure tooth substance. Sodium hexametaphosphate has been recommended to soften calculus, but careful tests indicate that calcium can also be withdrawn from tooth substance by using this agent. Other agents containing an enzyme of one type or another have been recommended periodically as safe agents that will soften calculus. Further study must be made before these can be recommended unreservedly.

OTHER ABNORMALITIES

Most of the other abnormalities of the oral cavity can be included in five categories: inflammatory lesions, tumors, congenital and acquired deformities, physical injury (trauma), and abnormalities produced by chemical and physical agents.

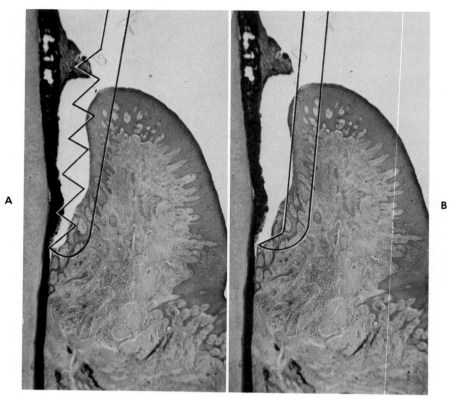

Fig. 6-7. Outline of prophylactic file, **A,** and scaler, **B,** drawn to scale and placed at the base of a gingival pocket. (From Orban, B.: J. Periodont. **27:**130, 1956.)

Inflammatory lesions

Certain bacteria, viruses, and fungi live within the oral cavity and seemingly produce no disease manifestation. These organisms are considered to be the "normal oral flora." Needless to say these same organisms under certain conditions, such as increased numbers and decreased resistance of the host, may produce disease.

Certain individuals harbor bacteria that produce no disease in themselves, but these same bacteria, when introduced into another person by respiratory droplets or body contact, may produce their disease. Such persons are the "germ carriers," "Typhoid Marys," or "staphylococcus carriers." Most highly contagious diseases—for example, syphilis—have no immune carriers.

If the person has the bacteria, he has the disease. The symptoms or lesions may not always be obvious to the dental hygienist; therefore, she should protect herself from acquiring disease bacteria by working a reasonable distance from the patient's respiratory outlets—18 inches is suggested—or by wearing a surgical mask when indicated. The hygienist also must be cautioned that bacteria from infections in a patient's mouth may invade her circulatory system through a cut in her finger, even a very tiny one. Rubber gloves or finger cots may be worn when injuries are present on the hands or fingers.

Inflammation. Inflammation is defined as the reaction of tissue cells to injury. The injurious agents may be bacterial, viral, fungal, chemical, or traumatic. The outstanding signs of inflammation are heat (calor), redness (rubor), swelling (tumor), pain (dolor), and loss of function. Inflammation is frequently a sign of disease. An inflammatory lesion may be defined as a structural tissue change caused by injury or disease.

Gingivitis. The most common inflammatory disease that the dental hygienist will encounter is gingivitis. This group of conditions is usually first seen in the adolescent and is thought to be a result of bacteria and lowered host resistance. The gums are usually red, swollen, and painful and truly seem to be inflamed. Microscopic examination of this inflammatory tissue shows the presence of large numbers of white blood cells, which are phagocytic (they engulf and destroy) in purpose.

The pathologist has no difficulty in recognizing inflammatory tissue microscopically. Another method that frequently is used to diagnose an inflammatory lesion is the examination of the bacteria themselves. This is done by taking some of the exudate from around the necks of the teeth and placing it upon a glass slide. It is then stained, usually with Gram stain, and examined microscopically. This method reveals the type of bacteria present, but specific classification requires further staining and laboratory technics by the bacteriologist.

Inflammatory diseases such as gingivitis may be acute, subacute, or chronic. Acute inflammation usually manifests a sudden rise or reaction and a short duration. The subacute condition is slower in developing and may take 2 or 3 days for its symptoms to appear. It may require several days for its symptoms to subside.

Chronic inflammation is produced over a long period of time and usually requires a long convalescing period. The most commonly seen form of gingivitis is the chronic form. Bacteria in dental plaque and in contact with the gingival tissues

are the initiating cause of gingivitis. Usually the process is an insidious one rarely noticed by the patient because of the absence of pain. Bleeding of the gingival tissues upon function (or during toothbrushing) may be the first sign of a problem to the patient.

A change in color of the gingiva to redness and slight changes in the form and contour of the gingiva are early signs of gingival involvement. If the bacterial irritants are allowed to remain and the progress of the disease continues, more obvious changes—increased ease of bleeding, increased redness, and obvious contour deviations—become apparent.

Other factors may now become contributors to the course of the disease. The bacterial plaque may mineralize and the resulting calculus then becomes an irritant. A slight aspect of the irritation from calculus may be from its physical presence, but the primary source of irritation is in the increased capacity for bacterial plaque retention. At this stage of the gingivitis, removal of the local irritants by removal of the bacterial plaque and calculus usually results in the return of the tissues to normal. However, the institution of effective mouth care practices to prevent the return of the bacterial plaque must be accomplished or the disease will continue because its cause will continue.

Periodontitis. When gingivitis continues untreated, the inflammation progresses into and involves the supporting tissues immediately adjacent to the tooth. The tooth is supported in its socket by the periodontal ligament attached to the alveolar bone of the socket wall and the cementum of the tooth.

When inflammation involves these structures, the disease is known as periodontitis. Thus periodontitis has its beginning in an untreated gingivitis. Because the progression of the disease is slow (chronic), its advanced form is frequently not seen until the third decade of life, although its true beginning may have been as early as age 5 or 6.

More teeth are lost as a result of periodontal disease than from all other causes. However, treatment can be effective if it is instituted in the early stages of the disease and before extensive loss of the supporting tissues occurs.

Other inflammatory reactions. Inflammation of the gingivae and mucous membranes is called gingivostomatitis.

If the mucous membranes of the buccal pads are inflamed but the gingiva appears to be in normal limits, the condition is called *stomatitis*. Stomatitis may be a widespread, evenly distributed redness of the mucous membranes, or it may appear as individual lesions separated by a normal-appearing mucous membrane. An example of the second type is herpetic stomatitis.

The *gumboil* (parulis) is an inflammatory condition of chronic nature. This usually appears on the buccal or lingual surface of the gingiva below the necks of teeth and is a soft, raised mass of tissue. When pressure is exerted with a dull instrument, pus is usually found to be present.

Pus is frequently taken from such lesions, and the bacteria are grown on media in the laboratory. This is known as a culture. As these bacteria are grown, various drugs are introduced into their colonies in order to determine which drug has the greatest bacteriocidal effect. This is known as a sensitivity test. The hygienist may be asked to take a sample of pus for a culture and sensitivity test.

Tumors (neoplasms)

Tumors or neoplasms are often discovered upon a routine dental examination because they frequently exist without symptoms. Tumors may be benign or malignant (cancerous).

Benign tumors usually grow very slowly, frequently become arrested, and produce their damage by mechanical or anatomical displacement of the tissues of the host. Malignant tumors grow rapidly, are seldom arrested, and may spread with devastating effects to vital organs, such as the liver, remote from their original site.

The more commonly seen benign tumors of the oral cavity are described here.

The fibroma is a raised mass of tissue that may have a diversity of appearance; some may be soft and red while others may be firm and pale or white. They may be located on the gingiva, lips, palate, or buccal mucosa (Fig. 6-8).

The papilloma is also a raised mass of tissue. It frequently appears to be hard and warty. It is found in the same areas as the fibroma but is most common on the lips, gingiva, and soft palate.

These two growths may appear in the same oral cavity. If a differential diagnosis is to be made, the pathologist must have a biopsy. This is usually a surgical wedge of tissue taken from the tumor growth. By microsectioning the tissue and staining it the oral pathologist may view the cells under the microscope. The cellular characteristics identifying the fibroma and the papilloma are more diagnostic than the clinical, visual, and digital examination.

The hemangioma is a raised, bluish growth usually located on the tongue or mucous membrane. The bluish color is caused by massive engorged blood vessels. A slight cut, abrasion, or tearing of the tissues by accident, such as by scaling instruments used for dental curettage, may produce hemorrhage.

The giant cell tumor, or epulis, may be seen frequently by the dental hygienist. They are usually located on the attached gingiva but may arise from the periodontal membrane. This tumor will appear to be raised, soft, and red, and it has a tendency to bleed. Biopsy and microscopic examination are necessary for differential diagnosis.

A tumor-like mass may appear on the gingiva of the pregnant patient. This has

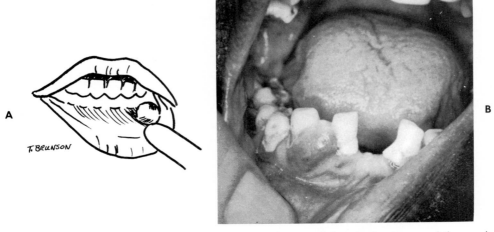

Fig. 6-8. A, Fibroma of the buccal mucosa. **B,** Fibroma of the gingiva (tumor of the gum).

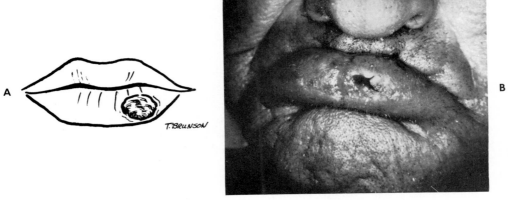

Fig. 6-9. Carcinoma (cancer) of the lower lip. (Courtesy University of Tennessee College of Dentistry, Memphis, Tenn.)

been termed *pregnancy tumor* or pregnancy hyperplasia. This mass of tissue will frequently regress some weeks after delivery.

There are certain anatomical variations that will suggest tumor. The most common example is a hard, raised mass of tissue varying in size and form and located on the hard palate or sometimes on the lingual surface of the mandible. These structures are known as tori, or bony protuberances.

They cannot be classified as tumors or abnormalities. They are anatomical variations. Tumors may arise in these locations associated with tori and may mislead the clinician in assuming their innocence. Years of experience are necessary before one can make the "snap diagnosis."

Oral cancer, or carcinoma (malignant tumors), may develop on the lower lip, tongue, gingiva, floor of the mouth, cheek, or palate. These lesions on the soft tissues may present a deceptive picture of innocent ulceration and may manifest themselves in a variety of forms. Occasionally a sublingual anomaly will escape close visual scrutiny.

The beginning carcinoma of the lip may appear as a tiny, slightly raised, strawberry-like lesion and may be referred to by the patient as a chronic "cold sore" (Fig. 6-9). Whenever ulcerations of the oral cavity or lips are detected, biopsy is recommended.

The normal oral cavity may present variations that may, because of inexperience, excite the examining clinician. If this impression is instilled into the patient's mind, unnecessary and sometimes irretractable fears may give mental discomfort to the patient. An attitude of "We will find out" is the key to answering the patient's query of "What do you think it is?"

Congenital and acquired deformities

The tongue, more than any other structure of the oral cavity, demonstrates variations in size, shape, and form. Some of these variations may be manifestations of some local or systemic condition or disease. One cannot imagine a complete physical examination without an inspection of the tongue.

The so-called fissured tongue is a congenital manifestation that usually has no significance or relationship to disease. Upon close inspection of the tongue and spreading of the top surface (dorsum) one will note deep fissures or irregular, trench-like furrows.

Ankyloglossia is thought to be a congenital condition in which the tongue is held fast to the floor of the mouth by a band of tissue called the lingual frenum. In such cases the patient is unable to thrust the tongue from the mouth. Speech impediments may be associated with ankyloglossia.

Many congenital abnormalities involving the lips and palate will not be seen as such by the dental hygienist because these conditions have been detected early and have been surgically corrected. Scars may be detected that may give some indication of the original deformity.

Surgical correction of clefts of the soft palate is not always successful and sometimes result in a short soft palate. Ordinarily the soft palate will rise and touch the back of the throat, which acts as a valve to close off the nasal passage. If the soft palate is insufficient in length to perform this action, deficient speech is noticed. The individual's phonation (sounds) will demonstrate hypernasality.

Persons with underdevelopment of the mandible (lower jaw) present a rather noticeable profile because the chin is receding while the nose and upper half of the face appear more prominent. This underdeveloped mandible is called micrognathia. The condition of overdevelopment of the jaws is called macrognathia.

Frequently when one sees an undeveloped maxilla (upper jaw) or mandible, the teeth appear to be unusually large, but this is because of a comparative relationship. There are instances when teeth are measurably larger than normal, and this is called macrodontia. The condition wherein teeth are measurably smaller than normal is called microdontia. The so-called peg lateral is an example of microdontia.

The teeth may present a variety of congenital abnormalities. Some examples follow.

Hypoplasia of the enamel is a condition wherein the enamel is poorly developed and the crowns of the teeth appear white and rough with an eroded surface. If calcification is disturbed only slightly, small white spots may appear. If the hypoplasia is more severe, the white spot will become infiltrated with a brownish stain, resulting in a condition called mottled enamel. If the disturbance is severe, pits or grooves in the enamel will be noted. These malformations are unsightly and result in the collection of debris, which makes it difficult to keep the area clean.

Poorly formed enamel is called amelogenesis imperfecta. Poorly formed dentin is called dentinogenesis imperfecta.

Gemination is a condition wherein the tooth bud in its developmental process divides and forms two crowns, usually with a single root. When two teeth grow together, the condition is known as fusion; the roots may or may not be joined. If two teeth are united by cementum only, the condition is called concresence. Excess amounts of cementum are known as hypercementosis.

When teeth are completely missing, the condition is called anodontia. This may be caused by a hereditary or developmental disturbance or may result when a tooth bud is inadvertently extracted with a tooth.

The condition known as dilaceration results from an injury to the developing tooth, which later calcifies in a bent position.

Enamel pearls are round, pearl-like enamel structures that usually are located on the roots of teeth.

Supernumerary, or extra, teeth are fairly common. They interfere with the ordinary growth and development of the normal teeth in their arches.

Hutchinson's teeth appear to be narrow, spaced apart, and notched in the center of the incisal surfaces. They are associated with congenital influences. The molars have a rough, pebbled occlusal surface and are often called mulberry molars.

Malocclusion, or the improper relationship between teeth, in the same arch or in opposite arches, may be a result of hereditary influences. Teeth, in order to function properly, have to come together in a prescribed manner. This requires proper alignment of the jaws with each other, and the arches must be in proper relationship with the skull. For example, a protruding upper arch results in the familiar "buck teeth." A prognathic jaw results in a protruding lower arch. Even individual teeth that are out of proper alignment constitute malocclusion. All dental examinations should include a study of bite relationship in the open and closed positions. Study models are of great assistance in studying and classifying occlusion.

There are hundreds of variations and abnormalities of the oral cavity. Adequate reference books kept readily at hand will be of great help to the dental hygienist as she attempts to become familiar with the more freuqently seen conditions. The patient can be helpful also. His answer to such questions as "Are you in good health?" or "How long have you been aware of this lump on your tongue?" can be valuable to the clinician in diagnosing the condition.

Trauma (physical injury)

Various abnormalities of the oral cavity will be related to trauma. Injury may have been received with or without the patient's awareness. In questioning the patient bring his attention to any possible traumatic abnormalities and ask whether he recalls having received any injury in this area.

Habitual cheek biting may produce a whitish raised area on the buccal mucosa, and the only clue to trauma might be that the white raised ridge follows the line of occlusion. Lip biting is a habit that has been known to produce severe sequelae (results).

Children frequently injure their oral structures and lips by biting themselves after a local anesthetic (Fig. 6-10). The wounds produced by teeth have been misdiagnosed and treated improperly. Gaping, open wounds produced by biting should be considered a serious matter, and patients should be encouraged to seek good care.

Fractured incisor teeth are among the most common examples of trauma. They are most likely to be seen in the dental

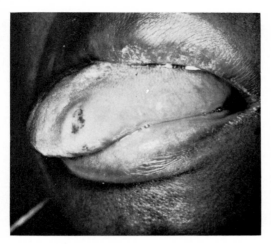

Fig. 6-10. Bite wound following local anesthesia. (Courtesy University of Tennessee College of Dentistry, Memphis, Tenn.)

office as an emergency problem. Careful diagnosis is in order, since the obvious crack of the fractured crown may be only a part of the entire problem. Since the pulpal horns of the central incisors extend toward the dentoenamel junction, it is possible that the pulp tissue is exposed, allowing contamination and subsequent infection. In such a case immediate cleansing and dressing of the wound or exposed pulp is indicated.

It is possible for a patient to have fractured teeth for a number of years without their function being impaired. Many teeth are literally split by exerting unnecessary biting force as might be used when cracking ice, nuts, or hard candy. As long as the pulps of these teeth do not become infected it is possible for the patient to be symptom free and often unaware of the condition.

Trauma of the gingiva. Examples of trauma may be seen in the gingiva. During mastication of food, lacerations of the gingiva and other soft tissues are sometimes inflicted by certain crunchy, hard, rough foods or by foreign bodies in food such as bits of eggshell. These mucosal

tears may be invisible to the naked eye; nevertheless, they are large enough to allow bacteria to invade and infect the tissue. Ordinarily bacteria lying on the surface of the mucous membrane and gingiva do not have an invasive power.

It may be noteworthy to consider the trauma to soft tissues that may be produced by toothbrushing. The design of the toothbrush and the technic of its use should be such as to prevent this injury.

It is also possible for undue trauma of the gingiva to result from the rubber cup used by the hygienist in performing dental prophylaxis. Instruments for scaling and curettage also may produce lacerations of the gingiva. These unwarranted insults to soft tissue are best prevented by demanding the highest degree of skill from the hygienist.

Postinjection complications as a result of needle trauma are unlikely; however, knowledge of recent injections made in the oral cavity is important, since the sites of needle injections may simulate pathological lesions.

Dentures may produce injury within the oral cavity. The combination of improperly seated dentures and tremendous masticatory forces may traumatize the gingiva and oral mucosa. It may be interesting to note that a person may exert biting pressure from 10 pounds up to 300 pounds per square inch. Injury from dentures also may occur when the patient is subjected to external trauma, such as results from altercations or auto accidents.

Trauma to temporomandibular joint. The temporomandibular joint is a frequent site of stiffness, soreness, and pain. This joint is formed by the condyle head of the mandible and the temporal bone of the skull. It is similar to other joints of the body and suffers the same reactions to such conditions as arthritis and trauma. Trauma to this joint usually manifests itself as pain in the joint or in the area of the ear, and it is common for patients with this symptom to seek advice from the ear, nose, and throat doctor, who will recognize readily the possibility of joint trauma and refer the patient to the dentist for assistance.

Patients subject this joint to a certain degree of trauma by persistent yawning, chewing in abnormal positions, and exerting unusual masticatory forces, as in taking large bites of very thick sandwiches. Similar stress to the joint might be incurred during certain extensive dental procedures that require the patient to hold the mouth in a wide-open position for long periods of time. This can be prevented by occasionally allowing the patient to close his mouth and rest the joint.

Other sources of trauma to this joint may be ill-fitting dentures, improper restorations, and clenching of teeth as a result of tension. Occasionally the joint will make noisy popping sounds. This is caused by physical irregularities of the condyle head or of the meniscus, the disk or membrane within the joint. Limited mandibular movements called trismus may be related to infections. The symptoms are soreness, stiffness, or muscle spasms.

Abnormalities produced by chemical and physical agents

The abnormalities that we have been discussing in general have been the result of accident or disease factors beyond our control. However, the chemical and physical agents we will be discussing in relation to their effects upon the structures of the oral cavity are almost completely under the control of the personnel of the dental office or of the patient who may be using them. There are several chemicals commonly found in the dental office that are escharotic (caustic) or produce injury to tissue. Silver nitrate, alcohol, phenol, eugenol, and trichloroacetic acid are a few examples.

Injuries from chemical and physical agents will, in many instances, mimic disease manifestations such as blisters, ulcers, white areas on pink mucosa, and red or raw bleeding surfaces. Mild irritation, as might be caused by alcohol, may produce redness of the soft tissues, called hyperemia (excessive blood accumulation). However, mild injuries from these agents do not always produce visible signs of damage.

Developing and fixing solutions from wet dental roentgenograms or their hangers may be accidentally introduced into the oral cavity and initiate tissue response. Even if the patient is unaware of injury, he will be displeased by the foul taste and odor of these chemicals.

When cold sterilization solutions are used that might be injurious to the tissues of the oral cavity, it is wise to rinse off this solution. This can be done with sterile water without interrupting the sterile chain.

In the dental office there are a number of ways patients can receive electrical burns in the oral cavity. In the event that electrical shock is incurred and the patient recoils from the unpleasant sensation, examination should be made to find any evidence of burns. Needless to say the equipment should be checked.

Caustics in the dental office should be kept in containers with labels that are clean and readily show the contents. Caustics should be used under careful supervision or in collaboration with other professional personnel. Neutralizing agents or antidotes for each chemical should be immediately at hand and well labeled, and their purpose should be kept well in mind.

When the more caustic agents such as phenol and silver nitrate are used, the antidote should be placed beside that agent for immediate access. For instance, in the event that phenol is accidentally placed on mucous membrane, a dilute solution of alcohol should be available for immediate application. By thoroughly washing the area with the alcohol solution the phenol is dissolved out. The affected

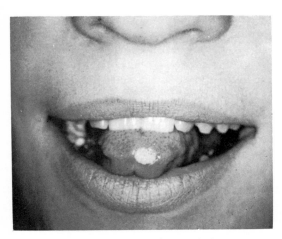

Fig. 6-11. Silver nitrate burn of the tongue. (Courtesy University of Tennessee College of Dentistry, Memphis, Tenn.)

surface then can be covered with a bland ointment. After chemicals have been allowed to do their damage very little benefit will be derived from application of their antidotes.

It is common practice for lay people to paint certain lesions of the oral cavity with silver nitrate. Since this is a strong caustic, further tissue damage may result from this practice, with little or no therapeutic value to the lesion and with the possibility of severe consequences. Cases of severe mucosal sloughing and of ulcers that will not heal have been attributed to silver nitrate burning of undiagnosed lesions (Fig. 6-11).

The mucous membranes of the oral cavity seem to demonstrate a high tolerance to heat. This may be shown by the fact that extremely hot foods are ingested and masticated that would be quite uncomfortable if they were placed on the hand or arm. It is thought that these mucous membranes gain this tolerance by conditioning.

During the process of taking impressions with wax or other impression compounds, injury to the tissues may be produced because of the high temperature of the fresh-

ly prepared materials and because these materials adhere closely to the tissues and must remain in place for several minutes to secure a sharp impression. The result may be redness, swelling, and even ulceration.

One interesting reaction to dental materials is the "tattooing" of the gingiva. This occurs when fine particles of amalgam are accidentally introduced into a fresh wound of the gingiva, as when a tooth receives an amalgam restoration, and the adjoining tooth is extracted. These particles are incorporated in the healing tissue, producing a tattooed effect.

Irritations of the mucous membranes are occasionally the result of allergic reaction to the materials in prosthetic appliances such as dentures. However, this is often incorrectly diagnosed, since the irritation is as likely to be caused by certain bacteria or fungus growing in the space between the denture and the tissue.

One patient with such a problem wore her dentures for several years with comfort. She then consulted her dentist with a rather sudden onset of discomfort, complaining of a burning sensation of her palate. The fit of the denture was found to be satisfactory, and the patient had not received any trauma to the oral cavity. However, the fungus that causes moniliasis, or thrush, was discovered on the denture and palate in large numbers. The fungous condition was treated, and the patient resumed wearing her original dentures. Since the area of irritation corresponded with the area covered by the denture, this could have been mistaken for allergic reaction to the denture.

Many chemical and physical injuries of the oral cavity are tolerated over long periods of time without symptoms. It is only when a secondary infection or a debilitating systemic condition occurs that painful symptoms appear in these areas.

Some people have the ability to adjust to dentures or to mild injuries, while others cannot tolerate even mild irritation. Since protein is essential for growth and repair of tissue, patients who do not obtain the daily protein requirements may be the first to notice a lessening of cellular maintenance and repair in areas where tissue is receiving even slight trauma. It has been found that patients who consistently demonstrate lack of proper protein metabolism show a severe retardation of tissue repair and regeneration.

At the present time there is overwhelming evidence relating the use of tobacco to gingival and mucosal abnormalities. These tissue changes may not demonstrate clear-cut and easily diagnosed conditions; therefore the dentist welcomes the assistance of the oral pathologist clinically and microscopically. The presence of heavy tobacco stains on a patient's teeth should alert the hygienist to continue her examination onto the gingiva and mucous membranes. Chronic use of tobacco may produce whitish plaques on the tissues or ulcerative areas. If such areas are discovered, they should be called to the attention of the dentist immediately.

Lesions and irritated mucous membranes from any cause must be viewed with concern. A patient may accept a postoperative complication as a normal consequence and fail to seek further care; therefore, it is wise to instruct the dental patient to "Let us know if you have any unusual troubles following your dental treatment."

SUGGESTED READINGS

Anderson, W. A. D.: Synopsis of pathology, ed. 6, St. Louis, 1971, The C. V. Mosby Co.

Burnett, G. W., and Scherp, H. W.: Oral microbiology and infectious disease, Baltimore, 1962, The Williams & Wilkins Co., chap. 25.

Kerr, D. A., Ash, M. M., Jr., and Millard, H. D.: Oral diagnosis, ed. 3, St. Louis, 1970, The C. V. Mosby Co.

Netter, F. H.: Digestive system: Part I. Upper digestive tract, Summit, N. J., 1959, The CIBA Collection of Medical Illustrations, pp. 104-136.

Orban, B., and Wentz, F. M.: Atlas of clinical pathology of the mucous membrane, ed. 2, St. Louis, 1960, The C. V. Mosby Co.

Shafer, W. G., Hine, M. K., and Levy, B. M.: A textbook of oral pathology, Philadelphia, 1963, W. B. Saunders Co.

Sicher, H., and Bhaskar, S. N., editors: Orban's oral histology and embryology, ed. 7, St. Louis, 1972, The C. V. Mosby Co.

United States Naval Dental School: Color atlas of oral pathology, Philadelphia, 1956, J. B. Lippincott Co.

chapter 7

PREVENTIVE DENTISTRY

Richard E. Jennings, D.D.S., M.S.D.

The dental profession has an obligation to maintain an adequate state of dental health. The dental hygienist is a recognized member of the dental health team, and one of the objectives of this chapter is to aid the hygienist toward an understanding of prevention and how it can be applied to a modern dental practice. The dental hygienist can and must fulfill her role in a preventive dental practice.

Fundamentally, there are two ways in which one can cope with any disease or health problem: treat it or prevent it. Most dental practices in the past have been oriented toward treating the damage resulting from disease, and little emphasis was placed upon efforts to prevent dental diseases from occurring. In a 1960 survey by the National Opinion Research Center of the University of Chicago, the majority of 757 dentists interviewed did not apply topical fluoride solutions to their patients' teeth, did not use a patient recall system, and did not use salivary tests to determine susceptibility to dental caries. The Survey of Dentistry,[1] impressed by the potentially overwhelming magnitude of the prevalence of dental disease in the United States, estimated in 1960 that the people in the United States had accumulated at least 700 million unfilled cavities. One out of every ten 5-year-old children had eight or more cavities. Advanced periodontal

disease affected half of our population by the age of 50 and almost everyone by age 65.

It would be totally impossible today to correct all damage that has been produced by dental disease in the United States. It is extremely doubtful that present dental manpower could ever cope with this amount of disease as long as the sole emphasis in practice is placed upon a reparative or restorative attitude. A continued increasing emphasis toward the prevention of these diseases offers hope for a future time when preventive technics will reduce the amount of dental disease to a manageable level. The dental hygienist can and must play a major role in a preventively oriented dental practice.

With a comprehensive consideration all procedures performed in a dental office are oriented toward prevention. The placement of a restoration in a tooth is preventive as well as reparative in that it is performed *to prevent* further damage to that tooth. A pulpally involved tooth is treated endodontically *to prevent* the subsequent development of periapical infection and loss of the tooth. The prosthetic replacement of a missing tooth is *to prevent* harmful and disease-producing drifting of teeth adjacent to the edentulous area. The removal of all the teeth in a patient with severe untreatable periodontal disease is to *prevent* potential harm to his health by systemic infection initiated orally, and the placement of complete dentures is *to prevent* any serious effects occurring functionally, nutritionally, or emotionally as a result of the lack of teeth. All dental procedures are *to prevent* something more serious after disease has occurred, but modern dentistry's concern is to place more emphasis upon all those procedures that can be effected *prior to* the occurrence of disease, thereby reducing the amount of reparative procedures needed.

The utilization of preventive practices has been arbitrarily divided into three distinct phases: primary, secondary, and tertiary. *Primary prevention* refers to those procedures applied prior to the inception of a disease. It perhaps could be aptly designated as "prepathogenic prevention." The goal of *secondary prevention* is to diagnose and stop a disease in its early stages so that damage and subsequent repair are minimized. Secondary prevention can also be considered "pathogenic prevention." *Tertiary prevention* refers to the utilization of restorative procedures in such a way *to prevent* any further damage from disease. Perhaps a label of "postpathogenic prevention" is suitable for this tertiary stage.

Fig. 7-1 illustrates this concept for prepathogenic, pathogenic, and postpathogenic stages of prevention during patient treatment. It is interesting to note that following the arrest of a disease process (pathogenic stage) and the repair of its damage (postpathogenic stage), the patient now has completed this circle and is in the "no disease" category. Prepathogenic (primary) prevention now becomes the major goal of treatment for this patient.

PREPATHOGENIC PREVENTION
Promotion of dental health

It is the responsibility of the dental health team to educate every patient in the importance of good oral health and the

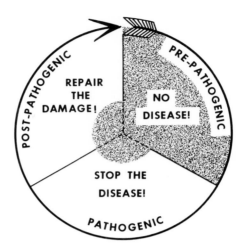

PATIENT TREATMENT

Fig. 7-1. (Courtesy University of Texas Dental Branch at Houston, Houston, Tex.)

methods available to obtain and maintain it. The dental hygienist has a unique opportunity in the dental office for patient education. Since practicing dentists must utilize most of their office hours in delivery of dental treatments, the dental hygienist becomes the main source of dental health information for the patient. Numerous articles helpful in patient education for prevention are available from such organizations as the American Dental Association and the American Society of Dentistry for Children. A dental office responsibility to disseminate dental health information outside the office also exists. National Children's Dental Health Week is a good example of a public information program that was initiated by dentists (A.D.A.) and is promoted each year by all local dental organizations. During this period of time, many dental hygienists and dentists are called upon to talk at schools or other special programs. Sponsoring newspaper articles, supplying speakers to service clubs and P.T.A. programs, and supporting science fair projects are also examples of dental health promotion at a community level.

Specific treatment procedures

Many specific treatment procedures to aid in the prevention of a disease before it occurs (prepathogenic prevention) are available today. Some of those more commonly used will be discussed.

Dental prophylaxis. Most patients today accept without question the routine dental prophylaxis as performed in the professional office. This is the procedure whereby the dental hygienist uses hand instruments (scalers) to remove calculus from the teeth and then "polishes" all surfaces of the teeth with a polishing compound. Dental plaque and surface stains are also removed during this scaling and polishing procedure so that the teeth are left clean and highly polished.

Since calculus develops and accumulates at different rates of speed in different patients, the decision regarding how often a patient's teeth need to be "cleaned" is determined individually. Immediately following the dental prophylaxis (scaling and polishing) is an ideal time to treat the teeth of caries-active patients with a topical fluoride solution.

Oral hygiene. Tooth decay affects over 95% of the population of the United States. Most people age 65 years and older suffer from advanced periodontal disease. These are rather startling statements when one considers that both diseases are produced by microorganisms that live on the teeth and that with thorough and complete oral hygiene procedures it is possible to remove them! The problem, of course, rests not only with our abilities or inabilities to teach correct oral hygiene procedures but also to motivate patients to practice these procedures faithfully. Motivation becomes a part of teaching.

Microorganisms live on the surfaces of the teeth in almost invisible colonies known as dental plaque. Arnim describes

dental plaque as "an adherent colonized microbial mass consisting of motile and non-motile bacteria, protozoa, leucocytes, desquamated epithelial cells all enveloped and permeated by a thick, viscous, serous exudate that helps hold these elements and their noxious end products in contact with the tooth and the gum."[*] Certain of these bacteria are capable of producing acids that will cause dental caries to occur on the tooth surface under the plaque and also toxic poisons that damage the gingival tissue and tooth-supporting membranes, causing periodontal disease. Removal of this dental plaque daily by every patient will greatly reduce, if not eliminate, both of these diseases. The dental hygienist's task then becomes one of teaching patients correct oral hygiene procedures in such a way as to motivate them to practice these procedures faithfully. Additional information about "home cleaning procedures" and about toothbrushes and dentifrices is also included in Chapter 8 and should be studied along with the information contained in this chapter.

Disclosing wafers. One past difficulty in motivating a patient to practice correct oral hygiene procedures rested in his inability to see dental plaque on his own teeth. Dentists and dental hygienists have for years applied chemical solutions (disclosing solutions) to a patient's teeth in the dental office to color the dental plaque and make it easy to see for removal during a dental prophylaxis. Only in recent years, however, have disclosing wafers become available for patient use at home. Refer to the section on p. 137 that describes these disclosing wafers and their use in prevention.

Toothbrushes. Details of construction for a toothbrush may vary, but it is generally agreed that it should have a straight

---

[*]Arnim, S. S.: Thoughts concerning cause, pathogenesis, treatment and prevention of periodontal disease, J. Periodont. **29**:217-223, 1958.

handle approximately 6 inches long, with a small in-line head not over 1 inch long. The bristles should be trimmed in a straight line, vary in stiffness from medium to soft, and be *round* and *smooth* on the end. Uneven and jagged bristles may scratch and injure the gingival tissue around the teeth as dental plaque growing on the tooth next to the gingival tissue is removed. The bristles of a toothbrush can be examined with a low-power microscope to determine whether the ends have been polished during manufacture.

Many technics have been described in the literature to ensure adequate tooth-brushing. Charles C. Bass, a physician teacher at the School of Medicine of Tulane University in New Orleans, designed and described a method of personal oral hygiene after years of concern with the causative factors of dental caries and periodontal disease. Bass' method of tooth cleansing utilized a brush with polished and round-ended bristles so that the ends of the bristles could be forced into the gingival crevices without damaging the soft tissue. He also recommended the use of dental floss (unwaxed) that consisted of many fine nylon threads twisted together.

With the use of a soft brush with round-ended bristles, the following technic (modified Bass) is recommended. When brushing the facial and lingual surfaces, the brush is placed against the junction of the tooth and the gingival tissue at approximately a 45-degree angle. Using firm pressure, a vibratory motion is started and the brush rotated so that the vibrating bristles move toward the occlusal surface of the teeth. This stroke should be repeated until the tooth surface is clean. By using a disclosing wafer after brushing, one can determine how many strokes are required. All the facial and lingual surfaces of all the teeth are cleaned in this manner. The occlusal, or chewing, surfaces can be cleaned with a forward and backward stroke, permitting the ends of the bristles to more or less "scrub" these surfaces. Regardless of the particular technic utilized, as long as the prime objective of removing dental plaque without damaging the teeth or soft tissues is achieved, the method should be satisfactory.

Electric toothbrushes. Electric tooth-brushes are becoming more popular each day. It should be emphasized that they can clean the teeth as well as a manual brush, but they offer no particular advantage to patients who develop a satisfactory hand-brushing technic. However, for some individuals, such as a child with cerebral palsy, who do not have the capability for manual dexterity, the electric brush has definite advantages. It may also have some appeal to people who are fascinated by "gadgets" and in this way serve as another motivational device.

Flossing. Even the most efficient tooth-brushing technic fails to remove all dental plaque from the surfaces of teeth adjacent to each other, since it is physically impossible for the bristles to reach deep into interproximal spaces. Unwaxed dental floss is supplementally used for oral hygiene to aid in removing dental plaque from approximating sides of the teeth beneath the contacting area. The floss is passed gently between the teeth and underneath the edge of the gingival tissue. While being held tightly against the proximal surface, it is pulled slowly toward the occlusal surface of the tooth. Both sides of every tooth should be cleaned in this manner with dental floss. Cleanliness is readily evidenced by a "squeaking sound" as the floss slides along the tooth surface.

It must be pointed out that the incorrect or careless use of floss may be harmful to the patient. It must be emphasized to patients that it be placed carefully and not moved in labiolingual directions in a "sawing fashion." *The correct use is exacting and must be taught thoroughly to patients.*

Mouthwashes and irrigators. Following the use of the toothbrush and dental floss, the mouth should be rinsed thoroughly to remove any loose dental plaque or food particles. A mouthful of tapwater should be satisfactory for this purpose. In special cases, the dentist may wish to recommend one of the irrigators available today. In recent years these devices have become increasingly popular, although the use of forced water irrigation to clean debris from subgingival spaces has been recommended for over 50 years. Irrigators may vary from simple hose and nozzle devices that fasten to a water faucet to relatively expensive electrical pump machines that pulsate water from a storage reservoir. All, however, have a small nozzle to permit the patient to direct the spray alongside and between the teeth to remove *loose* debris. Forced water irrigation is not suggested as a routine procedure for all patients but is valuable where mouthrinsing is not effective. Irrigators may help to rinse debris from under bridges, around fixed orthodontic appliances, or between the teeth of patients who have undergone periodontal surgery. Mouthwashes may be used for their pleasant taste although they should be considered as mechanical cleansers only.

Dentifrices. Regardless of the many claims made in dentifrice advertising, any dentifrice must still be considered principally as an aid in the toothbrushing procedure. The toothbrush bristles actually do the cleaning, but patients generally find the pleasant taste of dentifrices to their liking. Dentifrices are presumed to be effective in helping the brush to remove stains and to keep the mouth clean and pleasant tasting.

The use of a toothbrush and water alone will remove stains from some individuals' teeth. The addition of a mild abrasive, such as sodium bicarbonate, will be more effective. Most of the dentifrices on the market today contain some sort of abrasive, and ability to remove stain is thought to be related to the harshness of the abrasive used. The type of flavoring agent and detergent used will also affect the cleaning capability. For certain patients whose teeth are sensitive to hot or cold foods, a dentist may wish to recommend one of the desensitizing dentifrices available. In children and adults whose teeth are susceptible to dental caries, most dentists will recommend one of the fluoride dentifrices that has been approved by the American Dental Association.

Fluoride. Dentists learned many years ago that people who drank water containing fluoride compounds had much less tooth decay than those where the water contained no fluoride. The U. S. Public Health Service studied many communities where water did and did not contain this element and concluded that the presence of the fluoride ion during the tooth-forming years of children reduced tooth decay about 65%. Over 25 years ago, studies were undertaken in several large cities where fluoride was added to the drinking water. Control cities of approximately the same size and in the same area where water did not contain fluoride were also studied, and the results were conclusive that tooth decay could be reduced 60% to 65% by adding 1.0 p.p.m. of fluoride to a community's water supply. Since that time 4,834 communities with 80,096,860 residents have taken advantage of this prevention method. Adding the 8,378,824 people who use drinking water with fluoride naturally present, a total of 88,475,684 people now are receiving this benefit. Some 23% of the people in the United States live in areas without a central water supply where the addition of a fluoride supplement would be difficult.

Controlled fluoridation can be described as a conscious maintenance of the optimal concentration of fluoride in a water supply. This can be achieved by adding the chemicals to a water supply that is deficient of fluoride or by removing fluoride where the concentration is in excess of the optimal level. It is also possible to blend two different water supplies that contain natural fluoride to achieve the optimal concentration. The optimal concentration will vary from 0.7 p.p.m. to 1.2 p.p.m., depending upon the annual average of maximum daily air temperature in the community.

The fluoride ion combines chemically with the forming tooth structures to produce a tooth that is more decay resistant. Maximum benefits are received by the child who drinks this water throughout his tooth-forming years, but some benefits are thought to occur in adults (who did not drink fluoridated water as a child) from a topical effect of the water passing over the teeth. Community fluoridation programs have been described as "a classic example of a public health procedure since it serves the entire population, requires no conscious and sustained effort on the part of the individuals within the community and automatically restricts individual consumption of the fluoride supplement to levels which have been shown to be safe."*

Topical fluoride. Other ways have been sought to bring the benefits of fluoride to all people. In the late 1940's the use of topically applied fluoride-containing solutions was investigated. Since that time, it has been generally believed that the topical application of a fluoride solution at regular 6-month intervals can reduce tooth decay approximately 50%. The fluoride ion will form a loose chemical bond with the outer enamel layer. Over a period of time, however, the fluoride leaves the tooth. Because of this it is recommended that fluoride be reapplied at frequent intervals. Two fluoride solutions are commonly used today, and both require that the teeth be thoroughly cleaned just prior to application.

---

*Muhler, J. D.: Current evaluation of fluoride therapy, J. Amer. Pharm. Ass. NS3:133-135, 1963.

The cleaned teeth are isolated, dried, and kept free of saliva while the solution is painted on them. An 8% solution of stannous fluoride (SnF_2) applied for 30 seconds or a 2% solution of sodium fluoride buffered with phosphoric acid (A.P.F.) applied for a 4-minute period seem to be equally effective. Shannon[2-4] has recently reported a method using 2% stannous fluoride in a water-free prophylaxis paste for polishing the teeth, followed by a mouth rinse containing 0.5% stannous fluoride. In laboratory tests this seems to be as effective in combining with tooth enamel as the two previously mentioned topically applied solutions. The addition of fluoride compounds to polishing pastes and the development of self-applied fluoride pastes or solutions for daily patient use at home hold much promise for the future. Even though a patient is drinking fluoridated water, it has been demonstrated that the use of regularly applied topical fluoride is still of benefit.

Fluoride dentifrices. The Council on Dental Therapeutics of the American Dental Association granted approval a few years ago to a toothpaste manufacturer to use the following statement in advertising: " ——————— has been shown to be an effective decay-preventive dentifrice that can be of significant value when used in a conscientiously applied program of oral hygiene and regular professional care." The endorsement was granted after the review of research data from clinical trials of the dentifrice. The results indicated that this dentifrice imparted anticariogenic benefits to the patients in these study groups. Since that time, the same approval has been granted to four other dentifrices.

Fluoride prescriptions. Fluoride supplements have been suggested for the child who lives in an area where little or no fluoride is present in the drinking water. The suggested daily allowance for fluoride administration is 1.0 mg. for children 3 years of age and older. Between 2 and 3 years of age one half this dosage level is suggested. However, the procedure for fluoride supplement administration is not quite as simple as prescribing 1.0 mg. each day.

The dentist must be positive that the drinking water contains little or no fluoride. If this information is not available from the local health department or the state board of health, a sample of drinking water must be collected for fluoride analysis. Most city and state health departments are prepared to assist the dentist in this procedure. If it is found that the water contains at least 0.7 p.p.m. fluoride, supplemental fluoride is not recommended. If the drinking water contains from 0.2 to 0.6 p.p.m. fluoride, the amount prescribed must be adjusted accordingly to arrive at a maximum daily intake of 1.0 p.p.m.

Once a recommended daily level has been determined, the dentist must write a prescription. If the amount desired is exactly 1.0 mg. per day, any of the tablets that have been approved by the Council on Dental Therapeutics may be prescribed. However, if less than 1.0 mg. is desired, it is necessary to prescribe a liquid supplement. The parent is then instructed to add a specified number of drops of the solution to reach the desired dosage level. It is usually recommended that the tablet be dissolved in a glass of water or fruit juice for administration to the child. If drops are used, they are added to water or juice also.

For children under 2 years of age, no recommended daily dose level is suggested. A dentist may help this parent prepare water that contains fluoride at a concentration of 1.0 p.p.m. to use in making the formula or to use as the child's drinking water. Administration of dietary fluoride supplement must be consistent and continuous from birth until 12 to 14 years of age if presumed benefits are to be realized. Very few clinical studies are

available reporting the effectiveness of this method of fluoride administration.

Preparations containing sodium fluoride and vitamins in fixed combinations are *not* recommended by the Council on Dental Therapeutics. The effect of a fluoride-vitamin combination on dental caries has not been adequately studied. Also, any alteration of the amount of fluoride ingested to adjust it to the intake of fluoride from natural sources would also produce an alteration in the vitamin intake. It is not felt to be a logical method of administration for fluoride.

Caries susceptibility tests. Many dental offices are using tests to determine the state of current caries susceptibility for a particular patient in an attempt to predict future incidence of dental caries. The Snyder test is a colorimetric method for determining acids formed in a carbohydrate medium by oral microorganisms. It measures the quantity of oral microorganisms present in the patient's mouth capable of converting carbohydrates to acids. Since the number of these microorganisms increase in proportion to the frequency of eating freely fermentable carbohydrates, the test also becomes a valuable tool for monitoring a patient's diet.

The Snyder test as modified by Albans[5] makes it more practical for routine office use. The patient drools unstimulated saliva into a test tube containing Snyder's media. This test tube is then incubated (37° C.) for 4 days and daily observations made. The depth of color change from blue-green to yellow and the speed with which this occurs evaluates the ability of this saliva to produce acids. Other caries activity tests that have been suggested are the lactobacillus colony count, enamel solubility test, Wach test, and amylase test. Even though the degree of correlation of the results of these tests with the caries activity found in patients' mouths is not always reliable, many dentists are finding them use-

ful as a motivational tool in an office patient education program.

Dietary counseling. The knowledge that
dental health is greatly influenced by food
habits is generally well accepted today.
It is always a good health practice to encourage proper eating even though there is
no apparent deficiency that is causing
either general or dental disease.

Since new knowledge is not easily acquired with only one exposure, the dental
team is in a unique position for dietary
counseling in that patients are usually seen
in a series of appointments over a period
of time and information can be given at all
these appointments. A repetition of education exposures over a period of time
allows for greater assimilation of new
knowledge.

It is agreed that two facets of the diet
are important for good oral health: nutritional adequacy and frequency of sugar
ingestion. During the period of childhood
when the teeth are forming (birth to 12
to 14 years of age) an adequate diet is
necessary. This is true not only for the
teeth but for all other growth that is taking
place. A very good method for counseling
is to utilize the National Dairy Council's
Guide to Good Eating[7] in which all foods
are divided into four basic groups. It is
relatively simple to compare a patient's
food record with the recommended serv-
ings for these groups. A 5-day food record
can be kept by the patient and then evaluated for nutritional adequacy. Several studies using this approach have been reported
and it was found that less than 50% of all
the children studied were receiving a nutritionally adequate diet. In one of these
studies (in a high socioeconomic group)
only 13% of the children were found to be
eating a diet that could be considered
good.

Of particular interest to dental hygienists is the relationship of the refined carbohydrates (sugars) eaten and the amount of
tooth decay present in the mouth. A direct
relationship definitely exists between the
number of between-meal snacks containing sugars and the incidence of tooth decay. Since a person normally eats three
meals each day, this results in three exposures to refined carbohydrates and represents a certain amount of acid production in the dental plaque. If this same
individual "snacks" another three times
each day with a refined carbohydrate food,
the number of exposures has been doubled.
The repeated eating of foods containing
a high degree of refined carbohydrates
furnishes more material for dental plaque
to use and changes the microflora balance
of the mouth. As more of this food is eaten,
more of the microorganisms thought to be
involved in dental caries can be found.
The frequency of exposure is felt to be
more important than the total amount consumed in 1 day. The nature of the sugar-
containing food is also of importance. A
liquid form of sugar does not seem to
produce an increase of dental caries activity as readily as sugars that are combined with sticky or other highly reten-
tive food forms.

If the dental hygienist can aid patients
in selecting the foods necessary for a nutritionally adequate diet, there should be
less tendency for between-meal snacking.
For those patients who do snack between
meals, foods low in refined carbohydrate
content should be recommended.

Mouth protectors

Another facet of a dental practice frequently overlooked as a preventive element
is the recommendation to wear a mouth
protector for contact sports, since a very
serious and frequent problem in children
is the fracture of teeth during rough activity. Starting in 1962 the National Al-
liance Football Rules required that a player
wear a tooth and mouth protector. It is
interesting to note that during the first
year this rule was in effect, Texas high

school football players displayed a 48% reduction in dental injuries.

Three types of mouthguards are available for use: stock, mouth-formed, and custom-made. The stock guard fits all mouths and is held in place by keeping the jaws closed. The mouth-formed is fitted over the upper teeth directly in the mouth, whereas the custom-made is fabricated over a cast of the teeth made from a dentist's impression. Needless to say, the latter mouthguard is by far the most satisfactory. Many college and professional football players use mouth protectors routinely.

Pit and fissure sealants

Just recently new materials have been introduced to seal precarious pits and fissures. For many years methods have been suggested to treat those teeth that have deep fissures on the occlusal surface. These open pits or fissures occur most commonly in permanent and primary molars and result from an incomplete fusion of enamel during tooth development. Since it is impossible for the patient to adequately clean within these pits and fissures, dental plaque forms relatively undisturbed and dental caries begins soon after the teeth become exposed to the oral environment. The new method suggested is for application *prior* to the inception of dental caries. The pits and fissures are thoroughly cleaned and the tooth (or teeth) isolated. An acid is applied to the pits and fissures to decalcify and roughen the enamel surface. Following thorough rinsing and re-isolation, a plastic solution is applied and allowed to cure on the teeth. The excess plastic is removed by thorough polishing. The pit or fissure is now sealed and impervious to mouth fluids, bacteria, and debris, and thereby to dental plaque and subsequent dental caries. Although these materials have been studied in the laboratory, available clinical trials have been limited. The exact role that these fissure sealants will fulfill in a preventive program

for the practicing dentist is as yet undetermined.

PATHOGENIC PREVENTION

Pathogenic prevention (secondary prevention) is composed of those phases of prevention (Fig. 7-1) that are utilized during the early diagnosis and prompt arrest of a disease process. The concept of this stage is that since a disease already exists, the earlier the diagnosis can be made, the sooner treatment can be started. Early treatment in most situations will be more simple, expeditious, and satisfactory than if treatment is delayed.

The earlier a carious lesion is discovered, the smaller and simpler will be the restorative procedure necessary to replace the damaged tooth structure. Compare if you will the placement of a simple occlusal amalgam restoration in a first permanent molar with the placement of a full cast-gold crown on that same tooth. The amount of the tooth that has been destroyed by the caries process is the principal determinant of the type and size of the restoration placed.

Development of the x-ray machine and its subsequent refinements and newer technics for its use have been major aids in the early diagnosis of carious lesions. Routine and regular use of cavity-detecting (bitewing) x-rays is among the major tools in the dental office for prevention in the pathogenic phase.

It must be remembered that the treatment of dental caries goes much farther than just its discovery, removal of the damaged portion of the tooth, and its replacement by a restoration. Massler stated: "If the mouth harbors cariogenic flora, the most beautiful restorations will break down."* Dental caries must be treated as an infection as well as a restorative problem.

---

*Massler, M. M.: Changing concepts in pedodontic education, J. Dent. Child. 33:157-161, 1966.

Correct application of prepathogenic (primary) prevention is as important for the tooth with a restoration as for a tooth that has never suffered a caries attack. In cases of rampant dental caries, temporary anticariogenic restorations are placed (rather than permanent restorations) until such time that oral hygiene procedures and dietary changes have affected the oral environment to preclude the continuation of this rapid and severe caries attack upon the teeth. Another consideration of dental caries that should be stressed is the recommendation that all children receive their first dental examination *prior to* their third birthday. Most authorities will agree that the usual starting time for dental caries is during the second year of life. Again, early diagnosis and prompt treatment leads to the most simple and satisfactory result.

Recall appointment system. One of the more important preventive principles is to ensure that a patient visits a dental office regularly and routinely. Following the completion of any treatment necessary for a particular patient, it is good preventive policy to advise that patient when to return for another examination. The time interval should be determined individually and will vary according to the patient's needs. A recall system can vary from advising the patient when to return to actually scheduling the appointment months in advance. Some dental offices prefer to mail a reminding card or letter, yet others telephone the patient at the suggested time.

Procedures to be performed at the recall appointment will vary according to the patient's needs. A typical recall appointment may include a dental prophylaxis, topical fluoride treatment, and bite-wing radiographs for the patient susceptible to dental caries and periodontal disease. Personal oral hygiene practices can be evaluated and the previous teaching reinforced. Nutritional advice and other patient information procedures can also be reemphasized. The objectives of recall appointment are to reinforce patient information programs and to prevent disease. If disease already exists, early diagnosis may make the treatment more simple.

See p. 183 in Chapter 12 for a discussion of the methods by which recall systems can be developed by the dental hygienist.

Periodontal disease. Most cases of severe periodontal disease existed at some earlier time as a simple gingivitis. This could have been treated by a routine dental prophylaxis (scaling and polishing) and the institution of good personal oral hygiene procedures at home. Both office treatment and home care are the important treatment procedures that will prevent the continuation of damage to the periodontal tissues. Poor dental restorations and poor functional occlusion of the teeth can add to the severity of the disease. Again, early diagnosis and prompt treatment, followed by the development of good home preventive practices, can eliminate the continuing development of periodontal disease to a state of damage so severe it results in loss of the teeth.

Prevention of malocclusion. The prevention of malocclusion in child dental patients is a new and rapidly growing area of dental responsibility. As more is learned of the normal growth processes, dentists are better able to "intercept" a developing malocclusion by instituting some form of relatively simple correction and then maintaining this altered pattern until dental maturity. The most important area to consider is the maintenance of space for permanent teeth.

Many functions have been noted for primary teeth in a child's mouth. One is to preserve space in the dental arch for the permanent teeth that will replace the primary teeth. Premature loss of primary teeth plays a major role in the resultant lack of sufficient space for the permanent teeth. Space maintainers are used in the child's mouth to prevent unwanted migration and tipping of the adjacent teeth following premature loss of the primary molars. With few exceptions, the early removal of a primary tooth requires that space maintenance procedures be instituted.

Another important area for preventive orthodontic treatment is the diagnosis and early treatment of a functional disorder in a child's mouth. Most commonly this is manifested as either an anterior crossbite, a posterior crossbite, or sometimes a combination of both. The etiological factors that may produce this malposition of the mandible during occlusion are many and varied. Among the known factors are deficiencies in proper exfoliation of the primary teeth or abnormal eruption patterns of the permanent teeth, both of which may result in occlusal interference. The child will then "shift" his mandible forward or sideways to achieve a comfortable occlusal position. Differential diagnosis must confirm that it is truly a functional malocclusion and not a skeletal growth problem. Once the functional diagnosis is confirmed, treatment should be instituted promptly, since these malocclusions are seldom self-correcting.

Many malocclusions cannot be prevented. Most notable are the abnormal skeletal growth patterns (Class II and III malocclusions) or those cases where a discrepancy exists in the size of the permanent teeth (arch size, tooth mass discrepancy). Careful use of those diagnostic aids available to dentistry today must be utilized by the dentist in general practice, in determining which cases he can treat and which should be referred to the orthodontist. A set of well-trimmed study casts is an important diagnostic aid in the analysis of a patient's occlusion.

Examination and history. It has been said many times that the mouth is the mirror of systemic health and disease. A major part of prevention is early tentative diagnosis by a dentist of local and systemic diseases discovered by a careful and thorough examination of the soft tissues of the mouth and surrounding areas. Adding a well-taken history to this clinical examination, a dentist may uncover the beginning symptoms of many different systemic illnesses. Prompt referral to a physician may contribute to early and life-saving treatment.

Early detection and prevention are the most effective weapons for combating oral malignancies. It is the dentist who bears the principal responsibility for this early detection, since he is working constantly in the oral cavity and is familiar with normality and abnormality of the soft tissues in the mouth. In its early stages oral cancer does not exhibit pain, swelling, or bleeding. The American Cancer Society feels that the dentist's role is crucial in discovering the lesions early so that prompt treatment can be effected. In some countries of the world, oral cancers represent as much as 47% of all cancers, but in the United States oral lesions comprise approximately 6% of all cancers. At the present time 14,500 cases of oral cancer are diagnosed annually. Of these 38% will show a 5-year survival rate. The earlier the diagnosis and treatment, the higher the incidence rate of survival will be.

The exfoliative cytological smear (Papanicolaou test) may be used as a screening test for oral lesions. If a suspicion of oral cancer is present, microscopic examination of a biopsy section of tissue is mandatory.

Other diseases display symptoms in the mouth that can be detected during an oral examination. The oral findings in congenital syphilis may be the only clinical signs of the disease in a child. The permanent incisors may look like screwdrivers and be notched on the biting edge. These are known as Hutchison's incisors and result from a hypoplastic defect during an acute infection period shortly after birth. The first permanent molars may also be affected and are described as mulberry molars. Acquired syphilis displays a variety of signs in the mouth. The lower lip and tongue are frequent sites of syphilitic chancres. In the secondary stage of syphilis, mucous patches are seen in the mouth. If untreated tertiary syphilis is present, gummas are commonly seen in the oral cavity. Perforation of the hard palate, resulting in a communication between the oral and nasal cavities, may result from a gumma.

All the common forms of the blood dyscrasia diseases have definite oral signs and symptoms and, in most cases, a careful oral examination and adequate history will result in early detection. Icterus (jaundice) signs in the oral mucosa are common early diagnostic findings in sickle cell anemia. Osteoporosis, osteosclerosis, and a ladder arrangement of interseptal bone can also be seen on dental radiographs. Enlargement of gingival tissue with edema and hemorrhage is an early sign of leukemia. A smooth, red, and painful tongue may be indicative of pernicious anemia. Spontaneous bleeding from the gingiva is common in thrombocytopenic purpura.

Diabetes mellitus is yet another disease with definite oral signs. Dryness of the mouth, coupled with intense thirst and a sweet smell to the breath, are typical signs. The lack of protective secretions that produce the dry mouth lend a greater susceptibility of the soft tissue to local irritants. Periodontal abscesses and putrescent exudates occur more frequently in diabetic patients with periodontal disease than in nondiabetic persons. Marked destruction of the tooth-supporting alveolar bone may result in extreme loosening of the teeth.

If bone destruction in the maxilla or mandible in a "punched-out" pattern is discovered in a routine dental x-ray examination this may be the first clinical sign of one of the reticuloendothelial diseases.

Gaucher's disease also displays large destructive bony lesions on dental x-rays.

Even though the dental office is planned to facilitate the diagnosis and treatment of diseases of the oral cavity, the dental hygienist is a member of the total dental health team. History and examination of all patients must include a consideration of diseases other than those just occurring in the mouth. As Hine has so aptly stated: "Failure to locate a small area of dental caries may result in the loss of a tooth, but failure to locate a small cancer may result in the death of a patient."

POSTPATHOGENIC PREVENTION

The postpathogenic concept of prevention occurs during the restoration of the damaged portions of the teeth, dental arches, or mouth in such a way that function of these structures is maintained in a healthy manner. This process can be as simple as the occlusal amalgam restoration of one tooth or as complicated a procedure as placing immediate complete dentures.

The term *iatrogenesis* should be introduced here. Iatrogenesis is defined literally as "generated by a physician." It can be interpreted dentally as the use of poorly executed reparative procedures so that they themselves are capable of producing disease. All restorative dental procedures in this postpathogenic stage of patient treatment must be performed with the prevention of future disease in mind. A proximal amalgam restoration that is not extended sufficiently into self-cleansing areas will be more susceptible to recurrent caries. An overextended denture flange will produce a sore spot and ulcer of the soft tissue.

Prevention of future dental disease must be foremost in mind when restorative procedures are being performed. It is again noted that following the postpathogenic stage of patient treatment (Fig. 7-1) the patient has returned to the prepathogenic stage. All tissues are now healthy and primary prevention is again of first importance.

SUMMARY

Prevention utilization in a dental practice is principally a philosophy of the method of approach to the treatment of dental disease. In the past the dental practitioner waited until a disease was clinically visible and then concentrated his effort to correcting the damage that had occurred. However, since it is possible today to prevent most of the common dental diseases, a preventive concept must be used in a modern dental practice.

Patient education programs explaining the causes of dental caries, periodontal diseases, and malocclusion can be conducted by the entire dental health team, including the dental hygienist. These may be formal programs in the dental office that utilize audiovisual aids or casual conversations while treating patients in the dental chair. Dietary counseling and oral hygiene teaching may be performed by the dental hygienist. Most dental offices today perform prepathogenic procedures, and the dental hygienist has primary responsibilities in this area.

Prevention during the pathogenic stage depends upon early diagnosis of an existent disease. An efficiently functioning recall system with the routine use of bitewing x-rays is a major factor in early interception of carious lesions and periodontal disease. Proper home oral hygiene procedures and dietary counseling can be re-emphasized at these visits. In this way, damage correction is accomplished rapidly and with the greatest ease to both the dental office and the patient. Treatment procedures today are so easily and satisfactorily accomplished for the patient that an ever-increasing amount of time can be spent in patient education procedures, urging both the use of all prevention practices that are known today and dental visits often and early to minimized disease development.

REFERENCES

1. American Council on Education: Commission on the Survey of Dentistry in the United States, The survey of dentistry, the final report, B. S. Hollinshead, Director, Washington, D. C., 1961, American Council on Education.
2. Shannon, I. L.: Water free solutions of stannous fluoride and their incorporation into a gel for topical application, Caries Res. 3(4):339-347, 1969.
3. Shannon, I. L.: Preventive dental services in Veterans Administration hospitals, J. Public Health Dent. 30:156-162, 1970.
4. Shannon, I. L.: A pumice zirconium silicate prophylaxis paste containing 2% stannous fluoride in water free solution, J. Pharmacol. Ther. Dent. 1:24-30, 1970.
5. Albans, A.: An improved Snyder's test, J. Dent. Res. 49:64, 1970.
6. National Dairy Council, Chicago, Illinois.

SUGGESTED READINGS

American Dental Association: Teeth, health and appearance, Chicago, 1957, The Association.
Arnim, S. S., Diercks, C. C., and Pearson, E. A.: What you need to know and do to prevent dental caries (tooth decay) and periodontal disease (pyorrhea), J. N. Carolina Dent. Soc. 46:296-305, 1963.
Bass, C. C.: An effective method of personal oral hygiene, J. Louisiana Med. Soc. 106:100, 1954.
Blayney, J. R., and Hill, I. N.: Fluorine and dental caries, J.A.D.A. 74:234-301, 1967.
Bohannon, H. M.: Oral physiotherapy. In Goldman, H. M., and Cohen, D. W.: Periodontal therapy, ed. 4, St. Louis, 1968, The C. V. Mosby Co., p. 446.
Cartwright, H. V., Lindahl, R. L., and Bawden, J. W.: Clinical findings on the effectiveness of stannous fluoride and acid phosphate fluoride as caries reducing agents in children, J. Dent. Child. 35:36-40, 1968.
Culpepper, R. T., and Jennings, R. E.: Extradietary fluoride, Texas J. Med. 60:482-485, 1964.
Leavell, H. R., and Clark, E. G.: Preventive medicine for the doctor in his community, ed. 2, New York, 1958, McGraw-Hill Book Company.
McClure, F. J.: Fluoride drinking waters a selection of Public Health Service papers on dental fluorosis and dental caries; physiological effects, education, and welfare, Bethesda, Md., 1962, Public Health Service, National Institute on Dental Research.
Muhler, J. C.: Current evaluation of fluoride therapy, J. Amer. Pharm. Assoc. NS3:133-135, 1963.

STUDY QUESTIONS

1. A water fluoridation program produces maximum benefits for a child born and reared in this environment. Why?
2. Would you recommend the application of a topical fluoride solution to the teeth of a child living in a city with an optimal fluoride level in the drinking water? Why?
3. What would you suggest is the most important fact to know prior to the prescribing of a fluoride supplement for a child?
4. Would a fluoride tablet be prescribed for an adult? Why?
5. Discuss the possible uses of disclosing wafers (solutions) in a dental office during patient treatment and also in the patient's home.
6. You live in a community with 0.5 p.p.m. of fluoride in the drinking water. How would you answer the parent's question regarding possible benefits from using a fluoride-vitamin combination for her 3-year-old child?
7. Would you recommend an electric toothbrush for a cerebral-palsied child? Why?
8. How can you readily determine the shapes of the ends of the bristles in a toothbrush?
9. Describe the shape and size of the recommended toothbrush.
10. Unwaxed dental floss is a valuable adjunct to the toothbrush for the removal of dental plaque. Why must the technic for its use be carefully taught?

chapter 8

ORAL PROPHYLAXIS

Sam W. Hoskins, Jr., D.D.S., M.S.D.

Although in its broad application oral prophylaxis may encompass all of the treatment procedures directed toward the prevention of dental disease, its use in this chapter will be confined to those specific procedures directed at the removal of soft and hard deposits and the smoothing and polishing of the tooth surfaces. The patient's role in the prevention of dental disease as it applies to mouth care technics and procedures will be discussed and the proper technics described. Detailed information as to sterilization technics will be found in Chapter 15.

ROLE OF BACTERIA IN DENTAL DISEASE

In recent years epidemiological studies have focused attention upon the role of bacterial plaque and the bacterial content of the gingival sulcus as the primary etiological factors in tooth decay and periodontal disease. Mineralization of the bacterial masses and dental plaque to form calculus creates a secondary irritant that becomes an important etiological agent in the progression of periodontal disease.

In tooth decay, it is the presence of the bacteria in the plaque retained in close contact with the tooth surface that initiates the caries process by acting upon sugar-containing foods to produce the acid substance that decalcifies the tooth. In periodontal disease, it is the bacteria in the soft plaque deposit and on that surface (ad-

jacent to the soft tissue) of the hard mineralized calculus deposit, as well as the bacteria found in the gingival sulcus or pocket, that are the initiating factors. Toxins and enzymes produced by the bacterial activity initially affect the soft tissues of the attachment apparatus of the tooth. The supporting tissues, the periodontal ligament, bone, and cementum, become involved with extension of the infection.

The bacteria in the portion of the mineralized deposit immediately adjacent to the tooth surface do not produce acids, toxins, or enzymes and are not directly involved in the disease process. The mineralized calculus does act to some degree as a physical irritant, but this is of much less significance than the bacterial irritants present on its uncalcified surface.

It is primarily the responsibility of the patient, through daily oral hygiene efforts, to remove soft deposits from the teeth and the gingival sulcus area. However, the hygienist will usually find that soft deposits are present in the average mouth, and they should be thoroughly removed as a part of the prophylaxis procedure.

OBJECTIVES OF ORAL PROPHYLAXIS

The technical objectives of effective oral prophylaxis can be considered to be:
1. Removal of soft deposits from the teeth and gingival sulcus area
2. Removal of hard deposits from the teeth

3. Smoothing rough or irregular areas of the teeth
4. Removal of stain from the teeth
5. Polishing the tooth surfaces to make them less susceptible to plaque and stain accumulation and to facilitate the patient's oral hygiene efforts

Stains on the crowns of the teeth or in the plaque or calculus itself (extrinsic stains) affect the teeth primarily from the cosmetic viewpoint. Stain in itself does no damage to the tooth nor does it contribute to the periodontal lesion. These extrinsic stains are readily removed by routine prophylaxis procedures. Those intrinsic stains that occur within the tooth substance cannot be removed by routine prophylaxis approaches.

INSTRUMENTS FOR ORAL PROPHYLAXIS

Although hand instrumentation provides the basic oral prophylaxis armamentarium, there are additional mechanical instruments that can be used. The most commonly used and the most effective of these are any one of several designs of an ultrasonic scaler, which utilizes high-frequency vibrations in the range of 25,000 microscopically small strokes per second in a total range of approximately 0.001 inch. (See Fig. 17-34.) These instruments provide a water spray that acts as a coolant and creates a flushing action to remove dislodged debris from the operative field. The flushing action of the spray provides some cleansing and stimulation to the gingival tissues, but it does create a visualization problem. The tip of the instrument, which for scaling and stain removal is rounded and blunt, is used in a light paintbrush stroke and "vibrates" both calculus and stains from the tooth surface (Fig. 8-1). Primarily an instrument for the removal of gross calculus, it is less effec-

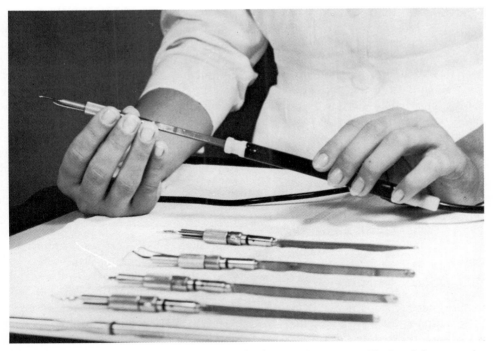

Fig. 8-1. Assembling one of the high-speed vibrating instruments (Cavitron) for removing calculus. (Courtesy University of Tennessee College of Dentistry, Memphis, Tenn.)

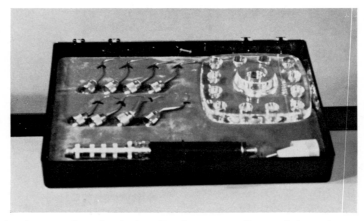

Fig. 8-2. Another set of mechanical scaling instruments (Dynocaire) can be attached to the control unit that drives the dentist's ultrahigh-speed turbine handpiece. (Courtesy University of Tennessee College of Dentistry, Memphis, Tenn.)

tive for root smoothing or polishing operations.

Another type of instrument, the Dynocaire, which depends upon vibrations created by the attachment of a special handpiece and tips to the ultra high–speed dental turbine handpiece, also provides a water spray as a coolant and flush (Fig. 8-2).

Both of these vibration instruments provide some advantage to the patient, since less forceful instrumentation is required, and to the therapist, particularly in terms of less fatiguing instrumentation. However, neither of the instruments is as effective in the removal of subgingival calculus or in root planing procedures as the conventional hand instruments. Use of a vibration type instrument for the initial debridement actions and finishing with hand instrumentation offers a practical combination.

Hand instruments

There are many groups of hand instruments with apparently wide differences in design that are utilized in scaling procedures. However, the differences in instruments are not so great as might be expected considering the number. Since the procedure of scaling is basically a scraping action, all instruments are designed to accomplish this purpose. Scalers fall into broad categories of chisels, hoes, sickles, curettes, and files.

Instruments can be designed to be used with either a pull or push stroke. The basic and most frequently used instruments are designed to be used as pull instruments. It is important in the procedures of scaling to avoid forcing calculus particles or root surface shavings into the gingival or periodontal tissues. When push type instruments that tend to do this are used, copious irrigation by means of a washed field technic can be employed to reduce the possibility.

Probably the simplest form of a scaler is the *chisel* (Fig. 8-3). Usually with a right-angle blade edge, it is used with a push stroke to split or flake off calculus. It may be used effectively in the mandibular anterior segment to pass horizontally through the interproximal embrasure in a facial (labial or buccal) to lingual direction (Fig. 8-4). Modifications of the basic chisel design have been made for utilization in an apical direction; however, they

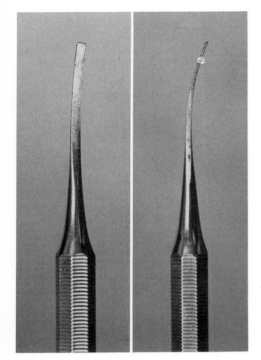

Fig. 8-3. Working surfaces of a chisel type scaler (Darby-Perry).

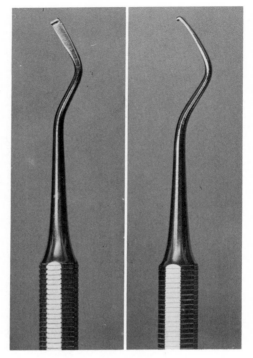

Fig. 8-5. Working surfaces of a hoe type scaler (McCall).

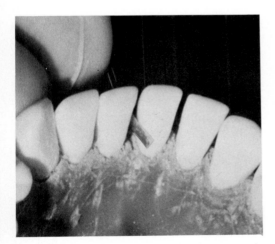

Fig. 8-4. Application of a chisel type scaler (Darby-Perry) to the interproximal space of the lower anterior teeth. Note the adaptation of the curve of the blade to the tooth surface.

are difficult to use properly and offer little advantage over more versatile instruments.

The *hoe* is similar in its method of action to the chisel except that it is used as a pull instrument (Fig. 8-5). It splits or crushes the calculus mass but has a limitation in that it tends to gouge root surfaces unless the blade is well seated against the tooth.

The *file* functions like the hoe in that it is in reality a series of fine hoe blades and is used with a pull stroke (Fig. 8-6). Because it is usually designed as a small flat instrument, it is more versatile than the hoe since it can be used more effectively subgingivally. Because of its small size it is particularly valuable in constricted areas. The file is extremely difficult to sharpen.

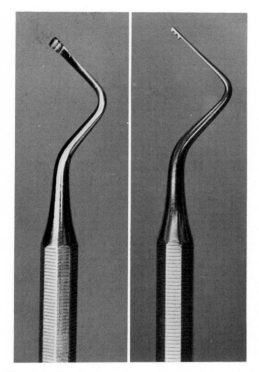

Fig. 8-6. Working surfaces of a file (Schraeder).

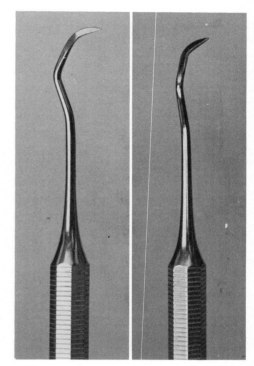

Fig. 8-7. Working surfaces of a sickle scaler (Jaquette).

The *sickle* is probably the fundamental scaler design (Fig. 8-7). A hook-shaped instrument, its primary use is for supragingival application; however, small and fine designs of the instrument can be effective subgingivally. The sickle is most frequently triangular in cross section and designed for use with a pull stroke. Some versions may be rectangular so that there are actually four cutting edges, and this instrument can be used with either a push or pull stroke. The blade tip usually is pointed, which permits the instrument to be used interproximally as well as on the facial and lingual surfaces. The sharp point restricts its use subgingivally, where damage to both soft tissue and tooth surface can easily result.

Of all the instruments designed for scaling, the *curette* is the most effective for both supragingival and subgingival appli-

cations (Fig. 8-8). The instrument is basically spoon shaped with two cutting edges along the elongated spoon edge. It may be designed as either a pull or push instrument, but it is most versatile when used with the pull stroke. By variation in instrument size, the curette (or curet) can be designed to remove heavy supragingival deposits or to smooth and plane root surfaces subgingivally in areas of difficult access.

Instrument design

Regardless of the type of instrument or of the variations in design, each instrument is composed of (1) a handle or shaft, (2) a shank that connects the handle to the working area and permits various angulations of the working area to the handle, and (3) the working area, which includes the cutting edge and point (Fig. 8-9).

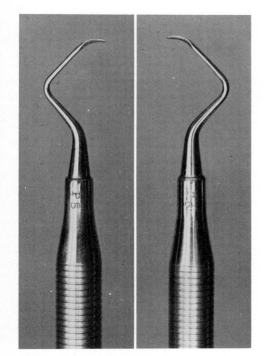

Fig. 8-8. Working surfaces of a curette (Gracey).

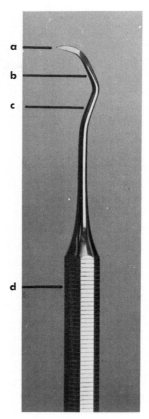

Fig. 8-9. Parts of a scaler: *a*, point of working surface; *b*, shank; *c*, lateral bend; *d*, handle.

Basic requirements of all instruments include: (1) a suitable design for the specific anatomical areas of proposed use, (2) a size to permit use in the constricted mouth areas but rigid enough to convey tactile sense to the user, (3) a handle design that is easy to grasp and comfortable in use, and (4) a working area of good quality metal that can be quickly and easily sharpened and that maintains a cutting edge as long as possible. Instruments can be designed with single end or double end working areas. The obvious advantage of two different working points on a single handle is a reduction in the number of instruments in use and the convenience of manipulation of a single instrument rather than having to repeatedly put down and pick up separate instruments. The double-end instruments require care in use to avoid injury to the user or the patient, but

this is true of any instrument. A slight cost saving is also realized when double-end instruments are used.

The instrument *handle* should be of adequate length for proper reach, approximately 100 to 130 mm. It should be light in weight to avoid tiring of the hand of the user; hollow handle designs to reduce weight are frequently used. It should be large enough in diameter (6 to 8 mm.) so that it can be held without strong finger pressure and so that it will not rotate in the hand in use. An instrument that is octagonal or round in shape and that has a knurled or roughened surface provides for a more positive grasp and is easier to manipulate.

The shank should taper from its junction with the handle to the working area. The different bends or angulations produced in the shank provide for versatility in access for the instrument. Regardless of the angulation produced in the shank, the working area of the instruments should be in line with the long axis of the handle and the cutting edge of the instrument presented parallel to the long axis of the tooth where it is to be employed.

At the working area, the size and shape of the blade are the determining factors in where the instrument can be used. Large bulky instruments or those with excessively sharp points cannot be used in subgingival areas.

The curette can be designed to provide the most optimum compromise instrument that can be used both supragingivally and subgingivally. Since it is advisable to reduce the number of instruments required, both from the viewpoint of speed and ease of manipulation and of cost, the use of a minimum number of double-end instruments seems to be the most practical approach to the total instrument requirement. This does not preclude the use of single-end instruments nor is it the intention to condemn any instrument because it may have limitations in its use in the hands of some therapists. Individual preferences and habits will be the determining factors in which instrument a given therapist employs and by its careful and skillful use attains the desired objective.

Minimum instrument set

A minimum set of instruments effective in both supragingival and subgingival scalings can consist of the Goldman-Fox Nos. 1 to 4 (Fig. 8-10). The No. 21 may be substituted for the No. 1 to provide a smaller sickle instrument or may be added to the set (Fig. 8-11). These five double-end instruments provide four sickle working points of various size and three pairs of curettes. The curettes are heavy enough

to function well supragingivally but are still small enough to be used in subgingival applications.

The No. 1 has a small straight sickle blade at right angles to the instrument shaft at one end; the other end has an offset in the shank with a similar working blade. The No. 21 is a smaller sickle blade with a straight shank at both ends. These blades are small enough to be used in constricted areas, but because the working blade is a pointed sickle, it is used primarily in supragingival procedures.

The No. 2 is a curette primarily intended for use on incisors, canines, and premolars.

The No. 3 curette has an increased contra-angle of the shank that permits its use for both premolars and molars. The No. 4 has an additional bend of the shank that provides for increased access in difficult areas.

Many other excellent designs of instruments are available and may be required in specific instances for access and manipulation in some mouths and in some specific therapeutic approaches (Fig. 8-12).

Explorers are useful in locating calculus deposits subgingivally and in determining defects in tooth surfaces. They are also useful in the final evaluation of the tooth surface to determine whether all calculus deposits have been removed (Fig. 8-13). A periodontal probe can also be used to locate calculus deposits as well as to determine the extent of sulcus or pocket depth (Fig. 8-14).

Instrument utilization

Although careful design and variation in instument size and shape improve the function of the instrument as a tool, it is not the instrument that accomplishes the objective but the skillful use of the instrument by the therapist. Knowledge of the objective to be attained and of the anatomy of the teeth and surrounding structures and the skillful application of the instrument

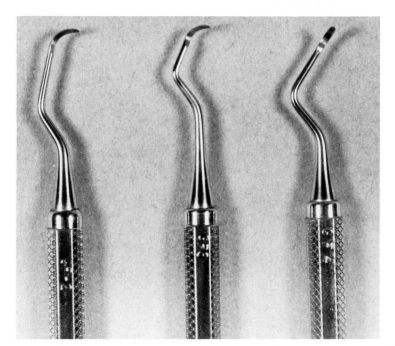

Fig. 8-10. Goldman-Fox curettes Nos. 2, 3, and 4. These are double-end instruments with a right contra-angle at one end and a left contra-angle at the other. They are fine enough to be used subgingivally and yet have adequate strength for removal of heavy supragingival deposits.

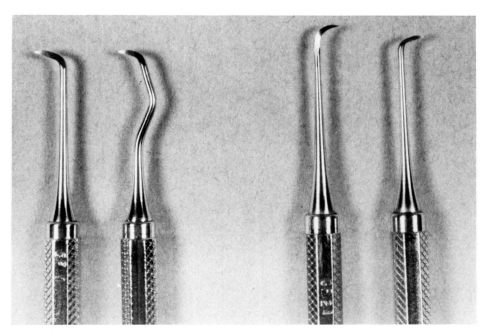

Fig. 8-11. Both ends of the double end Goldman-Fox No. 1 *(left)* and the No. 21 *(right)* are shown in this view. The No. 21 is a smaller and more delicate instrument and can be used with either a vertical or circumferential stroke.

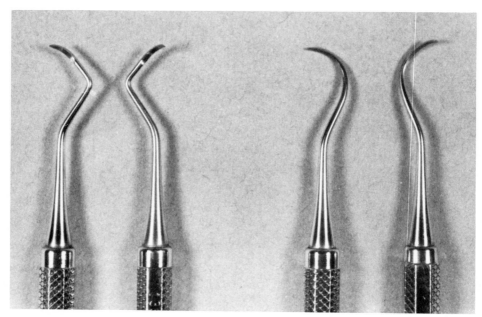

Fig. 8-12. Paired McCall 13S-14S and 17S-18S curettes. These excellent and versatile instruments can be used for both supragingival and subgingival procedures.

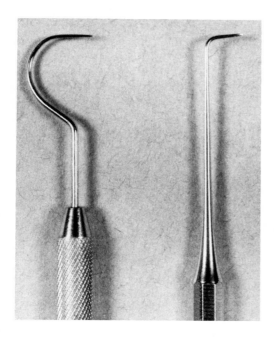

Fig. 8-13. The No. 21 explorer *(left)* and the No. 6 *(right)* are useful instruments to determine the presence or absence of subgingival calculus and of tooth surface defects.

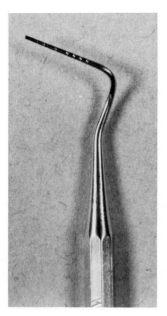

Fig. 8-14. The calibrated periodontal probe is used to measure sulcus or pocket depth and can be used to determine the presence or absence of subgingival calculus deposits. This Williams probe has calibrations at 1, 2, 3, 5, 7, 8, 9, and 10 mm. The absence of the calibration at the 4- and 6-mm. points makes for ease of reading of the markings.

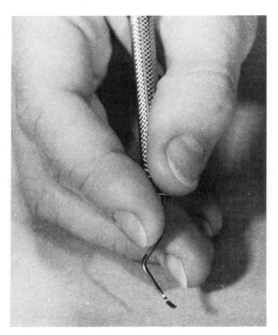

Fig. 8-15. True pen grasp. Note that the instrument rests on the middle finger and that the primary grasp is provided by the thumb and first finger.

are fundamentals for effective scaling procedures that must be mastered by the dental hygiene student.

Skillful utilization of instruments requires both control and stability of the instrument as well as the proper application of the instrument stroke. This means both effective grasp of the instrument and establishment of a firm fulcrum or finger rest.

Instrument grasp. The two basic instrument grasps used in dental practice have been described as the pen grasp and the palm grasp. Although the palm grasp is useful in some dental technics, it is not frequently utilized in scaling procedures.

The pen grasp is frequently misunderstood. Actually there are two methods of pen grasp, one of which should probably best be described as a modified pen grasp. In the true pen grasp the tips of the thumb and forefinger contact the shaft of the instrument. The middle finger lies alongside or under the instruments and may be utilized as a fulcrum or rest. This positioning gives maximum flexibility in instrument manipulation but may not provide the tactile sense desired (Fig. 8-15). In the modified pen grasp, the tips of the thumb, forefinger, and middle finger all contact the shaft of the instrument. This grasp may provide slightly less instrument maneuverability but increases the tactile sense of the therapist (Figs. 8-16 and 8-17). Both pen grasp methods have logical application in the scaling procedures. Most therapists find that they move from one grasp to the other to meet the demands of exploration or power stroking and the availability of finger rest areas.

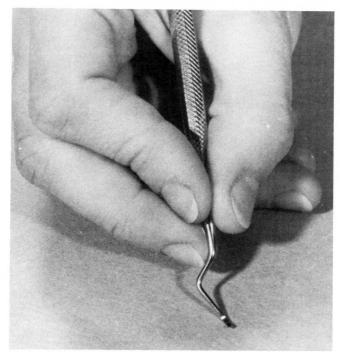

Fig. 8-16. Modified pen grasp. The ball of the middle finger contacts the shank of the instrument and provides both grasp and support. The middle finger may be used as the fulcrum finger with this grasp, or other fingers may provide the rest.

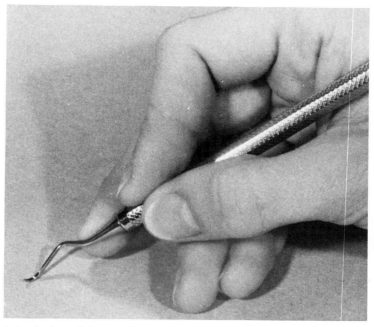

Fig. 8-17. Lateral view of the modified pen grasp showing the position of the ball area of the middle finger on the shank of the instrument.

When the palm grasp is used the instrument is cupped in the palm and held by the four fingers with the thumb serving as the fulcrum point.

Fulcrum or finger rest. The finger rest provides the stable base from which instrument activation is controlled. Where possible the rest should be on a firm tooth or teeth, generally as close as possible to the area of operation. Ideally the rest should be in the same arch as the point of instrumentation. Frequently, however, because of missing teeth or areas of particularly difficult access, it may be necessary to use the patient's chin, cheeks, or other soft tissue area as the rest area. Fingers of the therapist's free hand may be used to bridge from areas of the patient's teeth or other areas to increase the stability of the rest position.

Regardless of the actual site of the rest, the objective should be to establish and maintain as much control over instrument application as possible.

In the pen and modified pen grasp, at times the middle finger may provide the only finger rest or may be supported by the ring and little finger, or the ring and little finger alone may provide the rest. The actual fingers utilized will be determined by tooth position, size, and shape of the mouth and the location of the rest point.

Instrument stroke. The application of the scaling instrument uses two basic strokes. One, an exploratory stroke, is used to locate and define the size and outline of the deposit. This stroke requires the maximum tactile sense. The instrument is lightly grasped, usually in the modified pen grasp.

The actual working stroke, or power stroke, of the instrument requires a firm finger rest and may utilize either the true or the modified pen grasp, depending upon the preference of the therapist and the location of the finger rest or fulcrum in relation to the site of instrument application.

While the exploratory stroke is a feather-light feel with the instrument to transmit the tactile response, the working stroke is a short but powerful application of the instrument to break up or dislodge the deposit.

The cutting blade of the instrument should engage the root surface at an angle somewhere between 45 to 90 degrees. Many technics will specify that the instrument is to approach the tooth at a specific angle of, for instance, 60 or 88 degrees. Theoretically, although such an angle might be the optimum angle for efficiency of a given instrument, it is impossible to be so precise clinically (Fig. 8-18). Practically, the feel of the bite of the sharp instrument against the tooth surface or the deposit when the instrument is activated is a more logical measure of its correct angle application. If the blade slides or slips over the deposit, either the angle application or the instrument stabilization is incorrect.

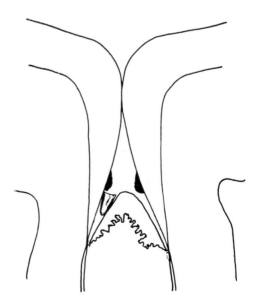

Fig. 8-18. The instrument is slipped gently below the most apical portion of the calculus. With firm pressure, a rocking motion, and an occlusal movement, the calculus is removed.

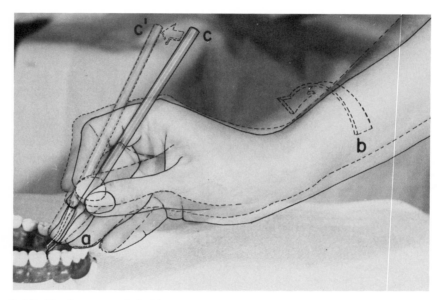

Fig. 8-19. The instrument is held as one would hold a pen or pencil, with the fingers immobile, close together, and slightly curved. *a*, The third finger is used as a rest or fulcrum and should be placed on a tooth close to the tooth being worked on. *b*, One of the basic scaling strokes is a lateral rocking arm motion. The solid line indicates the starting position and the broken line the terminal position of the arm. *c—c'* indicates the movement of the handle of the instrument.

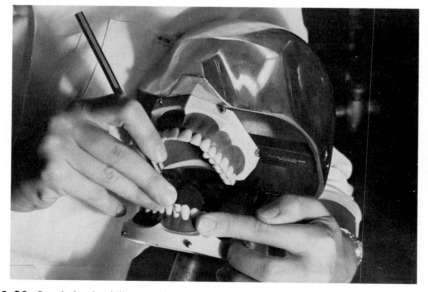

Fig. 8-20. Prophylactic skills can be learned on a manikin. Note the use of the fulcrum point and the use of the left hand to depress the lip.

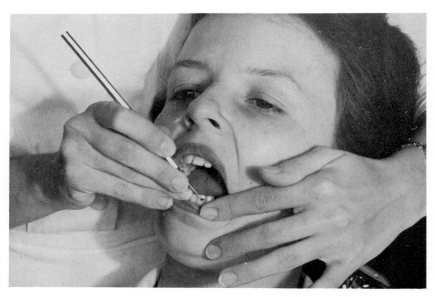

Fig. 8-21. Skills learned on a manikin may be transferred to a patient. Note that the fulcrum point, the use of the instrument, and the use of the left hand are the same as illustrated on the manikin in Fig. 8-20.

Following the initial or, when required, repeated power stroke to dislodge the deposit, one or more additional strokes, which might be described as shaving strokes, are done in the same area. This shaving stroke may be less powerful and have a longer sweep than the short forceful power stroke. The effect of its use is to ensure the total removal of the deposit and to scrape the tooth surface to a smoother finish.

The instrument is next positioned laterally with a slight overlap of the previous area, and the series of working and shaving strokes is repeated to dislodge the deposit and then smooth this area. The series of overlapping strokes is repeated until the surface is free of deposit. Although the shaving strokes follow the application of the initial power stroke, it is not the intention to remove the deposit in layers. The objective is to remove the mass of the deposit in one stroke if possible and then to remove any remnants and smooth with the shaving stroke.

The strokes described are made primarily in an incisal or occlusal direction. However, a circumferential stroke can be used in the problem areas of the line angles of the teeth. Less power is possible with the circumferential stroke but it functions well as a shaving or finishing stroke.

Activation of the instrument. In the actual application of the instrument stroke, the fingers serve only to hold the instrument and to guide it into its position. The fingers are not used to apply the actual force. To do so will prove to be extremely tiring. The actual force applied is a combination of action of the hand, wrist, arm, and shoulder. The hand rotates about the rest fulcrum (Fig. 8-19). If the instrument grasp and rest position are correct, the result will be a short and controlled, yet powerful, stroke. The skills of instrument use may be initially learned on the manikin (Fig. 8-20) prior to the actual use of instruments in the mouth (Fig. 8-21).

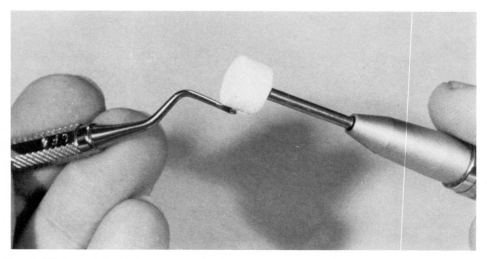

Fig. 8-22. Dental handpiece mounted stone showing the preferred sharpening of a curette. By sharpening the side of the working area rather than the face, the strength of the instrument in the line of the pull is maintained. As the curette is sharpened it becomes smaller and can be used in more constricted areas.

Instrument sharpness is essential

For calculus to be removed effectively and for smoothing of the surface to be accomplished, absolute sharpness of the instrument is essential. A dull instrument will habitually slide over deposits and give a false impression of a deposit-free surface. The dull instrument requires excessive force in its use, creating the potential of tissue damage, and is fatiguing to the therapist to attempt to use.

Instruments must be resharpened as often as necessary to maintain a truly sharp cutting edge. Frequently it is necessary in the prophylaxis procedure for one patient to resharpen several times or to have extra sets of instruments available. Probably no other single factor in effective deposit removal is as essential as the maintenance of a keen edge on the instruments being used.

Several types of mechanical instrument sharpeners are available. Some of these are discussed and illustrated in Chapter 17, where the sharpening of all kinds

of instruments is discussed in some detail. The hand-held or dental engine-driven sharpening stones offer many advantages. They can be readily sterilized and may be rapidly used at the dental chair during a treatment procedure to restore sharpness to the instruments being used (Fig. 8-22).

Many therapists prefer to sharpen curettes and sickle scalers on both *sides* of the blade rather than on the *face* of the blade. The basic strength of the instrument is maintained in the line of the pull stroke since no metal is removed in this dimension. It also produces an instrument that is made smaller laterally with each sharpening and becomes more suited for use in constricted areas.

It may be necessary occasionally to shape the face of the blade in order to restore the proper edge. This can be accomplished either with hand-held stones or with the dental engine–mounted stone. A hand stone may also be used to sharpen the sides of the curette blade.

The hard Arkansas stone is the most

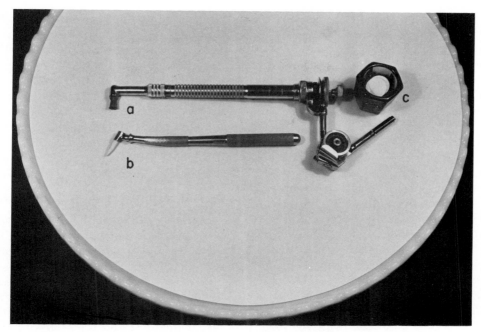

Fig. 8-23. *a,* Prophylactic handpiece on a dental engine: rubber polishing cup inserted in the handpiece; *b,* porte-polisher with wood point inserted; *c,* polishing agent.

nearly ideal of the stones for the sharpening of instruments because it produces the finest edge and removes the minimum amount of metal. The composition stones mounted for dental handpiece use are not as hard as the Arkansas stone but are sometimes easier to use.

Types of blade metal related to instrument sharpness. Cutting blades with a high carbon steel content are hard and maintain a cutting edge longer than other kinds under a given set of circumstances. However, they are brittle, tend to break, and discolor upon moist heat sterilization. Stainless steel blades are not as hard as high carbon steel and require sharpening more frequently, but they do not discolor upon sterilization. Blades of tungsten carbide have been developed that are extremely hard and do not discolor, but they retain the tendency toward brittleness.

Each type of blade has advantages and disadvantages, but regardless of the type used, it must be resharpened as often as necessary to maintain its absolute keenness.

POLISHING TECHNICS

Following the removal of deposits and stains and the smoothing of the tooth surface by instrumentation, the natural and restored tooth surfaces must be thoroughly polished. This is true for removable dentures also. The highly polished surface resists the accumulation of new stains and deposits, facilitates the oral hygiene efforts of the patient, and enhances the appearance of the mouth.

Polishing is primarily accomplished by the use of bristle brushes and rubber cups in the motor-driven dental handpiece, although a porte-polisher utilizing a wood point may be used in some instances (Fig. 8-23). The porte-polisher is useful in developing instrumentation technics, but the use of the motor-driven polishers is more practical and logical in the routine treatment of patients. Fine linen polishing strips and dental tape may also be used to produce the final polish upon the approximating tooth surfaces.

Many polishing (abrasive) agents are available for use, the most common of which is pumice. Pumice is a complex of aluminum, sodium, and potassium silicates of volcanic origin. The abrasiveness of pumice primarily results from the particle size. Four types are commonly available: flour or superfine, fine, medium, and coarse. Medium and coarse pumice should never be used on the natural teeth, and the use of fine pumice should be limited. Flour of pumice may be used for stain removal and for the first stage of the polishing procedure. The final polishing should be performed with chalk (precipitated calcium carbonate) or tin oxide or kaolinite.

Zirconium silicate is a special polishing and cleaning agent preferred by some therapists.

Cleaning and polishing agents may be mixed with water to produce a thick slurry or with an oil base such as glycerin to produce a paste that is more easily confined to the area being polished. All cleaning and polishing agents should be used moist and with a light touch of the rubber cup or brush. The motor-driven polishers should be run at low speeds. (See Fig. 17-28.)

Dry polishing agents, firm pressure, and high speed produces heat and discomfort and they excessively wear and abrade the tooth surface.

A flavoring agent may be added to the final chalk polish or a conventional toothpaste may be used as the final polishing agent to provide a fresh and pleasant mouth taste.

Following the polishing of the tooth surfaces that can be reached with the motor-driven brush or rubber cup, dental floss or tape should be used to put final polish on the proximal surfaces and to remove any remaining polishing agent from between the teeth.

If removable dentures are to be polished, extreme care must be exercised to protect them during the cleaning and polishing procedures. It may be more desirable to polish dentures in the laboratory, but when they must be polished at the dental chair they should be protected by polishing over a folded towel and held securely during the polishing procedure.

DENTAL CHAIR/THERAPIST POSITIONS

Because of the variation in dental equipment available today, it is difficult to attempt to describe therapist-to-patient positions for specific procedures. It would be necessary to consider the standing therapist and seated patient, the standing therapist and the reclining patient, the seated therapist and the seated or the reclining patient. This is impractical in a text, and this is left to the instructor or demonstrator.

The prime objective is that the therapist-to-patient position be such that it fulfills the concepts of work simplification and provides the greatest degree of comfort to both patient and therapist. The positioning must permit the therapist to perform the delicate and exacting technical procedures required. The ideal work positions may be a combination of both standing and seated positions to vary and interrupt a fixed working position and to reduce fatigue.

A reclining position may be contraindicated for patients with severe asthma, sinusitis, congestive heart conditions, and other physical problems.

The selection of operating positions will depend upon the factors of equipment availability, physical condition of the patient, and, last but not least, personal preferences of the therapist.

PERSONAL DENTAL CARE BY THE PATIENT

Although in some dental practices today other auxiliaries have been trained to be dental health educators, it remains one of the major responsibilities of the dental hygienist to instruct the patient in correct personal dental care procedures. Probably no area of dental practice has so many conflicting opinions relating to methods, armamentarium, and technics as does mouth care by the patient. In spite of the confusion, it is apparent that effective mouth care practices by the patient are essential to successful dental therapy. No restorative or periodontic treatment procedure can succeed if the basic cause is allowed to continue.

Role of bacteria

The patient must realize the role of bacteria as the primary etiological agent in both tooth decay and gingival and periodontal disease. The obvious contribution of high-sugar foods in the caries process must also be understood. Once these basic principles are grasped, the logic and objectives of mouth-cleaning procedures becomes clear.

The primary objective of mouth cleaning is the regular removal of the bacteria (microorganisms) contained in the adherent dental plaque on the surfaces of the teeth and from the gingival sulcus (gumline space) area. When the adherent bacterial plaque is removed on a regular and systematic basis, calculus formation is prevented since it is the mineralization of the plaque that results in calculus. Efforts directed at effective microorganism removal also removes any retained food and produces a frictional stimulation of the gingiva. Although this stimulation may be of value, there is no proof that it is necessary to maintain gingival health.

Methods

Regardless of the method recommended for mouth cleaning, it should meet the following requirements:

1. It must be effective.
2. It must be easy to teach and to learn.

3. It must not produce damage to the tooth or its supporting structures.

Of all of the methods suggested in the past or today, the methods of use of the disclosing agent, the toothbrush, and dental floss (or slight modifications of the basic concepts) as recommended by Bass and Arnim most nearly meet these requirements.

Disclosing agents

Disclosing agents have been used in the dental office for many years. Although effective, there were many limitations in their use. The development of the disclosing tablet by Arnim has eliminated many of the limitations and complications of use of a disclosing agent. Arnim incorporated a water-soluble vegetable dye (F.D.C. Red No. 3 or erythrosin) into a fruit-flavored tablet designed to be chewed by the patient. The solution resulting when the tablet is thoroughly mixed with saliva colors the accumulations of plaque on the teeth. It does not stain normal tooth structure or restorations nor does it permanently stain clothing, linen, or bathroom fixtures.

Since plaque is normally relatively colorless, it is difficult for the patient to identify its presence or location. The disclosing agent, used in the home as an aid in mouth-cleaning procedures, provides a positive identification of the bacterial plaque that the patient is trying to remove.

The use of disclosing tablets represents the most important single advance in mouth-cleaning methods in recent years. Not only is the problem identified as being present, but *where* it is, *what* to do about it (clean it off), and *when* it has been removed (the red is gone) is vividly visible to the patient.

Armamentarium

In addition to the basic tool, the toothbrush, many other items have been developed as adjuncts in mouth cleaning. Special wood and plastic toothpicks, rubber and plastic interdental stimulators, many forms of dental floss or tape, pipe cleaners, yarns, water irrigators, powered toothbrushes, mouthwashes, and many formulations of dentifrices have been recommended. Not only is the array of devices confusing to the patient, but rarely has there been an explanation of the correct use of the suggested device and rarely has the patient understood exactly what he was trying to accomplish.

To meet the objectives of bacterial plaque removal from the teeth and the gumline spaces, it must be realized that each tooth has five surfaces and four gumline spaces that must be thoroughly cleaned. The toothbrush can effectively clean three of the tooth surfaces (the biting surface, the cheek side, and the tongue side) and two of the gumline spaces (cheek side and tongue side). Dental floss is necessary to reach the two in-between (proximal) surfaces of the teeth and their gumline spaces.

Identification of the bacterial plaque with a disclosing agent and skillful use of both toothbrush and dental floss is probably all the average patient needs to do to effectively remove the bacterial plaque masses from their teeth and gums. If this is accomplished on a regular and systematic basis, the primary cause of both tooth decay and gum disease can be controlled. Obvious additional benefits are gained from a thorough regular cleaning of the tongue with the toothbrush.

Patients with special problems of fixed or removable prosthodontic appliances, orthodontic appliances, tooth malpositions, structural deformities, and the like may require additional and specific cleaning aids.

Dentifrices

The addition of various forms of fluoride to dentifrices has been effective in reducing the incidence of dental caries, particularly in children. However, there is no evidence to indicate that any specific dentifrice is effective in the prevention or treatment of periodontal disease. Dentifrices designed to reduce tooth sensitivity have produced sporadic results. No truly effective desensitizing dentifrice is known at this time.

The basic compositions of most dentifrices, paste or powder, is very similar. Each contains an abrasive (polishing agent), a binder (thickener), usually a preservative (to reduce bacterial growth), a softener in pastes, a coloring agent, and sweetening and flavoring agents. The more abrasive dentifrices may be dangerous in producing excessive tooth structure wear.

Although the average dentifrice may have some value in the removal stains and loose debris, it contributes little to the removal of adherent plaque. It functions primarily as a mouth freshener and stain remover. In fact, the removal of adherent bacterial plaque may be inhibited if the toothbrush bristles are matted or gummed together by the dentifrice. Probably the most effective approach is the use of the brush without a dentifrice initially to sweep away the adherent plaque. This permits visualization of the action of the bristles and of the disclosing agent–stained plaque so that effective removal is accomplished. Following this initial cleaning, a dentifrice can then be placed on the brush for its polishing and mouth-freshening action.

Toothbrushes

Hundreds of different designs of toothbrushes with variations in the bristles, head size, and handle length and shape are available. Almost all are relatively equal in price and there is little in price differential to recommend a particular brush. The 2 × 6 (two rows and six tufts of bristles) hard nylon or natural bristle brushes frequently recommended in the past are gradually being replaced by brushes with softer multituft nylon bristles (Fig. 8-24). Some of these brushes have rounded- or

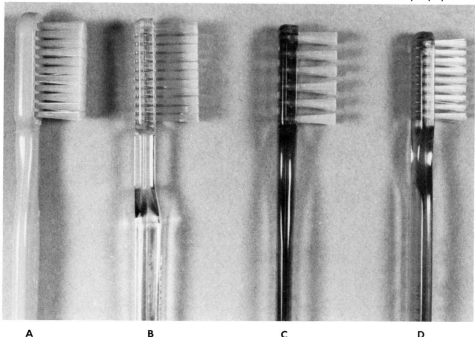

A   B   C   D

Fig. 8-24. Examples of soft multituft nylon toothbrushes. **A,** Lactona M-39. This contains forty-three tufts of bristles. The brush head is a little large, but the bristles stand up well in use. **B,** Dental H Periodontic. It contains thirty-three tufts of bristles. The head is small, the handle is comfortable, and the bristles stand up well in use. **C,** Right Kind Sub-G. This contains eighteen tufts of bristles. The bristles are soft and polished but do not stand up well in use. **D,** Butler No. 111. It contains twenty-seven tufts of bristles. The head is small, the handle is comfortable but a little short for some adults, and the bristles stand up well in use.

polished-end bristles. This may be of importance when the Bass technic or its modifications are used because the bristle ends are forced into a positive contact with the gingiva and gingival sulcus area.

The multituft brush with the soft nylon bristle (0.007 to 0.008 inch in diameter), usually set in three or four rows and trimmed level so that a flat brushing plane is produced, stands up well under normal brushing use and is less traumatic to both the tooth and the gingival tissues.

The important criteria for brush selection should include: (1) a handle long enough to reach all mouth areas and comfortable to hold, (2) a brush head small enough to be effective in all mouth areas, and (3) soft round-end bristles in the multituft design. These features should be incorporated into the toothbrush regardless of whether it is the conventional hand-manipulated or the powered toothbrush.

The powered or automatic toothbrush may offer a definite advantage for patients with physical restrictions in the use of their hands. Many children will use the automatic brush to some advantage because of its novelty or gadget value. However, most patients can do a more effective cleaning with the hand-manipulated toothbrush if they have been properly instructed and will expend the necessary time and effort. Careful instruction in the use of the automatic brushes is also necessary, and the patient

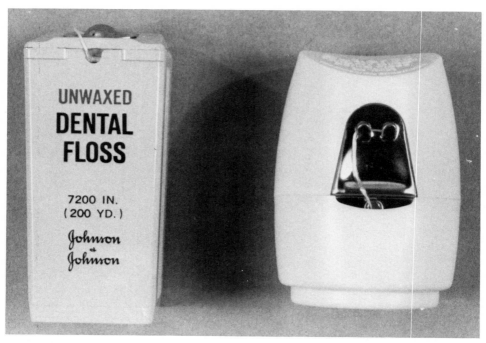

Fig. 8-25. Examples of unwaxed dental floss. The Johnson & Johnson floss *(left)* is specially treated to reduce fraying and shredding. The Butler floss *(right)* is a duplication of the original Bass floss.

must understand the basic objectives of brushing regardless of the type of brush used.

Most automatic brushes provide either a back-and-forth or an arcuate motion, although some powered brushes are designed to provide both actions. The back-and-forth motion is more effective in cleaning the critical area of the gingival sulcus (gumline space).

The rechargeable-battery automatic brush is adequate for individual or small family use since the charge is usually sufficient for several brushings. Electrically powered brushes may be more desirable for use in hospital wards or places where repeated uses must occur in a short period of time.

Dental floss

Although the facial (cheek side), lingual (tongue side), and biting surfaces of the teeth can be effectively cleaned with the toothbrush, the proximal (in-between) surfaces of the teeth and their sulcus (gumline space) areas are relatively inaccessible to the brush. The daily use of dental floss is mandatory if these areas are to be effectively cleaned.

For many years both dental floss and tape were provided only in a waxed form. Bass, in 1948, published specifications and a rationale for the use of a thin unwaxed dental floss. Many varieties of unwaxed floss are now commercially available (Fig. 8-25). Theoretically, the unwaxed floss is more effective in breaking up and removing the adherent plaque, since the filaments separate in use; each strand becomes an individual scraping tool, with the soft unwaxed floss readily conforming to the tooth contours. It does have the disadvantage of fraying or shredding easily, and at times the individual strands break and become lodged between the teeth. This is a definite disadvantage in that patients sometimes become discouraged and tend to discontinue floss use.

Waxed floss may be somewhat easier to learn to use, particularly if it is thin. Unfortunately, most waxed floss is thick and may be uncomfortable to insert between the teeth. This uncomfortable insertion also may prevent the patient from using the floss on a daily basis. Johnson & Johnson makes both waxed and unwaxed floss that is thin and excellent for patient use. It may be preferable to have the patient learn the skills and habit of floss use with the waxed floss and then, if desired, substitute the unwaxed floss.

ROLE OF THE DENTAL HEALTH EDUCATOR

To provide the motivation, information, and skill development necessary for the patient to develop effective mouth care habits, the dental health educator must perform two major functions: education and training. The patient must understand the cause of dental disease, what can be accomplished by mouth care practices to prevent disease, and the mouth care practices that are effective. He must develop the skills and the habits to perform these practices. For the patient to develop effective mouth-cleaning practices requires careful and repeated instruction and supervision of performance by the dental health educator.

At the initial appointment and prior to any dental treatment procedures, factual information regarding the role of bacteria and high-carbohydrate foods in the production of dental caries and periodontal disease must be presented to the patient. The fact that effective personal dental care practices used conscientiously on a regular and systematic basis can control and prevent the diseases must be established. The patient must realize that only he can

perform the procedures and that he must accept the personal responsibility for the prevention of dental disease. Careful prophylaxis by the dental hygienist or dentist every several months cannot, in itself, prevent disease. Although the hygienist and dentist can assist the patient in learning the proper methods, in training them to become skillful in performance, and in restoring the mouth to a state of health so that prevention of further disease is possible, it is the patient who controls or prevents dental disease in his own mouth.

Good personal dental care habits are difficult to establish, particularly when there are old ineffective habits to overcome. Although it is obviously easier to teach good health habits to the young child, and emphasis should be placed upon prophylaxis and mouth care instruction for the young patients, thorough instruction and training in effective personal dental care must be performed for *all* patients.

Instruction in mouth-cleaning technics

Identification. Following the initial education phase, the bacterial plaque masses must be identified in the patient's mouth by the use of a disclosing agent. Liquids or tablets may be used, but the use of the tablet in the dental office has advantages since this is the method that the patient will use during the home cleaning sessions.

Disclosing tablets (Butler Redcote or Amurol Xpose) are usually individually packed in plastic packets. The packets will tear easily if they are torn from the side rather than from the top or bottom. The tablet should be chewed thoroughly, mixing it with the saliva and swishing it around in the mouth to touch all the teeth. It should be retained in the mouth for at least 1 minute. The mouth should be rinsed with water. The rinsing may be swallowed since the dye is harmless or it may be emptied into a cup or other receptacle. The red areas visible on the teeth following rinsing are the stained plaque that must be removed by the patient's hygiene efforts.

Toothbrush. The toothbrush is used in the initial cleaning efforts. The brush usually can effectively clean the cheek side, tongue side, and biting surfaces of the teeth. A soft nylon multituft round-end bristle toothbrush (without dentifrice so that the stained plaque can be seen and the position of the bristles visualized) is used.

If study casts of the patient's mouth are available, they should be used to demonstrate the basic brush positions. Dentoforms or typodonts may be used. If none of these is available, the brush position should be demonstrated in the patient's mouth. Choose an area on the cheek side of the lower arch about the level of the premolar teeth, since this is probably the easiest area for the patient to see when learning brush position. Direct the bristles toward the gingival sulcus (gumline space) at approximately a 45-degree angle to the long axis of the tooth. Rock the brush gently back and forth and maintain a firm pressure against the tooth surfaces. After several motions, move to the adjacent area and repeat.

Demonstrate brush position on all cheek side and tongue side areas. Finally, demonstrate the position of the brush on the biting surfaces of the teeth. Point the bristles into the grooves on these surfaces and firmly scrub back and forth.

To ensure that the cleaning is thorough, a systematic pattern must be established. One effective way is for the mouth to be considered a circle. First, brush on the cheek side around the circle, then on the tongue side, and finally on the biting surfaces. Now, ask the patient to brush all areas using the circle pattern. Make corrections in brush position and usage at this time. When the patient seems to have grasped the fundamentals of the technic and has done an effective job of cleaning the cheek side, tongue side, and biting

surfaces, again inspect the mouth to see whether disclosing agent is visible. In most mouths, the brush can clean the three surfaces fairly well when properly applied, but plaque will almost always remain on the proximal (in-between) tooth surfaces.

Dental floss. Dental floss must be used to clean in-between surfaces. From the contact area of the teeth down into the interproximal sulcus is the critical area to be cleaned.

The use of floss is not a customary patient habit, and it is not easy for most people to learn without practice. However, when the patient sees the stained plaque that remains following brushing, he can usually appreciate the need for additional mouth-cleaning efforts.

If floss use is thoroughly demonstrated by the hygienist, most patients will be able to master its use. There are two methods of floss holding that may be helpful to demonstrate: the spool method and the circle or loop method, as suggested by Masters.

Spool method. In the spool method, use approximately 18 to 20 inches of floss and "spool" it onto the middle, ring, or little finger of both hands, leaving the thumbs and first fingers free to move the floss in the mouth. Hold one end of the floss between the thumb and middle finger (this is the easiest finger to use) of one hand and wrap or "spool" the floss around this finger for six or seven turns.

Wrap the floss around the middle finger of the other hand for two or three turns. Extend the thumb of this hand and continue to wrap the floss until the hands are the thumb's length apart. Slide the thumbs and first fingers along the floss until they are about 1 inch apart. The thumbs and first fingers control the direction of the floss while the "spooled" fingers control the tension.

Circle or loop method. Use about 12 to 14 inches of floss and put the ends together and hold between a thumb and first finger.

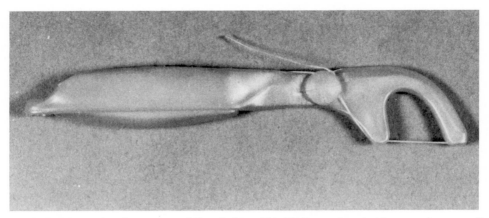

Fig. 8-26. Example of one type of floss holder. This EZ Denta-floss holder contains a small replaceable cartridge (10 yards) of unwaxed floss in the handle. It provides a practical aid for those patients who have difficulty in manipulating hand-held dental floss.

Tie two knots as close to these fingers as possible. This will form the loop and keep it from slipping. When the floss is tied into this circle or loop (about the size of an orange), it provides a handle to hold the floss with the middle, ring, and little fingers while the first fingers and thumbs are used to control the direction of the floss in the mouth.

Floss use in mouth. Using either the spool or loop method, the thumbs and first fingers should be about 1 inch apart and the floss introduced between the teeth with a gentle sawing motion. Push the floss firmly against one tooth and move up and down and into the gumline space several times. Lift the floss over the interproximal gum tissue, push it against this tooth, and move up and down and into the gumline space several times. Remove the floss from between these teeth with the same sawing motion used to enter, proceed to the next space, and repeat the cleaning motion.

When the floss becomes worn or frayed, move around the loop to provide a new area or release one turn from the "spooled" finger having the most turns of floss and take up one turn on the other finger.

In either floss-holding method, keep the elbows as close to the body as possible. This increases control of the hands and reduces fatigue. Keep the palms of the hands pointed toward the jaw that is being flossed—palms up for the upper jaw and palms down for the lower jaw.

For those people who have difficulty in manipulating the hand-held floss, there are several types of floss holders that may prove to be advantageous (Fig. 8-26).

For most patients, the effective use of the toothbrush and dental floss is all that should be required to thoroughly clean the mouth. The brush should be used to thoroughly clean the tongue. However, for patients with specific problems related to fixed or removable partial dentures and structural deformities, additional cleaning aids may be required. Following the actual cleaning procedures with the brush, floss, and other aids, if required, the teeth should be thoroughly polished with a small amount of a fluoride dentifrice applied with the brush.

Home cleaning procedures. When the patient realizes the actual effectiveness of the various hygiene devices, including the dentifrice, he is provided with several alternatives to the routine home cleaning procedures. Although mouth cleaning is best accomplished in the bathroom during the period of disclosing agent use and during the learning stages, effective toothbrushing and flossing can be accomplished in areas other than the bathroom while watching television or reading.

Many patients will prefer to alter the sequence of brush and floss use and floss first and then proceed to the bathroom for the final brushing and polishing. Either approach is satisfactory so long as the basic objective of effective mouth cleaning is accomplished.

One "thorough cleaning" each day is required to prevent and control dental disease in most mouths. However, during the learning phases and to ensure mouth freshness and promote esthetics, brushing following eating is highly desirable. Disclosing agent use should be continued frequently until the patient has reached a skillful level of mouth cleaning. At this time, the disclosing agent may be used approximately once each week as a check to reinforce the maintenance of an effective routine.

It is important to evaluate carefully the effectiveness of the patient's personal dental care upon return visits. The patient should be able to see an improvement in dental health as a result of his efforts but will require occasional reinstruction and remotivation to ensure that he realizes and appreciates the importance of those things that he does for himself.

Although the dental team can contribute much in assisting the patient in developing an effective personal dental care program, it is the conscientious daily effort by the patient in both food selection and mouth care practices that is the key to dental disease prevention.

SUGGESTED READINGS

Arnim, S. S.: Thoughts concerning cause, pathogenesis, treatment and prevention of periodontal disease, J. Periodont. 29:217, 1958.

Arnim, S. S.: Microcosms of the human mouth, J. Tenn. Dent. Assoc. 39:3, 1959.

Arnim, S. S.: The use of disclosing agents for measuring tooth cleanliness, J. Periodont. 34: 227, 1963.

Arnim, S. S., Diercks, C. C., and Pearson, E. S., Jr.: What you need to know and do to prevent caries and periodontal disease, J. N. Carolina Dent. Soc. 46:296, 1963.

Bass, C. C.: The necessary personal hygiene for prevention of caries and periodontoclasia, J. Louisiana Med. Soc. 101:52, 1948.

Bass, C. C.: The optimum characteristics of toothbrushes for personal oral hygiene, Dent. Items Interest 70:697, 1948.

Bass, C. C.: The optimum characteristics of dental floss for personal oral hygiene, Dent. Items Interest 70:921, 1948.

Bass, C. C.: An effective method of personal oral hygiene, J. Louisiana Med. Soc. 106:100, 1954.

Bohannan, H. H., Ochsenbien, C., and Saxe, S. R.: Preventive periodontics, Dent. Clin. N. Amer., July, 1965, pp. 435.

Goldman, H. M., and Cohen, D. W.: Periodontal therapy, ed. 4, St. Louis, 1968, The C. V. Mosby Co.

Masters, D. H.: Oral hygiene procedure for the periodontal patient, Dent. Clin. N. Amer., Jan., 1969, p. 3.

Merritt, S. W.: Periodontal diseases, diagnosis and treatment, New York, 1963, The Macmillan Co.

Wilkins, E. M.: Clinical practice of the dental hygienist, ed. 3, Philadelphia, 1971, Lea and Febiger.

part three

SUPPORTING BACKGROUND
OF OFFICE PRACTICE

chapter 9

PLANNING A MODERN DENTAL OFFICE AND SELECTING ITS EQUIPMENT

Charles O. Cranford, D.D.S., M.P.A.*
Shailer Peterson, B.A., M.A., Ph.D.

The dentist today depends upon his dental hygienist to help him in the planning of the new office and in selecting the new equipment that each will use. It wasn't many years ago that there were only a few manufacturers of dental equipment. All of the units and chairs were so similar that the decision on what to select was a case of choosing from a few colors in order to match the pattern of the office.

During the last decade, a virtual revolution has taken place in the equipment industry. Where there were once only a few manufacturers and all with similar ideas as to design and construction, now there are many. There is a host of different ideas and suggestions for improving the efficiency of office practice and the appearance of the total office image.

Whenever a practicing or a student dental hygienist has an opportunity to attend a meeting where there are commercial exhibits, she has a real opportunity to observe and inspect the new designs for

possible use in her own office. Fig. 9-1 shows one of the exhibit floors at a National A.D.A. Session where there were about 350 exhibitors. The Chicago Midwinter Meeting in February and the Greater New York Meeting in December have displays that are nearly as elaborate. All of the state dental association meetings have exhibits that are equally as interesting and informative but not quite so extensive and elaborate.

This extensive assortment of operatory equipment, office furnishings, and instruments is overhwhelming. Some potential customers find these exhibits confusing and almost frustrating merely because there is such a wide variety of items and each seeming to possess many unique advantages. These exhibits include lounge chairs with their heaters and vibrators that relax the tired dentist when he gets home in the evening, furniture for the reception room, bookkeeping systems and recall methods, visual aids to use in educating patients, books for keeping up to date, hand instruments, x-ray machines, and, finally, all of the different kinds of units and chairs for the operatory.

Other chapters in this textbook will make reference to bookkeeping systems, x-ray

---

*A portion of this chapter has been contributed by Dr. Charles Cranford. This was done in his own private capacity. No official support or endorsement by the U. S. Public Health Service is intended or should be inferred.

147

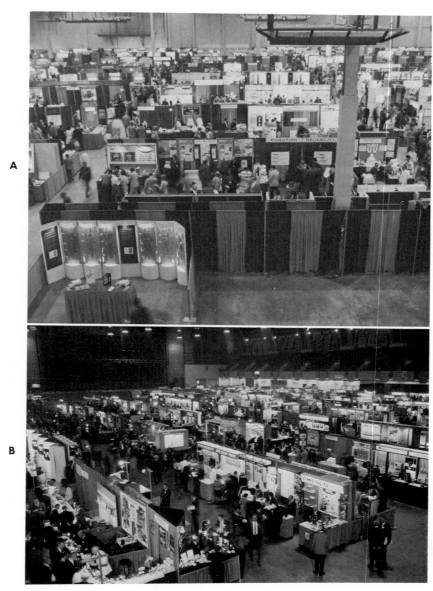

Fig. 9-1. Each year thousands of dentists and their dental hygienists study exhibits and examine new equipment at the annual meeting of the American Dental Association. **A,** The 1968 Session in Miami Beach; **B,** the 1963 Session in Atlantic City. (Courtesy American Dental Association.)

equipment, and hand instruments. In this chapter attention is directed to the equipment in the operatory that will suit the needs of the dentist and his dental hygienist.

The dentist and his dental hygienist should rely heavily upon the advice and suggestions of the dental dealers who serve their office. The dealer represents different brands of equipment, and each manufacturer in turn offers a variety of styles and models. Few local dealers have the space to stock many different models. This is why the dealers themselves advise the dentist and his dental hygienist to attend annual meetings where they can examine and inspect the several models that the dealer has described and that have been pictured in his catalogs and leaflets. The dealer deserves attention, for he will want the dentist to be satisfied with a fine piece of equipment that will serve him well. Every dealer wants to merit and earn the respect of the dentist and his dental hygienist, for he wants to serve their office for many years; he can do this only if he gives good advice and helps them to select good, trouble-free equipment.

Selecting the equipment is still something that should not be left completely to the salesman. He will advise and suggest. He should be able to answer the questions about the equipment or obtain the answers. However, most dentists and dental hygienists find that there are always several pieces of equipment having special merits and advantages, and no single one of them seems to possess all of the desirable features. Therefore, decisions must be made, and the dentist and his dental hygienist will want to be the ones who make the final selection for whatever piece of equipment is going to be placed in their office and that they are going to be using for a period of time.

Selecting the new dental equipment for the office is a bit like buying a new car. Sometimes it is probably too much like buying a new car, for statistics show that most motorists become accustomed to one kind of car and continue to buy new models of the make of car that they have owned previously. Certainly there is nothing wrong with buying a new model Buick when one has been very well satisfied with all of the Buicks that he has had over the past years. There is also nothing wrong with a dentist who has been well satisfied with his dental equipment, manufactured by company "X," to keep on wanting to buy new models of "X." Dental equipment has probably changed a great deal more than automobiles have in the last 10 years, and hence it is important for the dentist and his dental hygienist to make a list of the specific characteristics or functions that they are looking for in a new unit or in a new chair. The dental dealers themselves will help supply many of the characteristics that one needs to evaluate, for every salesman will talk about the various strong points of his product and sometimes even about the weak points of some of the competitive products. The dentist and his dental hygienist who make a list of the various points to be considered will be well prepared to attend a commercial exhibit and also well prepared to start making an evaluation of all of the equipment they examine and hear about.

The dentist and his dental hygienist should make a rational and objective approach to the selection of the equipment. There will be some who will want merely to update their equipment and get a new model of the item that has served them so well for so many years. However, most persons today feel that the drastic changes in equipment design have come about by the demands of the profession for improved equipment.

The name of the game today is to "find new and better ways to serve more patients and to serve them better." The proper equipment can help the dentist and his dental hygienist in many ways. It can:

1. Improve the patient's comfort and safety
2. Improve the comfort to the dentist and reduce his fatigue at the chair
3. Improve the comfort to the dental chairside assistant
4. Improve the comfort to the dental hygienist and reduce her fatigue at the chair
5. Improve the efficiency of the operator and his assistant by positioning the equipment so that instruments are within easy reach and fewer tiring motions are required
6. Improve the delivery of services needed by the patient, such as not requiring the patient to move to another chair for another service
7. Increase the ease with which the equipment can be kept clean and serviceable
8. Improve the adaptability of the equipment to serve the patient and the dentist in emergencies

Dentists today are coming to realize that they may have had some very fine equipment that has performed in an excellent manner, and yet "nothing is so good that there still cannot be an easier and better way of doing it." Dentists and their assistants are constantly looking for new and better ways of serving more patients faster and better. Dentists and their office colleagues are constantly wanting to find office equipment that will make the patient's trip to the dentist's office a surprisingly pleasant experience, free from pain and apprehension.

The dentist and his dental hygienist need to realize that when they decide on using some of the newer equipment, they may have to learn new ways of working. Many dentists learned to operate at a chair by standing all the time. Now the trend is to remain seated and to depend upon the chairside assistant to provide the instruments as they are needed. Some dentists find it difficult to learn to operate

in a seated position, but those who are able to make this change realize that they are adding years to their lives by this change, and they find that they can accomplish more work before becoming weary.

Some equipment is equally adaptable to working alone or in a "solo" type of practice, and other equipment or its arrangement makes it easier to use if one has an assistant. A dentist may use both a chairside assistant seated near him and a roving assistant. The modern dental hygienist is also finding now that she can use a chairside assistant to improve her work and the service that she renders.

When examining the different pieces of equipment, one immediately realizes that each piece of equipment has been designed with one primary method of use in mind. For example, a chair and a unit may have been designed for sit-down dentistry. If so, it may actually not be very comfortable or useful when used by someone who only stands at the chair while operating. Therefore, the dentist and his dental hygienist must either select equipment to suit the way they have been and intend to continue operating or to suit the new way that they have decided to use even though they will need to learn a new method and procedure. Or, of course, they may select equipment so that the transition from one method to another takes place over a period of time.

There are some practical considerations that need to be kept in mind, and the local dental dealer will probably remind the dentist of these matters also. A partial list of some of these factors is as follows:

1. Is the product manufactured by a reputable company?
2. Has the product been in production long enough and used by enough persons so that one can have assurance that it is reliable and trouble-free?
3. Can service on the equipment be secured locally and without delay?

4. Are spare parts for the equipment available locally or can they be obtained by air express in a day or two?
5. Is it necessary to have a standby piece of equipment to use in the event of an emergency?
6. Can daily or weekly servicing and cleaning of the equipment be done by the office staff?
7. Will the new equipment be compatible with the other equipment that will remain in the office (if that is essential or desirable)?
8. Can one talk with a dentist who owns and uses this product or who owns a product manufactured by this company?
9. Has the company been manufacturing products for the health professions for a long time?
10. If the product is a new one, where has it been tested, for what length of time, and under what kind of conditions?

It is important to note in this array of questions that there are several that might make it appear unwise to consider a new product or a new company. The fact remains that there are times when one wants to buy a new product and will accept it even though it has not been thoroughly tried and in spite of the fact that it is not manufactured and guaranteed by a dental manufacturer of long experience.

It is also important to realize that in the selection of equipment one cannot expect to rely solely upon the advice of friends and colleagues. These persons will be basing their judgments upon their own experiences and the way in which they want to practice. Each dental office has its individuality, and each dentist and his dental hygienist need to select the equipment and the furnishings that will permit the dental office team to operate at its optimum efficiency. Just because product "X" is suitable for Doctor "A" is no proof that

Doctor "B" could even make good use of the product, let alone want it as an important component in his office. Selection of equipment is a personal thing and the kind of equipment must be selected upon the basis of highly objective considerations.

The dentist should remember that in his clinical years in dental school he learned practice procedures that might be represented as

Dentist + Patient + Office equipment

When he started his practice he may have joined with another dentist, and it is possible that this office had the same kind of traditional equipment that he had used in school. In that case, the "equation" of his practice might still look very much like his dental school combination, namely:

Dentist + Patient +
        Office equipment like that in school

If the dentist were a graduate during the last 10 years, it is probable that he selected fairly modern equipment and also hired a chairside assistant at the outset of his practice. Or it could also be that the other graduate had decided to update his equipment, in which case either one would appear as:

Dentist + D.A. + Patient +
        Newer but still traditional equipment

The next logical step is for the office to have its own dental hygienist. It might be that this could be represented as

Dentist + D.A. + D.H. + Patient +
        Adequate equipment for entire dental team

The preceding diagrams show that the "dental practice" is dependent upon all of the members of the dental team *plus* the patient *plus* the equipment in the office. The dental team tries its best to make the best use of its own talents and abilities to serve the patient, but it is easy to understand that it must select methods that can be used with the equipment at hand. Methods of treatment and methods of practice depend upon the *team* and the *equipment.*

It is impossible to say whether the team, the method of practice, *or* the equipment is the most important. All three of these are dependent upon one another. It is difficult to change one without changing the other. It is obvious, though, that the dental team is limited in whatever method of treatment it is going to use *by* the equipment that is in the office.

Buying new equipment is not enough; the new equipment must be selected with a purpose in mind. This purpose must be one with which the members of the team are already very skillful, or the team must have decided that it is going to learn to operate in a new and different way and that for this it needs new and special equipment. Everyone knows that it is probably easier to continue to practice and to serve patients in the same way that was taught in dental school or the same way that one has been practicing for the past 10 years. It is obviously easier to keep in the same routine and not to be challenged into learning new things to do and how to operate new instruments. The modern dentist and the modern dental hygienist are inventive and resourceful. They thrive on change and challenge. Also, most of them have a tendency to be "gadgeteers," and they like the idea of having new equipment to master and new buttons to push.

The modern dentist and his dental hygienist know that just because a procedure has been done a certain way for 20 or 30 years does not mean that there is not a better way to do it. Every enterprising professional person is constantly wondering whether there isn't a better way of doing what they are now and have been doing. Basically, this is the difference between a professional and a nonprofessional person. The professional person is not content to follow a routine every day and every hour. The professional person

wants to put some ideas of his own into the operation and to invent the better way for his office team to get the job done.

In order to select a better method for conducting the office practice, one must first of all recognize that there are two things that have interraction: dental practice methods and kind and style of equipment. One cannot select equipment without knowing what methods of practice are going to be used. But, also, one cannot select practice methods without knowing whether one can procure the necessary kind of equipment that is demanded or whether one can have the special equipment designed and manufactured so as to serve these methods. Of course, almost anything can be manufactured, but most persons would prefer to use commercially manufactured products because of the servicing that is required and because they are more competitively priced. Therefore, even the most inventive person begins by using what is available commercially, but he may add his own touches of originality.

"Rational thinking" is an expressive key phrase to describe the kind of reasoning and diagnostic thinking required by the dentist and his team members when they are deciding upon the methods of practice that they are wanting to use. This might also be called a "scientific method" of approach because one digs out the facts, organizes them, and tries to draw conclusions from them. In other words, the dentist and his team must study the objectives and purposes of every operation and treatment that they give. Then they must enumerate and study every step of this procedure and analytically try to find out how they can improve upon it.

The team members ask themselves such questions as:

1. Have we been doing unnecessary things? Are there steps that can be eliminated?

2. Are there steps that can be combined?
3. Are there new methods that should be substituted for the old?
4. What methods depend upon the equipment that we use?
5. What methods depend upon the arrangement or positioning of the equipment?
6. Are there new steps that ought to be added?
7. Which of these steps will require special education and experience of the team members?
8. How will the patient react to the newer methods?

Rational thinking is comprised of subjective and objective elements. The subjective elements are the ideas, thoughts, and feelings of the individual that may not be observed by any other person. Therefore, the subjective elements do not lend themselves to be checked and verified by other persons. On the other hand, the objective elements of rational thinking are those factors whose characteristics and values can be verified by other persons.

In the past, operatory equipment has frequently been selected primarily on the basis of subjective judgments. Dentists today have become more conscious of the factors that need to be considered in evaluating the performance of dental equipment.

The dentist and his dental hygienist who have the responsibility for selecting equipment know which factors of performance and dependability lend themselves to objective measurement and evaluation. They also recognize that as the users of these pieces of equipment, it is up to them to assign weights of relative importance to each of the factors that they are studying. They recognize that these value judgments and the weights given to these measurable factors are somewhat subjective. However, even subjective evaluations can be based upon careful study and review.

There are other significant factors that affect the judgments of the dentist and his dental hygienist. For example, the dentist may identify the factors that he considers to be measurable and, hence, lend themselves to evaluation. He may also accurately appraise the fact that certain of his judgments are somewhat subjective. But if he lets his judgments be slanted or prejudiced by hearsay information or even by the fact that he once had an unsatisfactory product manufactured by one of the companies under consideration, then he may find that he is unable to judge the articles or the products fairly. This is not just a case of "fairness" to the company; it is possible that through this kind of unwarranted prejudice he may also have rejected a very fine product and hence he has been unfair to himself and to his office.

In order to understand exactly how one assigns a worth or value concept to a product or even to a method of treatment, it is well to consider and to study the following statements:

1. The value that one person assigns to dental equipment depends upon the degree to which this person feels that it satisfies his preference in a certain given situation.
2. The value assigned to a certain piece of equipment will probably be different for each of several individuals because each has different value judgments.
3. Preferences and value judgments may differ under different circumstances and under different conditions.
4. The assessment of value or worth is by definition "subjective" for the most part, and hence attempts to make these judgments appear to be based upon objectivity is usually a waste of time and not justified.
5. Worth or value judgments are in themselves "untestable" by ordinary scientific methods, although the separate and individual factors helping

one reach a conclusion may all have been very objective and factual.

The modern dentist and his dental hygienist train themselves to approach any problem in a systematic manner, just as they collect facts about the patient in order to reach a diagnosis and to plan a program of treatment. Today the dentist and dental hygienist also try to use this same scientific method in evaluating the time that they spend at the chair working on a patient and in evaluating the equipment that will help them improve their services.

There are a number of persons who are taking the scientific approach in studying how to improve one's practice procedures and also how to select equipment suitable for these procedures. Dr. H. C. Kilpatrick[1] has written many articles on the art of "work simplification." Dr. G. E. Robinson[2] and Miss Gertrude Sinnett[3] have written many articles and given many continuing education programs on this same subject. Dentists and dental school instructors often have cameras set up to record by elapsed time photography (or memomotion photography) the motions that take place during an operation. Wasted motions can be studied in this way, and resourceful operators welcome an opportunity to study ways and methods of improving their efficiency and avoiding the needless fatigue they have been experiencing. Even the Polaroid camera is often put to work in an office or a dental school clinic to snap a candid shot of a student dentist in an awkward position or a student dental hygienist using wasted motions.

When viewing either moving pictures of one's operations or elapsed time pictures with their jerky revelation of wasted motions, it is well to keep some of the following points in mind when trying to develop a new method or a new procedure:

1. Avoid sudden and sharp motion. Make motions continuous.

2. The two hands need never be idle at the same time unless completely at rest.

3. Develop a rhythm in the work, for it aids in providing smooth and flowing operations.

4. Keep motion to a minimum, for this reduces fatigue.

5. Position all needed instruments in advance so as to eliminate the need to search for instruments and to reduce reaching.

6. Instruments used in a particular sequence should be positioned in a way to reduce search time.

7. Provide adequate illumination for particular needs and requirements.

8. Arrange to work in a seated position with back support if possible, and select the stool or chair that will accommodate this.

9. Share the work normally done by the hands with other parts of the body, such as the feet, and by body movements.

10. Reduce the number of times that one needs to change instruments.

11. Use double-ended instruments when possible to reduce changing instruments and position.

12. Arrange to have someone pass and position instruments to one's hands as he works.

13. If patient cannot actually assist, then be sure that he does not hinder the operation.

The dental manufacturers know that the "name of the game" is a combination of:

1. Delivering more dental service to more patients

2. Delivering the service with a minimum of effort and fatigue to the dentist and his dental hygienist

3. Lowering the cost of dental care

4. Reducing the time required for each dental service

5. Producing trouble-free dental equipment

It has been said several times in this chapter that the dentist and his dental hygienist cannot go equipment hunting unless they know what it is that they need. They cannot know what they need unless they have analyzed what they now do or what they want to do. The expert dental health team has become so accustomed to working quickly and smoothly that the members often do not find it easy to analyze and to discover what specifically they do and what series of steps are involved. However, this is very essential; also, they may know what is done, but it is possible that they have almost forgotten why it is done. Every procedure needs to be analyzed, dissected, and studied under the microscope of "criticism" to determine:

1. Is time being wasted?
2. Are useless motions being used?
3. Are there better ways of doing the same thing or attaining the same objective?
4. Have new methods been discovered that have been overlooked?
5. What kind of equipment would be needed to improve the delivery of dental service?

The dentist and dental hygienist can prepare their own list of questions and answers to study their own particular office situation. The dental office team members should study this problem together. But they should not restrict their information to just what they can see around them. Also, while they can learn much from their dental dealer and his sales personnel, they should visit other offices and see how other people are doing things. They need to see what equipment is being used in these other offices. They should visit dental schools to see how students are being taught today. They need to attend continuing education sessions where people are discussing the building of a modern office with its modern equipment. They need to attend time and motion lectures and talk to the others attending the

dental meetings about their methods of practice.

The dental hygienist needs to be inventive and develop new ideas to help the office be effective and efficient. She should "steal" ideas wherever she can and put them into the framework that they deserve to have in her own office. One should never transplant another office to her own. One can transplant some of the basic ideas, but every office must have the personality of the dental team reflected in its equipment, in the furnishings, and in the total arrangement of the office.

The following is a partial listing of some of the criteria listed by a subcommittee of the Dental Student Training Advisory Committee, Division of Dental Health of the U. S. Public Health Service, and which in turn were based upon the opinions of various directors of Dental Auxiliary Utilization (DAU) Programs. This listing was produced because of the requests that had been made by schools wanting and needing to know what guidelines they should use in purchasing equipment for their own DAU clinic areas.

Dental unit should:

1. Be located so as not to occupy space needed by the dental team.
2. Position all instruments for easy delivery to the mouth and permit return with minimum motion and effort.
3. Be flexible enough for the use by both right- and left-handed operation. *Note:* This item has importance in a school where right- and left-handed students use the equipment, but this would have minimum importance to a dental team in a dental office.
4. Include high- and low-speed handpieces that are operated by a single, compact, and easily operable foot controller for variable speeds.
5. Include an air-water-spray syringe that is lightweight and easily managed.
6. Contain hoses and cords with sufficient length to permit all attached instruments to reach the operating zone easily.

The dental chair should:

1. Provide power operation for frequently adjusted parts.

2. Be easily operated by both the dentist and his assistant. *Note:* Similarly by the dental hygienist and her assistant.
3. Have thin, narrow back.
4. Provide complete body support for the patient in a full range of positions from upright to supine.
5. Place the operating zone (patient's mouth) at the seated operator's elbow level in all desired operating positions.

One can see from this that the members of the dental health team in any office could also develop a similar listing of desirable factors that they would like to see in any of the new equipment that is to be brought into the office. Most dentists and their dental hygienists will have many individual likes and dislikes that they will want to list, even though they do not want to be prejudiced about them. For example, some persons have had unfavorable experiences with various kinds of hoses and their retracting mechanisms. Some of these experiences might have been so traumatic that the dentist and his dental hygienist believe that they never would want to work with another unit that had a retracting system of any kind. Many manufacturers are the first to admit that certain systems did not prove to be very satisfactory, but there are many who now have developed systems that they now believe are practically troubleproof, and they are anxious to demonstrate them.

Similarly, there are some persons who feel strongly about electronic gadgetry, some who feel that pneumatic switches are to be preferred over solenoids, and so it goes with personal preferences. One must not disregard the personal preferences and even prejudices as long as one gives every manufacturer a chance to describe his new piece of equipment with its changes and modifications. This is where one can ask the dealer some of the questions mentioned earlier in the chapter that relate to how long the equipment has been in use, who has used it, how much trouble it has

given, how long it has taken to repair or adjust it, and so on.

The modern dentist and his dental hygienist have much more to say about the equipment that he and she will use than does the surgeon and his nurse. The surgeon usually must use equipment in a hospital where he has nothing to say about its selection. But the dentist, his dental hygienist, and his dental assistant are the ones who select the equipment that their team will use in their office. Therefore, there is no excuse for the dentist and his dental hygienist working in an office that is not properly equipped with the exact kind of equipment that they need for their special kind of practice and to suit their special needs.

There may be a dental hygienist someplace who will raise the question as to whether she can really expect to have any influence over the equipment that she will use in her office and the equipment that her dentist-employer will use. The concept of four-handed dentistry and the DAU program came about only about 15 years ago. But the concept of the dental health team came from the American Dental Association before that. One cannot say that every dental office gives all of its dental team members a chance to comment on the new equipment that will be ordered, but there is a tremendous number of offices that has been doing this for many years. The dental hygienist and the dental assistant who demonstrate their knowledge of equipment and who can show that they have studied these principles relating to the delivery of dental care are surely the ones who will be asked to aid in the selection of the new equipment and also in its placement and arrangement.

The modern dentist wants to be the administrator of his dental office, but he also wants to share the creation and the maintenance of this efficient dental office with the responsible members of the dental health team.

REFERENCES

1. Kilpatrick, H. C.: Work simplification in the dental practice; applied time and motion studies, ed. 2, Philadelphia, 1969, W. B. Saunders Co., p. 702.
2. Robinson, G. E., and others: Four-handed dentistry: the whys and wherefores, J.A.D.A. 77:573, 1968.
3. Sinnett, G. M., and others: Four-handed dentistry: a new mobile dental cabinet design, J.A.D.A. 78:305, 1969.

SUGGESTED READINGS

Anderson, J. A.: Dental office design and layout, J.A.D.A. 60:82-91, 344-353, 1960.

Anderson, J. A.: Efficient use of space to conserve time and energy, Dent. Clin. N. Amer. 5:185-195, 1961.
Clynes, J. T.: Planning makes maximum use of minimum space, Dent. Survey 44:46-49, 1968.
Coburn, D. G.: An environmental approach to office design, Oral Health 60:11-18, 1970.
Cutler, M.: Dental Office design, Dent. Assist. 37:16-18, 1968.
Cutler, M.: The well-planned dental office: form follows function, Dent. Student 48:26-29, 1970.
Green, E. J.: Efficient office design facilitating auxiliary training, Dent. Clin. N. Amer. 15:245-256, 1971.
Weinert, A. M.: An evaluation of the modern dental lounge chair, Dent. Clin. N. Amer. 15:129-144, 1971.
Winkler, N. D.: Time and motion studies in the dental office, Oral Hygiene 51:46-47, 1961.

chapter 10
EXPANDED DUTIES FOR THE DENTAL HYGIENIST

James L. Bugg, Jr., B.A., D.M.D, M.S.
Wade B. Winnett, D.D.S., M.S.D.
Shailer Peterson, B.A., M.A., Ph.D.

Never before in the history of the dental profession has so much attention been given to the utilization of auxiliary dental personnel. With the anticipated availability of private or federally supported dental health insurance, an immense problem confronts those responsible for the nation's dental health. Any worthwhile relief through preventive measures seems remote, at least for another decade.

Auxiliary personnel, in various capacities, have been employed in dentistry for almost a century. Originally the dentist carried out every phase of his work, but over the years he has delegated some of his clinical duties to the dental hygienist and the dental assistant. The medical profession delegates many aspects of treatment to trained personnel such as registered nurses, physiotherapists, x-ray technicians, laboratory technicians, and other individuals who carry out much of the actual treatment. However, some aspects of dental practice are very specialized, and the delegation of duties is sometimes more difficult. It is on this basis that the dental profession has been reluctant to support the concept of patient treatment by auxiliary personnel. But, because of a shortage of dentists and for economic reasons, an extension in the use of dental auxiliaries now appears expedient. The accepted standard still remains—although auxiliary dental personnel must serve as an integral part of the dental health team with appropriate status, they are complementary to, and not a substitute for, the qualified dentist.

The attitudes of practicing dentists toward auxiliary dental personnel vary widely, ranging from those who employ no auxiliaries and regard them negatively to those who "wouldn't be without them." Fortunately, the negative attitude is held only by a small number of dentists, and this percentage is growing smaller each day.

The gradual rise of the population-per-dentist ratio has created much discussion on increasing the scope of the duties of auxiliary dental personnel. Experiments such as those performed at the Louisville Manpower Training Center,[1, 2] Great Lakes Naval Training Center,[3] and the University of Alabama School of Dentistry[4, 5] have shown that some routine chairside duties being performed by dentists can be delegated to dental auxiliaries without a sacrifice in quality, thus increasing office production and causing dentists and dental educators to take another look at their old concepts of practice management and patient treatment.

Wider use of dental auxiliary personnel can also be attributed to the formation of courses in the dental schools dealing with dental auxiliary utilization at both the undergraduate and graduate level, as well as continuing education courses on this subject. Studies[6] have shown that the employment and correct utilization of one full-time dental assistant can increase the dental office patient load over 40%; two full-time dental assistants properly utilized can bring this average increase to over 65%; three full-time personnel to over 85%; and an increase of above 100% with four full-time personnel.

Until recently all the attention regarding expansion of responsibilities has been focused upon the dental assistant. Dr. Harold Hillenbrand[7] suggested in 1967 that emphasis be put on the expansion of the duties of the dental hygienist, because she is licensed in all states and legally and professionally qualified to perform intraoral services.

On any subject there can undoubtedly be two or even more different opinions or points of view. Some dental hygienists say: "We have enough to do now; we don't want any more responsibilities." Other say: "We want to be permitted to perform more duties and to have greater responsibilities."

Some dentists also want to have the duties and responsibilities of their dental hygienist expanded or enlarged, and still others think that they now have all of the responsibilities that they should be given. They envision their hygienist as an independent income-producing member of the office team. She is the prediagnostician of the office. While she is taking radiographs, performing oral prophylaxis, and doing other duties currently prescribed by state law, the dentist is performing highly technical duties that only he is qualified to perform. So, expanding the role of the hygienist will take time away from her duties where she is most effective.

In the last 10 years, increasing concern has been demonstrated on the part of both the public and the dental profession relative to the manpower that will be available to provide the dental service that will be sought by the public in the future. The number of dentists and auxiliaries now serving the public has been just about adequate in most areas of the nation, and yet there are many places where the patient must wait several months for an appointment. It is also a well-known fact that there has been a steady increase in the public's demand for and awareness of the need for dental care. This means, of course, that in future years more service will be demanded.

To prepare for this increasing demand, several methods are being used. New dental schools are being constructed and present dental schools are being expanded to enroll larger classes. Also, studies are being conducted to decrease the length of the dental school program to provide practicing dentists in a shorter length of time. But increasing the number of dentists is not enough. Therefore, the dental profession is advocating that the dentist reevaluate his own function and his own duties in his office so that he will make the very best use of his talents and delegate to other persons the responsibilities that he can let them perform under his supervision and with them working under his basic responsibility toward the welfare and safety of the patients.

Therefore, the dentist needs to delegate to his helpers those duties that they are equipped to perform or those that they can be trained to do. With a team approach, his office team can provide an optimum of dental service to his patients.

It has been suggested that as long as the dentist is responsible for the patients in his office, he should be encouraged to authorize his auxiliary personnel to perform any and all operations in that office that he feels they are qualified to perform and for which he is willing to be responsible.

This is basically the way that professional men view the operations in their offices. They will surely not permit any of their personnel to perform duties that they are not qualified to perform, for this would endanger the patient and the dentist would be liable and responsible.

However, it is really not enough that every dentist and every office have its own set of rules and regulations. Certain lists of responsibilities need to be agreed upon so that the schools educating the dental assistant and the dental hygienist can properly provide the education and experience for those responsibilities that the dentist expects those personnel to accept. Dentists do not have time to educate their own personnel, although all of them give freely of their time to add to the education of each person on their staffs. Also, the state boards of dental examiners need to recognize that there are certain groups of responsibilities that practicing dentists and the schools agree are appropriate for the curriculum of these trained personnel.

To date, most of the changes toward the expansion of the duties of the hygienist have been limited to "reversible procedures."

With changing concepts in almost all fields of endeavor, it should be no surprise that there are changing roles of dental auxiliaries along with a shifting emphasis in dentistry as a whole. Some of this change is the result of the modern concept of teamwork in the dental office.

Many studies have been conducted to demonstrate to the dentist and his auxiliary personnel the various responsibilities that can be delegated to the dental hygienist and assistant and the amount of time that this will save the dentist. Studies have also been conducted to demonstrate the length of education required to provide the level of competence that is judged basically essential or minimal.

There have been studies in which the auxiliary has taken on more difficult tasks and also those that were not "reversible." For example, some have been taught to cut hard tissue, such as in the preparation of cavities. However, most members of the profession are of the opinion that the auxiliary should only be given responsibilities that can be "reversed," which is to say, that anything the auxiliary has done incorrectly can be brought back to normal and redone correctly. Obviously, if tissue is cut and damaged or if a nerve is exposed during the preparation of a cavity, there is no way that the actual damaged tissue or part can be returned to its original state and the cavity prepared without the nerve exposed.

The dental nurse in New Zealand does prepare cavities in children's teeth and hence is permitted to perform irreversible operations. When discussions were first begun relative to the expanding functions of a dental hygienist and a dental assistant, there were some who were very fearful that any change in duties would create serious problems. People sometimes forget that everyone is making changes and adjustments in the way that they do things all of the time.

Some persons will say that it is still questionable as to whether dental hygienists and dental assistants will elect to take on new and added responsibilities that will update their usefulness. It is really not a questionable matter, for as long as the dental profession has already made the decision that the dentist must be relieved of some of the duties that can be performed efficiently by auxiliary personnel, it is only a question of who will perform them. If the dental assistant and the dental hygienist should resist or turn down this opportunity to become more adaptable, then the profession will immediately begin to educate and train a new auxiliary such as the "dental nurse" or a "dental therapist" or any other new name to distinguish this person from the present members of the team.

The question may be raised as to what will happen to the individual dental hygienist in practice today who tells her dentist-employer bluntly and forcibly that she will not take on additional duties; that she will not learn to perform any of the new duties; that she will not take on new and additional responsibilities. This is a question that only the specific dentist-employer can answer about that specific employee. It might very well be that he does not want this particular dental hygienist in his office to take on any new duties. It may also be that he may feel that she is not capable of learning new skills and hence would not want to be responsible for her taking on new tasks involving the patient's safety. On the other hand, he might encourage his dental hygienist to prepare herself for taking on new duties, or again he might decide to employ an additional dental hygienist who has already acquired this new education and experience.

The nurse in the medical profession has gone and is going through a history of learning new skills, adapting herself, expanding her functions; moreover, new kinds of auxiliary personnel have been created. New "kinds" of nurses have been created to divide the numerous tasks that the physicians and the public require. This is exactly the same approach or procedure that is now becoming a new "milestone" in the progress of the practice of dentistry.

Therefore, it is really not a question of: "Should the dental hygienist learn new skills so that she may expand her functions and her responsibilities?" Instead, if there are any questions, it is only: "How fast can we decide on what new tasks should be assigned to the dental hygienist?" and "How fast can we set up educational programs to provide these skills for our dental hygienist in practice and also for our new students?"

There are some dental hygienists who have resisted any expansion of duties because they are probably misunderstanding the urgency of this problem and the effect that it will have upon them and their friends. Expanding duties and expanding responsibilities mean permitting the auxiliary personnel to be eligible to perform a greater variety of tasks than they are now trained and permitted by law to do. Expansion of duties does *not* mean that every dental auxiliary is going to work hours that are twice as long and have twice as many different kinds of things to do during the day. For example, the fact that a prospective employee has the skill to use the typewriter doesn't mean that she will spend any significant amount of time typing or being a secretary. This skill is useful for even the chairside assistant to possess in emergencies, just as it is useful also for the dentist himself when he is working on a paper to deliver to his local dental society.

Added skills provide the dental hygienist with just that many more attributes that will make her useful and valuable in a dental office, particularly in one that already has a staff on hand that has become accustomed to do all of the ordinary and usual things. Also, just as dentists now tend to specialize, even though only a relatively few work solely in the specialty fields, so will the dental hygienist also find that she will be able to specialize and that a dentist will employ her because she possesses a special combination of talents in which she has become expert. She will *not* be hired just because she has learned to do a hundred things in a mediocre manner.

Those young women who are learning to become dental hygienists today are being educated at a very exciting period of time. They will have the unusual opportunity of being among the first dental hygienists to take on new and real responsibilities that have never been done before by anyone other than the dentist himself.

Dental societies and state boards of dental examiners are all becoming very concerned about the duties that need to be given to all of the auxiliary dental personnel. More than half of the states have already liberalized their state dental practice acts, and the rest are all working on it.

Dental hygienists need to be alert to the changes coming about in the new duties and responsibilities that will be assigned to them. They need to see that it is important for them to be able to take on these new tasks, and they should be glad that these opportunities for advancement do exist. It is in this way that dental hygiene will become even more important, and it is in this way too that the dental hygienist can show to her employer that she is increasingly valuable to that office and in the delivery of the dental health services of that office.

To increase the dentist's efficiency, who is going to assume the responsibility? Will it be the dental assistant, the dental hygienist, or both? Since studies have proved that personnel with less education and training than the hygienist or dentist can perform minor procedures satisfactorily, then these trained personnel should be given the right to perform these duties by law. Most of these procedures are routine repetitive chores that rob the dentist of productive time that could be spent in performing tasks requiring his professional judgment and skills. The auxiliary that seems to be the natural one to assume this task is the dental assistant.

Additional training could be provided to give the certified dental assistant this knowledge and ability. Her new title could be something quite different. Some have suggested the term *dental nurse*, but most persons would consider this to be an inappropriate title, for the Australian dental nurse is permitted to prepare cavities as well as to perform restorative work on children, and dentists in the United States do not wish to have anyone except the dentist cutting either hard or soft tissue.

Some have suggested that as long as the dental hygienist is licensed and is already permitted to work in the mouth, she should be the one who would have her duties changed so that she would place amalgams in the cavities prepared by dentists. However, others disagree and feel that this fairly simple operation of placing the restorative material in the cavity can better be given to the dental assistant and that the dental hygienist should have her work restricted to operations in which her more extensive education will aid her in making decisions and using sound judgment.

The solution as to who should perform this "cavity-filling" responsibility may be solved very simply by making it possible for either the dental hygienist or the dental assistant to acquire a special certificate to prove and attest to the fact that she is qualified to perform this task.

There are some who blame dental hygienists for not being more forceful than they have in trying to work out their own destiny and in determining their own future. However, dental hygienists could not be blamed for this in the past, for until just recently it was quite evident that most members of the dental profession did not want auxiliary personnel to be given very many duties or responsibilities. Even when dental hygienists would attend a meeting at which the duties and responsibilities were to be discussed, they themselves discovered that their duties in the different offices, in the different regions of the nation, and working for dentists with different specialties were basically fairly limited. When they found that there were differences, they also discovered that any expanded duties would depend upon the particular practice of the dentist in that office.

Dental hygienists have been loyal to the

profession of dentistry and have looked to the dentists for guidance and suggestions. They have not wanted to forge ahead independently for fear that this would be interpreted as rebellion and lack of respect. If anyone is to be blamed, this blame probably should be shared by both the dentist and his dental hygienist.

Until recently, not very many dentists had been given any education or experience in how to use a dental assistant or a dental hygienist in his own office. It was only a dozen years ago that the Dental Auxiliary Utilization (DAU) Program in the dental schools started giving every graduate some experience in four-handed dentistry, but even then no attention was given to the work of the dental hygienist. Therefore, the functions and the responsibilities of the dental hygienist in an average office have been the product or result of some system that has been worked out jointly by the dentist and the dental hygienist. It is little wonder that the responsibilities of the dental hygienist have been kept at a very conservative level. The dentist has been told that the dental hygienist has been educated in scaling teeth and in providing patients with dental health education information. He has not had time to teach her other skills, and the state licensure laws have also discouraged any extension of these duties.

While there is some general agreement finally today by the dental profession that the duties and responsibilities of dental hygienists and dental assistants should be expanded, there is very little agreement as to what these new duties should be. When one realizes that only a relatively small percentage of dentists has had the opportunity to work with a dental hygienist and to know what she can do, it is little wonder that the recommendations are a bit nebulous.

In order to understand why it is that the expansion of duties has come about so slowly, it is necessary to take a closer look at the practice of dentistry and perhaps some comparative examination of the practice of medicine. Most physicians are specialists, and only about 10% or 15% are general practitioners. In the case of dentistry, the situation is just reversed, with about 85% being so-called general practitioners. The term *so-called* is used because even the general practitioner is not and cannot be an expert in everything. He realizes this and patterns his own private practice in accordance with his special interests, his special skills, and his abilities. It is easy to understand that a dental hygienist working for a periodontist might have different functions than if she were working for a pedodontist. But actually her general practitioner employer might make just as many different demands upon her time as any specialist.

When dentists have gathered to discuss the educational programs or the office function of dental hygienists, the solutions have all been just as varied and different as the office practices of the dentists on these committees. It has been difficult to get agreement on these points at meetings of the American Dental Association's Council on Dental Education or at various committee meetings at which dental hygienists have been in attendance.

Just as the dental office practices are very different, the dentists themselves did not come out of the same mold. Even those who are graduated from the same dental school still have different backgrounds and interests, and this influences their mode of practice and their methods of utilizing auxiliary dental personnel. As one looks at all of the dentists on a dental school faculty, one can see very plainly that each faculty member has his own special interest. The dentist in operative dentistry demonstrates a different interest in the various parts of the curriculum than the dentist who teaches complete dentures, or the one who teaches oral pathology, or the one who teaches in the department of oral surgery. The sameness of their degrees and the fact that they are all dentists does not mean that they will easily reach a similar conclusion as to what the dental profession should require of a dental hygienist in the future.

Similarly, it is going to be a bit difficult for dental hygienists to come up with a solution or a conclusion because they are all the products of the offices in which they have been practicing and of the dentists who employ them.

Dean John A. DiBiaggio wrote an interesting article[8] in the *Journal of the American Dental Hygienists' Association* a short time ago. The title of the article, "Dental Hygiene at the Crossroads," is particularly significant. DiBiaggio points out the fact that the dental hygienists are being called upon to make some decisions right now about their future. This is true, for unless the dental hygienists do come face to face with the problem and invent a solution to it, they will be destined to a decaying type of existence and with a brand-new auxiliary being brought onto the scene to replace them.

As has been pointed out, it is going to be difficult to find a solution that is right, and it will be impossible to find one that will please any sizable number of persons. But it is important that something be done, and it is even better to do something that may not be perfect than *not* do anything at all.

There are several points that need to be made clear.

1. Some decisions need to be made immediately about the needs of the dental hygienist of the future.
2. No new trend is going to change all of dental hygiene practice immediately, for there are 18,000 practicing dental hygienists of which only a small number will want to take time to add to their education.
3. Practicing dentists need to be educated or reeducated in how to use the "new breed" of dental hygienist.
4. Perhaps there will always be more than one "breed" of dental hygienist. This will be determined best by the kind of a dental office in which she works and the kinds of demands that are made of her.
5. Perhaps the dental hygienist will be able to specialize the same as a dentist or as a physician. Some will have more training and experience in certain fields than will others.
6. Perhaps the dental hygienist will obtain special certificates for each phase of her educational and experience program either in place of a single degree or in addition to her certificate and degree.
7. Perhaps the dental hygienist will become intimately associated with one of the major functions in the dental office and basically assume complete charge of it, for example, the prevention program, the office management program, or the like.
8. Perhaps the dental hygienist will need to have her own auxiliary personnel in order to increase the efficiency of her functions.

The dental profession (that is, the organized dental profession) would welcome some well-constructed suggestions from dental hygienists relative to their future purpose and aims. It is one thing for the dental hygienists to sit back and wait for their present and prospective employers to dictate what they are going to be required to do in the future. The employers would frankly like to know what dental hygienists honestly believe they are competent to do when they are given an educational program with these objectives. When dental hygienists decided to make a statement on what they are sincerely interested in doing for the dental health team, this will give dentists some real assurance as to the true importance of these personnel to the practice of dentistry. When dentists give way to their auxiliaries certain functions and responsibilities that they have been guarding very zealously for over 100 years, these dentists want to have some assurance that they are giving them to a group that appreciates and understands the meaning of this responsibility.

It is not the purpose of a textbook to attempt to provide the readers with solutions to problems such as this challenge of the future. It is the responsibility of the authors to demonstrate to the reader the importance of taking a stand and developing a philosophy about the role of a dental hygienist in tomorrow's dentistry. Failure to assume this responsibility will be interpreted by dentists as reflecting the fact that dental hygienists today think of their profession only as a temporary "job" or position and that they are really not interested in the basic objectives of the dental profession.

There are some who will think that the licensed dental hygienist should be the auxiliary who will complete the restoration when the dentist has prepared the cavity by cutting the hard tissue. There are some who will think that the dental hygienist should be a super office manager. There will be others who will want the dental hygienist to take over the entire program of prevention in the dental office. This is fairly logical, for she already performs some level of scaling and provides dental health instruction. But there is much more than this, and the dentist in a well-organized office could beneficially use someone to take over this entire operation. There are others who feel that the dental hygienist could provide much support to the examining of the patient, collecting diagnostic information, and working closely with the dentist in regard to the diagnosis and the plan of treatment.

Perhaps it is correct up to a point to say that "dental hygiene is at the crossroads." This implies that there is a choice of routes

or roads and that one can travel merrily and happily over either one of them. Actually such is not the case, for an unwise choice could mean the destruction or abolition of dental hygiene as a profession.

REFERENCES

1. Lotzkar, S., Johnson, D. W., and Thompson, M. B.: Experimental program in expanded functions for dental assistants; Phase 1, baseline and Phase 2, training, J.A.D.A. **82**:101-122, 1971.
2. Lotzkar, S., and others: Experimental program in expanded functions for dental assistants: Phase 3, experimental dental teams, J.A.D.A. **82**:1067-1081, 1971.
3. Ludwick, W. E., Schnoedelen, E. O., and Knoedler, D. J.: Greater utilization of dental technicians: II. Report of clinical tests, Great Lakes, Ill., 1964, U.S. Naval Training Center.
4. Hammons, P. E., and Jamison, H. C.: Expanded functions for dental auxiliaries, J.A.D.A. **75**:658-672, 1967.
5. Hammons, P. E., Jamison, H. C., and Wilson, L. L.: Quality of service provided by dental therapists in an experimental program at the University of Alabama, J.A.D.A. **82**:1060-1066, 1971.
6. Baird, K. M., Purdy, E. C., and Protheroe, D. H.: Pilot study on advanced training and employment of auxiliary dental personnel in the Royal Canadian Dental Corps: final report, J. Canad. Dent. Assoc. **29**:778-787, 1963.
7. Hillenbrand, H.: Fact and forecast, J. Amer. Dent. Hyg. Assoc. **43**:207-209, 1969.
8. DiBiaggio, J. A.: Dental hygiene at the crossroads, J. Amer. Dent. Hyg. Assoc. **43**:131-136, 1969.

SUGGESTED READINGS

Abramowitz, J.: Expanded functions for dental assistants: a preliminary study, J.A.D.A. **72**: 386-391, 1966.
American Council on Education: Commission on the Survey of Dentistry in the United States, Survey in dentistry: the final report, B. S. Hollinshead, Director, Washington, D. C., 1961, American Council on Education.
Brown, W. E.: Dental hygiene stands on the threshold, J. Amer. Dent. Hyg. Assoc. **41**:133-135, 1967.
Dunn, W. J.: Manpower in dentistry—the dental hygienist, J. Canad. Dent. Assoc. **27**:19-23, 1961.
Fulton, J. T.: Experiment in dental care; results of New Zealand's use of school dental nurses,

Geneva, Switzerland, 1951, World Health Organization.

Hammons, P. E.: Accelerating dental education by utilization of auxiliary dental personnel, Alabama Dent. Rev. **10**:4-7, 1962.

Kerr, P. A.: Some additional duties for the dental hygienist—a regional experiment, Bull. Mich. Dent. Hyg. Assoc. **14**(4):3-6, 1968.

Stearns, P.: Dental auxiliary-itis, J. Amer. Dent. Hyg. Assoc. **42**:191-199, 1968.

chapter 11

UNDERSTANDING THE PATIENT

Jack Miller, B.A., M.S.W.
Shailer Peterson, B.A., M.A., Ph.D.

The dentist and his dental hygienist would each like to know the secret for getting along well with every patient. Both of them want the patient to desire to return regularly for treatment and to follow their home care suggestions to prevent dental disease. Both of them want to possess or to be able to develop those personalities that will attract patients so that their office practices will be a success.

Someone will quip glibly; "So what is new about that?" Or they may ask: "Isn't this true of everyone?" No, as a matter of fact this is not true of everyone. There are many persons who are not at all interested in operating a "popularity contest." Also, there are many patients who have never thought it very important that the dentist or his dental hygienist like them or get to know them. This is true not only of the youngster who hates everyone in a white jacket but also of some adults who hate the very thought of being forced to go to a dental office. And it is true of many others as well. Dentists and their dental hygienists would not rate very high in any popularity poll.

Someone is bound to say: "Everyone has to try to get along with the public, with the customers, and with the patients." No, there are some workers and even some employers who do not need to concern themselves very much about their "popularity" status with anyone else, or at least not with very many. At least, the need to be "liked" is relative. Some persons need to get along with their customers and with their patients more than others do.

The members of the health professions need their patients just as the patients should need them. The dentist and his dental hygienist need to work at the job of understanding their patients as well as understanding each other. (See Chapter 3.)

There are formulas and equations for almost everything, but there is no formula that will magically tell the dental hygienist how to be successful in understanding her boss or each of her patients. A dental hygienist may have earned a Phi Beta Kappa key in school and may have received straight A's in her dental hygiene courses but still may lose one job after another and be a failure at her profession. Intelligence, technical judgment, and physical attractiveness comprise a wonderful combination of traits, but in themselves they will not guarantee success in a dental office.

Someone will say: "The ability to understand the patient is the missing ingredient in the office success equation." This is only half correct, if that. The missing ingredients include (1) understanding the patient, (2) understanding oneself, and (3) understanding one's colleagues and co-workers. Perhaps the term *understanding* is too strong, for it is usually sufficient if one "wants to understand" and then if one "tries to understand."

The dental hygienist and her dentist cannot take the time to become philosophers, psychologists, psychiatrists, counselors, and public relations experts, but they must be a "junior-grade version" of each of them. When the dental hygienist reading this textbook was first making application to dental hygiene school, probably someone asked her: "Why did you choose dental hygiene for a career?" She may have answered in any number of ways, such as:

1. Because of its prestige
2. Because of the financial benefits
3. Because a health service can be rendered
4. Because of working with people

Some students become so consumed with the responsibility of passing courses and getting grades that they forget what their original reason was. Instead, each should be developing new and better reasons for wanting to enter a dental hygiene practice. Each should be crystallizing a philosophy of what she believes in and what she stands for.

It would be well for a dental hygiene student to define periodically what she thinks that a dental hygienist is, and also what a dentist is. The very way in which she will phrase her definitions will give a clue as to whether she understands what the profession stands for, and it will provide a prediction as to whether she will make a success of this career.

Someone has said: "Everyone has his own philosophy of life." Perhaps it should better be said: "Everyone should have a philosophy of life if they expect to succeed," for we know that there are many persons who have never given a moment's consideration to what they believe in and,

as a result, they wander aimlessly from one job to another.

There are many sample questions that one can ask herself in starting to arrive at a personal philosophy. For example, every dental hygienist should have her own personal idea of:

1. What is a patient?
2. What is your concept of "health" and "healthy"?
3. What is your responsibility to your patient?
4. When can you ignore your patient?
5. What loyalty do you owe to your doctor?

Such items could never be used in an examination for the responses could never be graded. No matter what a person were to answer, it would be "right" for that person. Also, what might be right for that person would not necessarily be right for everyone else.

Building and creating a philosophy is an exercise in thinking, in remembering, in association, in projection, in relating. It compels the dental hygienist to give meaning to her career and identity to her role in that professional career. The professional person who is concerned about her career, her patients, her employer, and her colleagues is bound to be more effective and more successful than the dental hygienist who takes her career for granted and who feels that the public owes her a living.

How many dental hygienists have ever stopped to ask themselves questions such as the following?

1. Give specific reasons why five of your patients come to the office.
2. Describe how each has accepted instruction on home mouth care.
3. Describe what you know about the home environment of each patient.
4. Describe the overall health condition of each patient and how each patient accepts or evaluates it.
5. Describe special fears or trigger points that each patient has acquired.

6. Describe special technics or methods that you have used successfully in obtaining the attention and/or cooperation of each patient.
7. Describe those technics or methods that you have tried but that you feel have failed and why.
8. Describe those personality or attitudinal factors in each patient that you have observed changed in intensity or direction on various office visits. Describe to what you attribute these changes, and choose some items of your own manufacture and design.

The next few paragraphs give some additional thoughts that the dental hygienist should ask herself as she learns to understand herself and her patients.

Have you ever wondered what constitutes an "easy patient"? Have you ever decided that it is your own attitude and worries on a particular day that make the reactions of your patients seem to change? Are there days or parts of days when you feel that it is the attitude and the approach of your dentist-employer or your dentist-supervisor that help to make the whole day move along better or worse? Have you been able to identify what these changing characteristics are? What are they?

How many times have you been able to detect that your instructor must have left home that morning with worries and concerns that he does not normally have? What enabled you to detect this or to suspect it? Do you suppose that your classmates are able to tell from your behavior in class or in the clinic whether you encountered problems at home or at the dormitory? If so, when does this happen? How do you "telegraph" this information to the persons who work with you?

No student or practicing dental hygienist can afford to *ignore* and to be oblivious to her own personality and attitude changes. Also, she must be *concerned* and *aware of* the nature of the attitude and personality changes of everyone around her—her fellow workers, her supervisor, her patients, and all others who come with the patients.

It becomes a bit difficult to advise a dental hygienist as to how much of "junior-grade psychologist" she should permit herself to become. For example, she must be warned against building mountains of serious problems and suspicions from molehills of unusual behavior. And she must be warned against ignoring an obvious observation and yet concentrating on a bit of minutiae. While the dental hygienist obviously can never be a substitute for a highly trained psychologist who has matured through experience, it is certainly true that many dental hygienists can train themselves to be very observing and also very analytical in their observation of patients and those around them. There are certainly times when the "expert" tends to overcomplicate his interpretation of a problem while a young dental hygienist will look for the simple manifestations of behavior and be able to understand the patient's fears or problems. Of course, it is also always possible for the untrained person to oversimplify matters. What is even worse, she may make an incorrect interpretation of a problem and hence handle it clumsily.

The dental hygienist and the dentist must not *look for* problems but instead they must be *concerned* so that when things do not move smoothly, each can be ready to make adjustments in his or her conversation and in the methods of approach. If the dental hygienist and her dentist always approached each patient with the expectation that this was bound to be a *crisis*, they would soon excite the patient and their practices would be destroyed. Some operators seem to know how to handle situations. It is not always easy to know whether this success is pure accident or whether it really resulted from a carefully planned mode of operation. Some persons think that conversation of the proper type can cure all problems and be a good therapeutic. This is not always true. There are times when the patient does not wish to have anyone *chatter* to him constantly just to be talking.

It must be repeated again and again that the operator's success is not the result of a simple equation or a simple formula. Some dental hygienist students are warned that they should not be overly talkative with their patients for fear that they will appear to be intruding upon their private lives. Obviously, a dental hygienist must be able to converse with her patients or she may appear to be aloof or even angry with the patient. It is true that the astute dental hygienist will want to choose her topics of conversation with care and must not "chatter" nonsense gibberish just to be talking. It should also be remembered that a patient usually wants to talk or to have an opportunity to visit. Sometimes this is for the purpose of relieving anxiety and sometimes just to be making conversation. Therefore, this is an additional reason that the dental hygienist must appear to be a good "listening post."

There is an art in listening. Even though the dental hygienist may not fully comprehend all of the patient's conversation, it is important that she train herself to make mental notes on what is said, for this may be useful later as she reports to her dentist. But in other instances, the patient's conversation will provide clues to continuing the conversation or attacking a new and related topic. Remember that one of the primary functions of the dental hygienist is that of being a teacher. She cannot teach unless she understands the student (patient) or understands his background of information. This requires conversation or communication.

Sometimes patients want an opportunity to put into words some of their own thoughts and interpretations about such things as dental health. They enjoy expressing themselves and even making errors in their statements so that they can see how their listeners are going to react. This then gives the dental hygienist an opportunity to praise the patient for his understanding or to give the patient a corrected view on the matter.

A patient must not feel that he is being judged, but the patient often feels an urging to express opinions so as to provide a stimulus for further enlightenment on a subject in which he has a special interest.

One must remember that learning is not the process of listening to someone else's version of a solution or an answer. Learning must be experienced. The learner must reinterpret what he has heard or even seen so that the experience becomes his own and he remembers the fact as his own experiencing of it and in his "own words."

Just as learning is much more than the listening to a fact being explained, it is interesting to note that behavior is not restricted to "movement." The mere fact that a person sits "frozen in fear" in his seat is a very meaningful behavior that cannot be mistaken. Therefore, do not expect your patient to move or emote just to "telegraph" messages to you.

In conversing with the patient, one of the first things that the dental hygienist will want to discover is why he decided to come to the dental clinic or the office. Maybe he came for a routine checkup, to have his teeth cleaned, because he was afraid that he had a cavity, and so on. He must have had a reason for coming, and it is important that the dentist and his dental hygienist discover his reasons for coming. First, the patient must feel that his purpose in coming is cared for. Second, the doctor can always use some clues from the patient. Third, the dental hygienist can always use information to help her in conversing with the patient.

The dental hygienist knows that she is

not qualified to diagnose their patient's condition, and yet the patients will want to know what the x-rays reveal or what the dental hygienist finds while she is scaling and cleaning their teeth. These are not easy questions to answer. Moreover, it is no answer to say: "I am not allowed to tell you anything about your teeth."

It is important that the dental hygienist appear neither mysterious nor stupid when she converses with patients. But she must be mindful that she must not try to give the patient diagnostic and interpretive information that must come only from the dentist.

In addition to asking "Why did you come," one needs to find out when the patient was last in a dental office and the answers to the following questions.

1. What did they do for him?
2. What was his reaction to what they did?
3. How did he feel about what they did?
4. What does he still remember about the experience?
5. Did they ask him to come back? Did he?
6. Did that first visit bother him? Did the second?

There is another point to be remembered before one becomes too unhappy with an unruly patient or even with a misinformed or impatient patient. Always remember that if there were no patients, the dentist and his dental hygienist would have no jobs. Neither one of them would be needed.

Earlier in this chapter it was pointed out that there may be a few persons who do not have to try to get along with their customers and their supervisors, but in dentistry and in dental hygiene it is most important that both the dentist and all of his auxiliary dental personnel bend over backward to try to understand and to get along with each other, with their patients, and with their associates in the profession. The total purpose of this chapter is to emphasize the great importance that must be associated with trying to understand all of those persons with whom the professional person must associate.

With recall patients, there are times when the dentist will not spend a great deal of time with the patient after the dental hygienist has taken the x-rays and performed the oral prophylaxis. While making this statement about an "oral prophylaxis," it might be a good time to suggest that the prophylactic treatment should *never* be referred to as a "prophy," even though this happens in 90% of all offices and all dental hygiene schools. The dentist objects to hearing about a tooth being "pulled" and wants to hear it referred to as "extracted." It is also good public relations for the professional dental hygienist to want to refer to her principal treatment by its correct name and not by a "slang expression" or "abbreviation."

When a dental hygienist treats her patient, it is customary for the dentist-employer in the office or the dentist-supervisor in the dental hygiene school to see the patient, even though it is only for a short time. It is during this brief or long period that the dentist can discuss the results of the x-rays with the patient, providing, of course, that the dental hygienist has also prompted him on what she has observed and perhaps alerted her dentist about the patient's special interest in what the films disclosed. When this question is asked in a dental office, it is easy for the dental hygienist to bring this to the attention of her dentist, who may wish to talk with the patient during that visit or set up another appointment for reviewing the results of the x-rays. When this question is asked in a dental hygiene school, it is handled in any one of a number of ways. There are always methods for handling the situation, but the dental hygiene student may not always be aware of these and hence she will need to inquire of her instructors about the procedure and the philosophy of the school or the department.

Every practicing dental hygienist should keep her own records on her patients. It is possible that her dentist will want a copy kept in the central files, but she will also want to work out her own method of learning to know her patients and how to understand them. She will probably develop a card index system or a filing system of some kind. She may develop a "history" form, or she may have a card with an "essay" report that she has written about the patient.

Depending upon the area in which one practices, one may come in contact with patients with quite a variety of dental backgrounds. This whole chapter could have been written from a standpoint of describing various kinds of patients who have found their way into a dental office. To name just a few:

1. Patient A's father forbade the mother to permit a dentist to examine their young daughter because the father insisted that the child should be treated only by a local "faith healer" in whom he had complete confidence.
2. Patient B (age 25) had only been to a dentist twice, and both times this was for an extraction. He had never had any restorative work done and had never been treated by a dental hygienist.
3. Patient C's mother insists on pampering the child (age 8) and will not permit child to have any treatment carried out without her presence. Child is known to be unruly in school and has been turned away from other dental offices.
4. Patient D (age 20) is a football hero at the university. He takes very poor care of his teeth, has very sensitive teeth, and visits the dental office only when an emergency requires it.
5. Patient E (age 20), female, was voted runner-up in a beauty contest

for a local Chamber of Commerce public relations program last year. She is very conscious of the relationship between facial beauty and care of her teeth.
6. Patient F (age 60), male, wears upper and lower partials and has eight teeth remaining that he would like to retain. He has many restorations. He is willing to schedule visits as required.

There is an interesting story behind every patient. With the flow of patients that the average dental office will have, it is not possible for the dental hygienist to make a complete study of or to write a lengthy report about each one. However, each patient is a challenge and each patient is a person deserving the best of dental health care and attention.

The dental hygienist will routinely have a scheduled office meeting with her dentist and with the other members of the office staff. However, she should also ask her dentist to give her a certain amount of time each week to talk about her patients and to compare notes with him as to what he has learned about them. This is very important to the dentist, the dental hygienist, and the patient. These discussions about patients should not be on the agenda of the weekly office staff meetings but should be done during a confidential session between the dental hygienist and her dentist.

At the end of this chapter there is a great number of suggested readings. While the dental hygienist doesn't have time to qualify as a psychologist or a psychiatrist, she is interested in many of the same kinds of special problems that concern these experts. Some of these articles are easy to read and others require considerably more time and care. But this is the kind of extra study that should intrigue the practicing dental hygienist as well as the dental hygiene educator. A great many persons have written on these subjects and their articles vary from excellent to very poor. Even this should be a challenge to the dental hygienist, for she will be able to differentiate between the worthwhile articles and reports and those that have less quality and validity.

The dental hygienist should never forget that *dental hygiene is a profession.* She must also remember that a profession can lose status and prestige if its members do not remember that they have obligations to keep up with the advances in their profession. Many dental hygienists will want to go further in their formal education and take additional courses in the university or even at the graduate level. There are many courses that deal not only with their own technical skills but also many more courses that relate to the problems of the public, the patient, and the colleague.

When the dental hygienist begins to study some of these new subjects, she will learn a completely new vocabulary. You will learn such things as:

1. Perception
2. Selective perception
3. Reflective thinking
4. Reasoning
5. Analysis of problems
6. Association
7. Discrimination
8. Differentiation
9. Evaluation
10. Deduction
11. Induction
12. Generalization
13. Synthesis

The student and the practicing dental hygienist should study these terms well, for they are becoming the vocabulary of the present and will be used more and more in the future. Unless she knows what these terms mean, she will not be able to keep up with the progress of the dental hygiene profession.

As one studies these background materials, it will become evident that the "concept of health" is composed of four links in the chain of health: Economic, sociocultural, biological, and psychological links. These four are related to one another by "adjustment" and "adaptation."

It is very important to understand, however, that the whole of a dental hygienist's practice depends upon a triangle of special knowledge, special skills, and philosophy.

It has been emphasized previously in this chapter that each person in the dental office has his own importance and significance. Each has his own personality. Therefore, when the dental hygienist considers and studies the various ways by which she can get along best with the dentist, her co-workers, and the patient, she must really be thinking about how she, with her personality, can adapt herself to get along with the personalities of all of these other persons.

Consider that each person's personality consists of two categories of traits, namely inborn traits and acquired traits.

Inborn traits include such thing as:

1. Basic physical structure, anatomy, functioning, physiology
2. Reflexes, drives, urges
3. Psyche: intelligence, emotions (undifferentiated potentialities at birth)
4. Temperament
5. Special talents, such as an "ear for music"

Acquired traits include such things as:

1. Learning and thinking—conceptual thinking, analysis, synthesis, reasoning
2. Perceptual skills
3. Knowledge, manual skills, dexterity
4. Misinformation, illusions (knowing the wrong thing is usually more damaging than the mere failure to know the truth or the fact)
5. Beliefs and disbeliefs
6. Frames of references
7. Sets of values
8. Needs, wishes, and motivations
9. Sense of identity

10. Philosophy of life, love, and work
11. Attitudes and biases
12. Feelings about others
13. Feelings about one's self, self-image, self-concept, self-worth, self-esteem, self-respect
14. Degree of insight
15. Accepting responsibility for one's acts (being able to take and to accept the blame for a mistake and not trying to make excuses)
16. Adaptability
17. Feelings of frustration, anger, fear, anxiety, security, and love
18. Defenses against anxiety—denial, rationalization, projection, regression, repression, compensation, displacement, reaction formation

One's recognition of the kinds of factors and qualities that contribute toward one's inborn traits and acquired traits cannot help but assist the person in understanding himself better but also in understanding the other persons and being somewhat tolerant of their actions and behaviors. One could easily develop a much longer list of traits. One could also attach a rank order of importance or significance to each list. And what would be true for one person's listing of his five most significant traits might be completely untrue for another person. The things that "rule" the personality and the actions of one person may be practically nonexistent in another person. This is why it is very difficult to understand some persons who are so very different from oneself, for it is difficult—if not impossible—to put oneself in "their shoes" and to try "to think as they do."

Not enough has been said about the patient and the patient's attitude about his face. If there is an explosion or an automobile accident or almost any frightening experience, a person's reflexes cause him to protect and to cover his face. Even the pianist or the violinist who depends upon his hands will use his hands to protect his face from harm. This should give the dental hygienist additional background knowledge as to why many persons come to the dental office and also why some fear coming. Some come for cosmetic reasons because they want to improve their looks. Others fear to come because they are more conscious of pain in the face and head regions than in any other part of the body.

Patients who fear pain would probably never come at all if, added to the fear of pain, these same patients realized that the dentist and his workers could disfigure them for life if they failed to use the utmost skill in guiding those disks that revolve at tens of thousands of revolutions per minute and that have sliced many a cheek and tongue by accident.

In conclusion, it should be said that the dentist and the dental hygienist owe their success not so much to their technical or biological skills and knowledge as they do to the fact that they do their best to understand their patients. These are special skills and abilities that cannot be learned from a book or even during the time that a student is in school. People and patients are not only the reason that there are dental offices and dental hygienists, but the fact that these people and these patients have complicated personalities makes the task challenging and exciting. An automobile mechanic can tune up an engine or reline the brakes, but this service requires about the same manual skill on every car that comes into his shop. When the setting is a dental office, every new patient involves a new story, a new script, a new set of scenery, new props. It is interesting to note that the dental hygienist is the first one to work with the patient and to set the scene for the entire new set of sequences, as a new and special story unfolds in the dental office.

Perhaps it is just as well that people and patients are as difficult to understand as they are. The dentist and the dental hygienist would surely never have chosen these careers and these professions if they had anticipated that it was going to be monotonous and "humdrum."

SUGGESTED READINGS

Bird, B.: Talking with patients, Philadelphia, 1955, J. B. Lippincott Co.

Bloom, S. W.: The doctor and his patient, New York, 1963, Russell Sage Foundation.

Cooley, C. H.: Social aspects of illness, Philadelphia, 1951, W. B. Saunders Co.

English, H. B., and English, A. C.: A comprehensive dictionary of psychological and psychoanalytical terms, New York, 1958, David McKay Co., Inc.

Fenlason, A. F.: Essentials in interviewing (revised ed.), New York, 1962, Harper and Row, Publishers.

Hollander, L. N.: Modern dental practice, chap. 2, Philadelphia, 1967, W. B. Saunders Co., pp. 13-24.

Kahn, R. L., and Cannell, C. F.: The dynamics of interviewing, New York, 1957, John Wiley and Sons, Inc.

Kegeles, S. S.: Why people seek dental care: a review of present knowledge, Amer. J. Pub. Health 51(9):1306-1311, 1961.

Leavell, H. R., and Clark, E. G.: Preventive medicine for the doctor in his community, ed. 3, New York, 1965, McGraw-Hill Book Company.

Maier, N. R. F.: Principles of human relations, New York, 1966, John Wiley and Sons, Inc.

Strauss, R.: Sociological determinants of health beliefs and behavior, Amer. J. Pub. Health 51(10): 1547-1552, 1961.

Szasz, T. S., and Hollender, M. H.: A contribution to the philosophy of medicine—the basic models of the doctor-patient relationship, Philadelphia, 1958, W. B. Saunders Co.

Theodorson, G. A., and Theodorson, A. G.: A modern dictionary of sociology, New York, 1969, Thomas Y. Crowell Company.

Weiss, R. L., and Swearingen, R. V.: Chairside psychology in patient education, Washington, D. C., 1969, U. S. Department of Health, Education, and Welfare.

Witmer, H. L., and Kotinsky, R.: Personality in the making, Palo Alto, Calif., 1952, Science and Behavior Books.

chapter 12
METHODS OF APPOINTMENT AND RECALL

Tillie D. Ginsburg, B.A., R.D.H., M.Ed.
Marilyn Moss Beck, B.S., R.D.H.

The dental hygienist is an integral member of the dental health team and should be familiar with the various types of appointments and appointment records. She will be particularly concerned with preventive procedures for patients because of her interest in providing measures for maintaining optimum oral health. It is imperative that the dental hygienist give utmost consideration to the patient through effective appointment planning and control.

APPOINTMENT CONTROL

Appointment control is the daily management of the scheduling of patients who will visit the dental office. It should facilitate a continuing flow of patients through the office, providing effective and efficient preventive maintenance for the greatest number of the population. It also serves to reduce undue emotional tension and physical stress for the patient and the members of the dental health team. Appointment control begins with the effective administration of the appointment book. If appointment control is to be effective, certain basic policies should be instituted and conscientiously followed.

1. The basic premise for effective appointment control should be the education of the patient through preventive maintenance programs.

2. Appointments should be controlled by one person who has full responsibility for all reservations, and the appointment book should remain at this person's desk and not in full view of the patient.

Appointment books

There are several types of appointment books available to members of the dental profession. The type of book to be selected will depend upon the policies of the particular dental office and the members of the dental health team for whom appointments must be scheduled. It is desirable that the appointment book show the schedule for all those who will provide a dental health service. However, a separate appointment book may be maintained for the hygienist.

Appointment books are usually organized on a yearly basis and may be bound or of the looseleaf type. The advantage of the looseleaf type of appointment schedule is that pages can be added as needed; at the end of the year this eliminates handling two appointment books, and the pages can be easily removed for changes or copying purposes.

Appointment books are usually arranged so that the entire week is shown at one glance (Fig. 12-1). The daily division of time in an appointment schedule will be

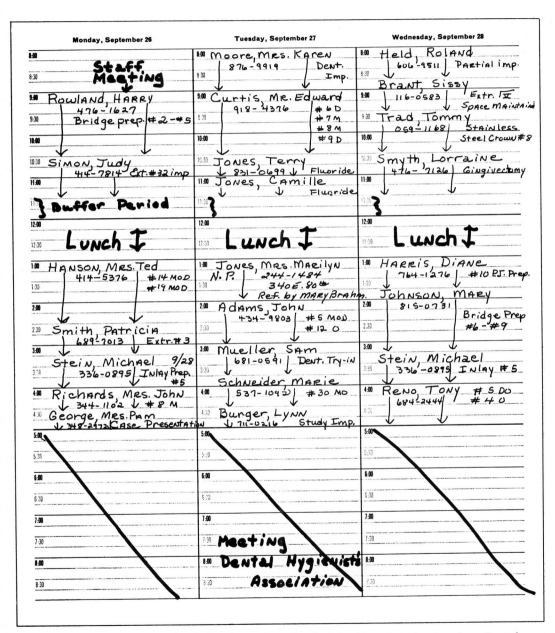

Fig. 12-1. Appointment book showing a 1-week schedule. (Copyright by American Dental Association. Reprinted by permission.)

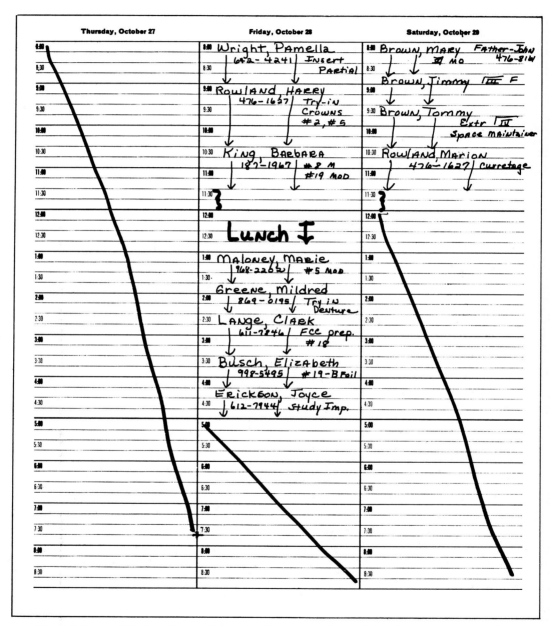

Fig. 12-1, cont'd. Appointment book showing a 1-week schedule. (Copyright by American Dental Association. Reprinted by permission.)

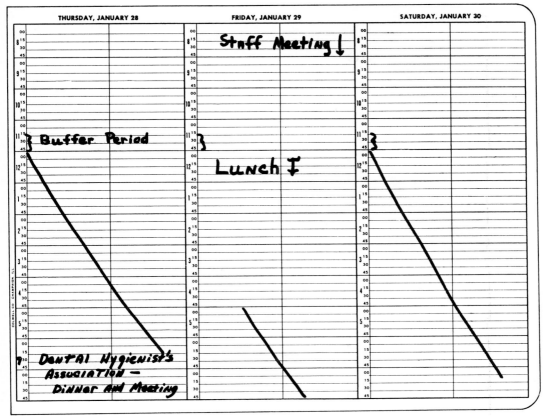

Fig. 12-2. Appointment book blocked off. (Courtesy Colwell Co., Champaign, Ill.)

arranged on an hourly basis subdivided into 15- to 30-minute intervals. The 15-minute arrangement is a very satisfactory one, since each 15 minutes can be considered a unit of time. Appointments are reserved according to the number of units required rather than the number of minutes. A reservation of one unit does not appear as insignificant as a reservation of 15 minutes.

Blocking off the appointment book. The person in charge of the appointment book is responsible to indicate clearly in advance the time not available for the routine scheduling of patients. A brightly colored pen or pencil may be used to block off lunch hours, buffer time, staff meetings, professional meetings, legal holi-

days, and vacations (Fig. 12-2). Buffer time is that period during the working day that is reserved for flexibility in the schedule and unforeseen situations that may arise in providing preventive care. Buffer time may be arranged in various ways. Ideally it would consist of two units of time both in the morning and in the afternoon, preferably at the end of each scheduling session. If there is only one buffer period per day, it should be scheduled immediately before or after lunch. The dental hygienist should have a buffer period in her daily schedule. This time would be reserved for the following situations:

1. For patients who need to be evaluated on their progress in home care

and for the follow-through on patient counseling, for example, plaque control programs

2. For patients who need additional time to complete a prophylaxis or whom the dentist wishes the dental hygienist to see immediately

Recording appointments. When recording reservation time for the patient, certain pertinent information should be considered. All appointments should be printed in pencil to permit erasure and rescheduling. The patient's full name is recorded on the appointment schedule, preferably last name first, which facilitates reading the schedule and removing filed records. The patient's telephone number should always be indicated. If the time reserved is for a new patient, the address and the name of the individual who referred the patient to the office should also be recorded. There are some appointment schedules that allow space next to the patient's name for the service rendered. When such an arrangement is not provided, this information may be entered immediately below the patient's name. The length of the appointment will be indicated by drawing a vertical arrow through the appropriate number of units of time. If there is a series of appointments, the dates of the next reservations should be recorded opposite each previous appointment for quick reference (Fig. 12-1).

Considerations in making appointments

There are several important factors to be kept in mind in maintaining appointment control.

1. Time reserved with the dental hygienist must be sufficient to allow for the necessary preventive maintenance procedures.
2. Morning appointments should be reserved for those procedures for which the operator and the patient must be at their best. This time is especially good for the child patient.

3. If possible, the appointment should be scheduled on the most convenient day and at the best time for the patient.
4. When it is necessary to schedule a series of appointments, an effort should be made to provide continuity on days and time of appointments.
5. Greater efficiency in appointment control can be rendered when:
   a. There is a standard office policy regarding units of time reserved for new patients.
   b. Time alloted for preventive maintenance procedures is recorded on the patient's records for ready reference.
   c. Patients needing extensive dental care have appointment planning that will include the treatment plan (Fig. 12-3).
   d. If the patient needs only one or two appointments, the dentist or dental hygienist indicates this before the patient leaves the chair. "Routing slips" may be kept in each operatory for completion for the appointment control desk (Fig. 12-4).

Appointment confirmations

Appointment cards or slips must be given to every patient who reserves future time while in the office. For patients who contact the office by phone, an appointment form should be mailed immediately following the telephone conversation. There are many types of appointment cards or forms in a variety of colors available to the dental profession. Colored cards are easily noticed by the patient, and the office will be identified by the color of the appointment card. Pads of appointment confirmations may be used in which a carbon copy of each appointment will remain in the office.

All appointment confirmations should in-

TREATMENT PLANNING FORM

PATIENT _Smith, Mrs. Robert S._

PREFERRED DAY _Mon. or Wed._   TIME _Mornings (Late)_

TREATMENT PLANNED	UNITS REQUIRED	APPOINTMENT	
Study Models Proph, Radiographs	6	8/20	10:30 A.M.
Consultation	2	8/22	10:30 A.M.
Preventive Program	4	8/24	10:30 A.M.
" "	2	8/29	10:30 A.M.
" "	2	8/31	10:30 A.M.

Fig. 12-3. Treatment planning form.

Smith, Mrs. Martin			
PREVIOUS BALANCE	NAME		

Please present this slip to receptionist before leaving office.

SERVICES RENDERED

EXAMINATION			
X-RAY			
EXTRACTION			
CLEANING			
FILLING			
BRIDGE			
DENTURE			
Brushing and Flossing Instr.		20 —	
TOTAL		$ 20 —	

N⁰ 17094   NEXT APPOINTMENT _Hyg. 2 units_

Fig. 12-4. Routing slip. (Courtesy Control-O-Fax.)

APPOINTMENT

FOR M _____

_____ AT _____ O'CLOCK

Dr. Robert H. Harder

DENTIST

MAYFAIR PROFESSIONAL BLDG.   TELEPHONE
2500 N. MAYFAIR RD.   476-7105
WAUWATOSA, WIS. 53226   BY APPOINTMENT

IF UNABLE TO KEEP THIS APPOINTMENT KINDLY GIVE US TWENTY-FOUR HOURS NOTICE, OTHERWISE A CHARGE WILL BE MADE FOR TIME RESERVED.

Fig. 12-5. Appointment confirmation or verification. (Courtesy Dr. R. H. Harder, Wauwatosa, Wis.)

dicate the dentist's name, address, telephone number, patient's name, the day, and the date and time of the next reservation. There should be an indication of the office policy regarding changed or broken reservations (Fig. 12-5). Some forms will have space for indicating more than one appointment.

Appointment reminders

To maintain an efficient appointment control, emphasis must be placed on handling the patient who is late or who disappoints. A review of the patient's orientation and follow-through to the preventive maintenance program is indicated.

Office policy and patient preference should dictate the method by which pa-

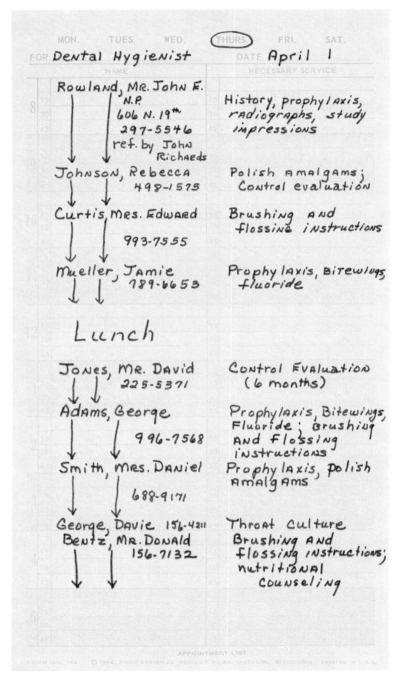

Fig. 12-6. Daily or appointment schedule. (Courtesy Professional Budget Plan, Madison, Wis.)

tients are reminded of their appointments. Postcards or telephone communication may be used. It is advisable to remind the patient 24 to 48 hours prior to the appointment; some patients prefer to be called shortly before the reservation.

Daily schedules

Effective appointment control requires that the reception desk, office, laboratory, and each operatory have a complete record of the appointments for that particular day. Each member of the dental health team should be aware of the schedules of the other members. If a looseleaf type of appointment book is used and a copying machine is available in the office, the daily schedules may be quickly made, or the schedules may be typed with the necessary carbons. These daily schedules will be posted in all the working areas (Fig. 12-6).

Emergency lists

For effective appointment control it is advisable to have a list of those patients who may be called to come and fill changed and/or broken reservations. The list will include the patient's name and telephone number, procedures and time needed, and preferred time for the patient. Patients who can be called on short notice may be indicated by checking their name with a red pencil. Two emergency types of lists may be maintained—the call list and the waiting list. The call list would indicate those patients who can be called on short notice; the waiting list would be for those patients who desire an earlier date or who have made a request that cannot be handled during the buffer period.

PREVENTIVE MAINTENANCE PROGRAMS

Our modern scientific knowledge provides the dental health team with the ability and responsibility to offer total preventive maintenance programs. These programs should reduce not only the incidence of oral disease but also ensure that dentistry is a basic human right.

The dentist who accepts a patient becomes responsible to provide that patient with dental care and preventive measures that will ensure optimum oral health. Traditionally, a recall system has been a methodical procedure whereby the patient has received periodic and systematic treatment. Often the emphasis of these programs has been placed more on the technical skills than on educational aspects.

The term *preventive maintenance programs* will be used to denote all preventive measures available to the patient. Preventive maintenance dictates a continuous on-going program and is all-encompassing. A recall program is a methodical means to schedule patients for periodic evaluation according to their individual needs.

Once the patient has been established on preventive maintenance and has demonstrated the effective follow-through of the control program, he is then scheduled for routine maintenance evaluations.

The preventive maintenance program encompasses all patients in the dental practice. Evaluation of the following is included:
1. Plaque control
2. Hard and soft oral tissues
3. Restorative and replacement dentistry
4. Occlusion/malocclusion
5. Diet and nutrition

Upon ascertaining that the patient has demonstrated his successful involvement in the preventive program, his name is then placed on a recall program.

Types of recall programs

It is difficult to indicate which type of recall program will be the most effective for any one office. This will depend upon the type of practice, the personnel in the office, and the accuracy of the recall records maintained.

Advanced scheduling. At the time of the

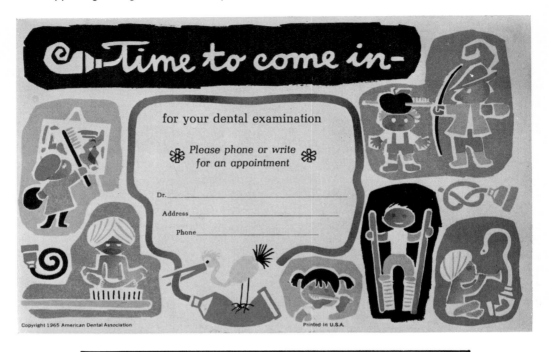

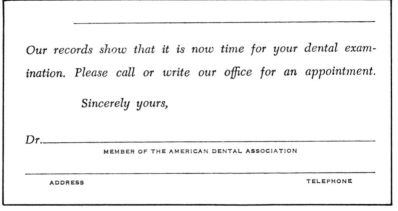

Fig. 12-7. Two types of recall cards. (Copyright by American Dental Association. Reprinted by permission.)

completion of the preventive maintenance procedures, the patient is given a definite reservation for the next evaluation. In this program patients must be reminded of their appointment by either postcard or telephone, depending upon the office's policy of notification. A double postcard may be used as a reminder. In some of-

fices, the patient addresses the card to himself. The card is then placed with the patient's recall record until 3 to 5 days before the appointment and then mailed. The patient will be quite surprised to receive his recall reservation addressed in his own handwriting.

The advanced scheduling recall could

prove to be the most effective program. However, the appointment book may become completely scheduled as far as 6 months in advance. Solid scheduling presents a problem in case of any change or illness in the office personnel, especially the dental hygienist; this reinforces the necessity for buffer time in the dental hygienist's schedule.

Letter or postcard recall. In the letter type of recall program, patients are notified, either by form letter or postcard, that it is time for them to make an appointment for evaluation of their oral health (Fig. 12-7). This may put the responsibility of arranging for the appointment on the patient and is therefore not consistent with the philosophy of a preventive maintenance program. This method may be the least effective in terms of response, but it is also the least time consuming for the office personnel. A definite appointment could be included with the recall message to avoid placing all the responsibility of the reservation on the patient. The reservation would be determined from the patient's recall record, where the patient has indicated his preference of day and time. A double postcard may be used. One card could relay the recall message with a given reservation; the other card would indicate the patient's confirmation of the appointment and would be mailed to the dental office by the patient.

Telephone recall. In the telephone recall the patient is contacted by telephone by the dental office and a definite appointment arranged. This method can be effective for the following reasons:

1. Verbal communication is immediate.
2. The dental office has the opportunity for further reinforcement of benefits the patient will receive in following the program.
3. Misunderstandings can be handled at this time.

For this method to function with maxi-mum efficiency, ample time and personnel must be available.

Recall records

No matter what type of recall program is established, its success will depend upon the orderliness and accuracy of the office personnel who maintain the recall records.

Double-file or cross-reference recall record. The double-file or cross-reference system has been found to be one of the most efficient and can be used for all types of recall programs. Under the double-file system, one card is filed alphabetically by the patient's name and the second card is filed under the month in which the patient is to be recalled.

The card in the alphabetical file should contain the following information: patient's name, home and business addresses, telephone number, and remarks concerning the day of the week and the time of day most suitable for dental appointments, the type of reminder desired (card, telephone call, or both), a record of previous preventive maintenance appointments, reasons for recall, and desirable recall time.

The other card, filed according to the month in which the patient is to be recalled, contains the patient's name, the method by which he is to be notified, and the exact appointments that may have been given previously (Fig. 12-8). Depending on the policy of the office, but usually a month in advance, the recall records are reviewed using the chronological file.

1. When recall appointments have been recorded at the time of the previous visit, double postcards are mailed.
2. If definite appointments are to be scheduled, they are recorded in the appointment book at this time and a double postcard is prepared for mailing.
3. Recall form letters are prepared for each patient when this method is being used.
4. For those recalls requiring telephone

Smith, Miss Nancy
340 North 72nd Street

Date of Next Recall

Sept. 1973 ✓
MAR. 1974 ✓
Sept. 1974

A

B

NAME *Smith, Miss Nancy*

ADDRESS *340 North 72 Nd St.* TELEPHONE *746·2448*

RECALL FREQUENCY *6 months* UNITS REQUIRED *3*

PREFERRED DAY *Tuesdays* TIME *Afternoons*

COMMENTS

NOTIFICATION	DATE OF APPT.	SERVICE
	9-6-73	*Prophylaxis, Radiographs*
	9-13-73	*Instr. - Brushing, flossing*
	9-15-73	" " "
2-1-74	*3-6-74*	*Control Evaluation*
3-15-74	*9-15-74*	*Prophylaxis, Bitewings*

Fig. 12-8. Double-file or cross-reference recall records. **A,** The card with the name and address of the patient is to be filed alphabetically. **B,** The record with the pertinent recall information is to be filed chronologically by months.

calls, the card will be pulled at the time of the call.

No matter what type of recall program is used, a note is made on the recall record giving the date of notification of recall or reminder and/or appointment.

At the time of the recall appointment both the alphabetical and chronological cards are removed from the file. On the alphabetical card, the date, service, and any pertinent information regarding the evaluation are recorded. The date of the next recall will be indicated on the chronological card and refiled. This card is refiled according to the month in which the patient will again be recalled.

Periodically the recall records that have not been removed from the present month's file must be examined to determine the patient's recall status. If the patient has a

---

I understand the benefits of the preventive program in Dr. Smith's office.

I do/I do not wish to continue this program.

Name _____ Date _____

---

definite appointment at a later date the recall card can be tagged to so indicate. For those people who have failed to respond or keep their appointment, postcards may be used to determine the patient's intentions regarding the preventive program. A postcard can be sent to be completed by the patient and returned to the dental office. The message could read as shown above. If time permits, a telephone call might be preferred, since telephone response is more immediate.

In addition to patient contact in cases of recall failure, it is the responsibility of the dental office to reevaluate the effectiveness of the preventive maintenance program.

SUMMARY

The dental hygienist is particularly concerned with preventive procedures for patients because of her responsibility to provide measures for maintaining optimum oral health. Preventive maintenance and appointment control are the core for providing dental health care for the greatest number of people. Many types of preventive programs and appointment records are available. The office policy will dictate the type of program and record selected. Because the dental hygienist is intimately involved with preventive maintenance, it is her responsibility to be familiar with appointment control.

SUGGESTED READINGS

Journal of Periodontology, American Society of Preventive Dentistry, Indianapolis, Ind.

Kilpatrick, H. C.: Work simplification in dental practice, Philadelphia, 1964, W. B. Saunders Co.

Mann, W. R., and Easlick, K. A., editors: Practice administration for the dentist, St. Louis, 1955, The C. V. Mosby Co.

Morrison, G. A.: In the dentist's office, Philadelphia, 1959, J. B. Lippincott Co.

Peterson, S.: The dentist and his assistant, ed. 3, St. Louis, 1972, The C. V. Mosby Co.

Rutledge, C. E., and Winsor, E. H.: The dental business office, Philadelphia, 1956, Lea & Febiger.

Schwarzrock, L. H., and Schwarzrock, S. P.: Effective dental assisting, ed. 3, Dubuque, Iowa, 1967, William C. Brown Co., Publishers.

Stinaff, R. K.: Dental practice administration, ed. 3, St. Louis, 1968, The C. V. Mosby Co.

REVIEW QUESTIONS

1. Define the dental hygienist's role in preventive maintenance programs and appointment control.
2. What is appointment control? What is its importance?
3. Discuss the various types of appointment records that will be maintained in a dental office.
4. What information should be recorded for every appointment that is made?
5. What information should be recorded for a new patient?
6. For whom should morning appointments be reserved?
7. How can the dental office avoid broken appointments?
8. Define buffer time. For what is it used?
9. Define daily schedules, emergency lists, call lists, and waiting lists.
10. Of what value is the recall program to effective appointment control?
11. What factors would determine the type of recall program used in a particular dental office?
12. Describe the major types of recall programs. Give the advantages and disadvantages of each.
13. Why is the "double-file" or "cross-reference" recall record the most efficient?
14. What information should be recorded on a patient's recall record?

part four

BACKGROUND INFORMATION

chapter 13

EXPOSING, PROCESSING, AND USING ROENTGENOGRAMS

Harrison M. Berry, Jr., D.D.S., M.Sc.
James E. Phillips, A.B., D.D.S., M.Sc.

On November 8, 1895, a discovery that was to have a profound influence on the scientific field and on the healing arts professions was made by Wilhelm Conrad Roentgen, Director of the Physical Institute of the University of Wurzburg. At the time of the discovery Roentgen was 50 years old.

For some years Roentgen had followed with keen interest the experiments of others on the effects of passing electrical discharges through glass-walled tubes. The current running between the two electrodes in the tube was called the cathode stream, and it produced beautiful luminous colors within the tube. The German physicist Heinrich Hertz had suggested the possibility that the cathode stream might pass on through the glass; Philipp Lenard, a Hungarian physicist, had placed an aluminum window in a tube and demonstrated, by the fogging of a photographic plate held close to the window, that the cathode stream actually could pass through the window.

Fascinated with these reports, Roentgen decided to go one step further and determine whether the cathode stream could pass through a thick glass wall without an aluminum window. Believing that the brilliant light within the tube might prevent observation of any light passing through the glass wall, he carefully covered a Crooke's tube with black paper and darkened the room completely. To satisfy himself that no light from within the tube was visible, he passed an electrical discharge through the tube. At this instant he noticed a faint greenish glow coming from a table near the tube. Striking a match, he saw that the glowing object was a piece of barium platinocyanide paper (a fluorescent material that under certain conditions can give off visible light). When asked later what he thought at that moment, he replied: "I did not think; I investigated." He noted that the paper glowed whenever the current passed through the tube and realized immediately that the energy causing it came from within the tube and, while invisible, was passing through the glass wall of the tube and the black paper as well. When held 6 feet from the tube, the paper still glowed, and when certain objects were held between the tube and the paper, a shadow image of the object was cast on the paper. While holding a metal ball, he could see a shadow of the ball, but he also noticed two other images on either side of the shadow. When he moved his fingers, these images also moved. He must have been awestruck, indeed, to realize that he was the first person to see a picture of his bones!

Roentgen took the mathematical symbol for an unknown quantity, X, and called his mysterious rays *x-rays.* For weeks he locked himself in his laboratory, experimenting feverishly and carefully documenting his observations in a paper entitled "A New Kind of Ray." When, on January 23, 1896, he read his paper before the Physical Medical Society of Wurzburg, the scientists arose as one and declared that henceforth these rays be known as *roentgen rays.*[1]

From this beginning the development of the use of roentgen rays has been wondrous, but in some instances tragic as well. Many of the early pioneers in medicine and dentistry who worked with these rays, unaware of their effects on living tissues, forfeited their very lives. We today, who use and benefit from roentgen rays in so many ways, owe a debt of gratitude to these men.

From the original suggestion that x-rays be called roentgen rays the prefix *roentgen* is now applied to all terminology in the field of roentgen rays. *Radiology* is a broad term meaning the science of ionizing radiations, encompassing radium and other radioactive materials as well as roentgen rays. *Roentgenology* is the science of roentgen rays solely and includes the taking of x-ray films, their interpretation, and the use of roentgen rays in the treatment of disease (therapeutic use.) *Roentgenography* is the art of producing x-ray films (*roentgenograms* or, as is sometimes used synonymously, radiograms or radiographs) and is the subject of this chapter. Although the production of roentgenograms is the main objective, members of the dental team must have a thorough understanding of the x-ray energy they are employing, from the point of view of both the patient who receives the roentgen rays and the operator who is in daily contact with them.

ELECTROMAGNETIC SPECTRUM

It may be said that roentgen rays are a form of invisible light. At first this is difficult to comprehend, since we are accustomed to thinking of light as something that can be seen (hence something visible) and of dark as anything that is not light and cannot be seen. It must be understood, however, that there are many forms of light energy to which the human eye is insensitive. The spectrum of electromagnetic radiations (Fig. 13-1) helps to relate the familiar visible light to the unfamiliar invisible forms. It is a series of radiant energies arranged in order of wavelength, and it becomes obvious at once that the visible portion (those wavelengths that a person can see) is a relatively small part of the entire spectrum. At first glance it also would appear that there are many forms of so-called *light* energy that we have never before associated with our usual concept of light. All of the types of energy listed in the spectrum have certain common properties: (1) all travel at the same speed (the speed of light), 186,000 miles per second; (2) all travel with a wave motion, and (3) as they travel through space, they give off an electrical field at right angles to their path of travel, and at right angles to this, a magnetic field (hence the name *electromagnetic*).

The basic difference between all the types of radiations is the wavelength—the distance from the crest of one wave to the crest of the next, measured in angstrom (Å) units for short waves and meters for longer waves. As wavelengths change, the properties change, and as certain properties become more prominent, we give names to the waves that are merely convenience terms. To illustrate: it would be correct to say, "I like the 3,600-Å ribbon on the hygienist's cap," but we have found

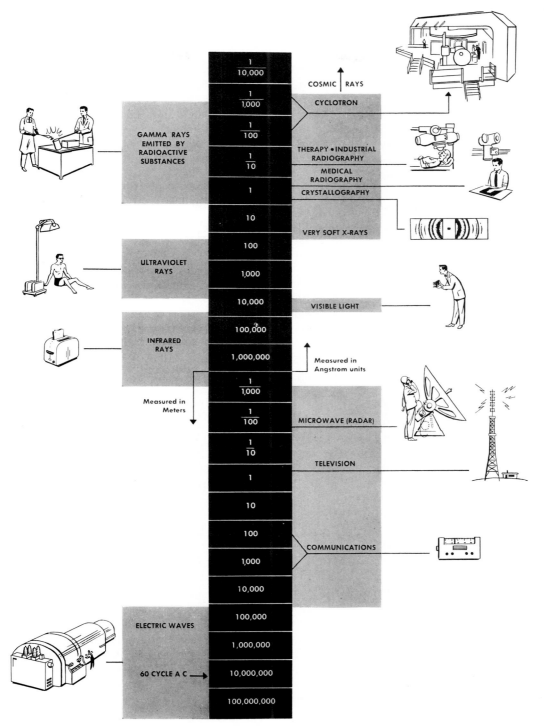

Fig. 13-1. Radiations as depicted by the electromagnetic spectrum. (From The fundamentals of radiography, ed. 9, Eastman Kodak Co., Rochester, N. Y.)

it more convenient to say, "I like the lavender ribbon on the hygienist's cap." Thus we have used the name of a color in place of the wavelength that produces it. Whenever the eye receives a certain wavelength within the visible portion of the spectrum (from 3,800 Å to 8,000 Å), we have been trained to call it a certain color: red, orange, yellow, green, blue, indigo, or violet. The order or arrangement of these colors is sometimes memorized by remembering the name Roy G. Biv, which is spelled with the initial letters of these colors.

As we progress from the color red of the visible portion to longer wavelengths, the eye can no longer detect them; however, these infrared waves are of such nature that we can feel them in the form of heat. As we pass from the waves that produce heat, we come to a group of longer wavelengths that we can neither see nor feel. These long waves are utilized for communication, for example, radar, television, and radio. In the standard broadcast portion of the radio waves the distance from the crest of the one wave to the crest of the next is as long as a football field. Below this on the spectrum are waves given off by electrical currents; one wave of 60-cycle alternating current would reach from coast to coast!

Going up the scale to shorter wavelengths, we encounter a group that is beyond the visible violet color, known as ultraviolet waves. Some waves of this length reach us from the sun and produce a biological effect on the skin commonly known as sunburn. This effect results from their ability to penetrate a short distance into the skin (they can penetrate materials up to the density of quartz), a property that the longer, visible waves do not possess. They also can cause certain salts to fluoresce (the basis for fluorescent lighting) and can darken photographic films.

The wavelengths shorter than ultraviolet are the ones produced in an x-ray tube.

These are extremely short waves that can penetrate materials up to the density of lead; dental roentgen rays have wavelengths that are shorter than 1 Å, which is 1/250,000,000 inch. Their penetrating power makes them capable of producing greater biological changes in tissue than ultraviolet light. This property is the basis for the use of roentgen rays in the treatment of tumors. They also can cause certain salts to fluoresce (the basis for medical fluoroscopy) and can darken photographic films (the basis for roentgenography).

Gamma rays emitted by radium have the same wavelength and the same properties as the short-wave roentgen rays. Cosmic rays from outer space are the shortest known waves and have a length of one hundred-billionth of an inch. Everyone is subjected to some cosmic radiation each day; this is known as background radiation and will be referred to later in this chapter.

BIOLOGICAL EFFECTS OF IONIZING RADIATION

Short-wave, high-energy radiations, such as roentgen rays, radium, and cosmic rays, can knock electrons out of molecules. This ionization of molecules causes them to become very active chemically and to form new combinations. A living cell is a marvelously delicate balance of interacting materials; each molecule must be just what it is to play its proper role. Any chemical change in a cell may destroy its normal life processes or even kill the cell. Every cell in the body contains a collection, passed down from the parents and their parents before them, of diverse heredity units called genes. These genes exist in all cells of the body, strung together in tiny threads called chromosomes, which can be seen under a microscope. The most important chromosomes are found in the germ cells of the reproductive organs, for they play the essential roles in reproduction.

It is known that genes can become altered or changed; this is called mutation. Mutation can be produced by heat, chemicals, and ionizing radiations. Thus it becomes apparent that roentgen rays have the capacity to alter genes and that if the genes should be those of reproductive cells, the rays could produce changes in offspring that would be passed on in the changed form from parent to children, to their children, and so on.

With the advent of the atomic age, mankind is being subjected to ionizing radiations from several sources. Because of the possible effects upon unborn generations, a study was instituted by the National Research Council of the National Academy of Sciences[2] to determine limitations of radiation exposure for the population. Since the average age of both parents by the time half of their children have been born is 30 years, the Council selected the period from conception to the age of 30 years as the basic period for determining limits.

The Council's first step was to determine the sources of ionizing radiations and the approximate amounts of exposure each would give in the 30-year period. Amounts of radiation are measured in roentgen units (R). Briefly stated, 1 R is the amount of x-ray energy that will produce approximately 2 billion ion pairs in 1 c.c. of air at standard conditions of temperature ($0°$ C.) and atmospheric pressure (760 mm. Hg). Modern dental x-ray units deliver about 1 R per second to the patient's face when the short pointer cone or open-end cone is used and the unit is operated at 65 kVp and 10 mA and with filtration equivalent to 2 mm. of aluminum.

Background radiation must be considered first, since each person is continually and unavoidably exposed to it every day of his life. It comes from cosmic rays from outer space and from naturally occurring radioactive elements in the earth (for example, radium, uranium) that continually disintegrate and shoot off radioactive particles. From conception to the age of 30 years each person would receive over the entire body about 4.3 R of background radiation.

Over and above the background radiation from which we cannot protect ourselves are the so-called manmade radiations.

One source of radiation exposure to the populace comes from radioactive wastes from atomic power plants that must be disposed of so they will not expose the populace. This problem is receiving serious attention, but no accurate estimate of the 30-year exposure can be made at this time.

Medical and dental roentgen rays for diagnostic and therapeutic purposes are another form of manmade radiation. These differ from the aforementioned types in that they are directed at a localized portion of the body rather than over the entire body; hence, the reproductive cells receive varying amounts of radiation. By present estimate the average accumulated exposure to the reproductive cells from this source in 30 years is 3 R. In a dental x-ray examination a relatively small percentage of the radiation delivered to the jaws scatters to the reproductive cells. Recent clinical research[3] has shown that approximately 1/10,000 of the radiation exposure directed to the face during a dental x-ray examination is scattered to the reproductive organs of an adult man. A full-mouth series of sixteen films, using a modern x-ray unit with a properly filtered beam of the recommended diameter, would expose the reproductive organs of an adult man to approximately 0.0005 R when a fast film is used. Women receive even less radiation to the reproductive cells than do men, since the ovaries are embedded more deeply in the body than are the male testes. An exposure of 0.0005 R is equivalent to about 2 days of natural background radiation. Since everyone is exposed every day by natural background radiation, the additional exposure resulting from a dental x-ray examination would appear to be relatively insignificant.

The preceding forms of radiation apply to the general population. For some specific individuals working with atomic energy and with equipment producing roentgen rays (including dentists and hygienists), an additional occupational hazard can exist, and precautions must be taken to prevent unnecessary exposure.

With the foregoing data as a basis for their deliberations, the Council made certain recommendations. For the general population it recommends: "The average exposure of the population's reproductive cells to radiation above the natural background should be limited to 10 roentgens from conception to age 30."* It also recommends that: "Individual persons [including dentists and hygienists] should not receive a total accumulated dose to the reproductive cells of more than 50 roentgens up to 30 years, and not more than 50 roentgens additional up to age 40. (About half of all U. S. children are born to parents under 30, nine-tenths to parents under 40.)"*

The foregoing is a general consideration of ionizing radiation; a discussion of the specific aspects of dental radiation as they apply to the patient and the operator is now in order. However, since the x-ray tube current and characteristics of the x-ray beam have a great effect upon the quantity of radiation delivered, a prior understanding of the operation of the machine and function of the tube is essential.

PRODUCTION OF ROENTGEN RAYS

Roentgen rays are produced when *electrons,* traveling at *high speed, strike matter* (Fig. 13-2). This collision of high-speed

---

*From National Academy of Sciences: The biologic effects of atomic radiation—a report to the public, Washington, D. C., 1960, U. S. Government Printing Office.

electrons with atoms of matter causes a disturbance within the material, which releases heat and radiant energy, which we call roentgen rays. The three steps in the production of roentgen rays and their means of generation are as follows.

Electrons

An atom consists of a central nucleus with surrounding rings of negatively charged electrons. In some atoms it is very difficult to dislodge electrons (such materials are called *insulators*), but in others (called *conductors*—chiefly metals) it is possible to knock them loose. One means of freeing electrons from atoms of metal wire is to apply heat, a phenomenon known as thermionic emission (emission of electrons by heat). Electrons will literally be "boiled" out of a wire when it is heated to incandescence (for example, an incandescent light bulb). The source of electrons for roentgen rays is a longitudinal coil of tungsten (Wolfram) wire mounted in the cathode (negative terminal) within a vacuum tube (Fig. 13-3). When current from a low voltage transformer passes through the coil, it creates heat, and electrons are boiled out. The number of electrons given off (measured in milliamperes: 1/1,000 of an ampere) is controlled by the amount of heat created, which in turn is controlled by the voltage applied to the transformer.

Imparting speed to electrons

Electrons, being negatively charged, will be attracted to a positive charge, and the greater the positive charge the faster they will travel toward it. Opposite the cathode filament in the x-ray tube is the anode (positive terminal). When a high voltage (the force that drives a current of electrons) is placed across the tube, the anode becomes extremely positive, and the free electrons are accelerated toward it. This high voltage current is supplied by a high tension *(step-up)* transformer, which steps

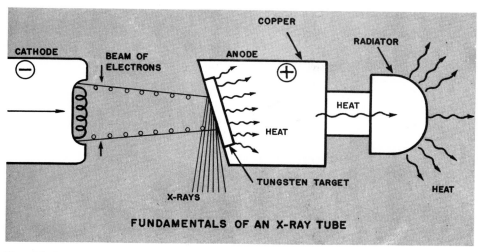

Fig. 13-2. Fundamentals of an x-ray tube. (From Principles of dental x-ray generation, General Electric Co., Milwaukee, Wis.)

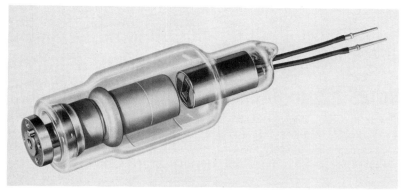

Fig. 13-3. A modern dental x-ray tube. (Courtesy General Electric Co., Milwaukee, Wis.)

up the line current from 110 volts to 60,000 to 90,000 volts (60 to 90 kVp). The force propelling the electrons, then, is a function of kilovoltage.

Target to stop electrons

Embedded in the face of the anode is a thin wafer of tungsten in the path of the electron stream. When electrons strike this target, a disturbance is created within the tungsten atoms that produces heat and roentgen rays. Tungsten is the metal of choice, since its high melting point prevents it from melting under the heat and its high atomic number is favorable to the production of x-ray energy. The tungsten wafer is embedded in a copper stem, which carries the heat out of the end of the tube to be dissipated in air, oil, or gas.

The tube and the high and low tension

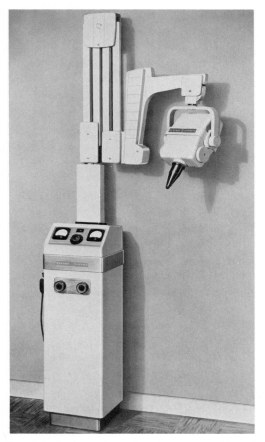

Fig. 13-4. A modern dental x-ray machine. A plastic pointer is shown; however, open-end cones are now recommended. (Courtesy General Electric Co., Milwaukee, Wis.)

transformers are encased in a metal casing called the tube housing. There is one small opening over the anode through which roentgen rays can pass, and over this is a plastic pointer cone used for aiming the x-ray beam.

BASIC CIRCUIT OF THE DENTAL X-RAY MACHINE (Fig. 13-4)

As the alternating line current enters the control stand from the wall plug, it enters the autotransformer, a device that picks off the proper amount of current required for the high tension transformer. It is regu-

lated by a dial called the voltage regulator, or voltage compensator. From the autotransformer the regulated line current passes, on one side, to the high tension transformer, which steps the current up to a high kilovoltage; this in turn is passed through the tube to provide the driving force for the electrons. On the other side the line current passes to the low voltage transformer, where it is stepped down to 8 to 12 volts. This low voltage passes into the cathode and heats the filament to boil out electrons. An interval timer switch is incorporated into the circuit that will terminate the exposure at a preset time (Fig. 13-5).

Many of the machines in use are the so-called standard type; they operate at a standard and constant kilovoltage (usually 65 kVp) and milliamperage (10 mA). Others are of the variable type, which have dials that permit variable selection of kilovoltage (anywhere from 60 to 90 kVp) and of milliamperage (0 to 20 mA).

Milliamperage

One definition of an electrical current is electrons in motion, and the quantity of the current is measured in amperes. In the x-ray tube the electrons in motion from the cathode to the anode constitute the tube current, and the quantity of this current, being small, is measured in thousandths of amperes, or milliamperes (mA). With a 20-mA tube current, twice as many electrons are traveling to the target as with a 10-mA current, and twice as many roentgen rays would be produced when they strike the target. Milliamperage, then, is an indication not only of the tube current but also of the quantity of roentgen rays. Milliamperes × seconds (MAS) indicates how many roentgen rays are being produced for how many seconds. If a given film would be properly darkened in 2 seconds at 10 mA (20 MAS), it also would be properly darkened in 1 second at 20 mA (20 MAS), or any other combination

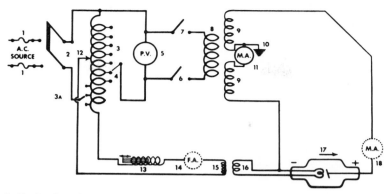

Fig. 13-5. Basic dental x-ray circuit diagram. (From Principles of dental x-ray generation, General Electric Co., Milwaukee, Wis.)

1. Fuses
2. Switch
3. Autotransformer
3A. Autotransformer line-voltage compensator
4. Autotransformer control
5. Prereading voltmeter
6. Circuit breaker
7. Automatic timer
8. Primary of high-voltage transformer
9. Secondary of high-voltage transformer
10. Ground
11. Milliammeter
12. Circuit connector for cathode filament
13. Voltage control for cathode filament with adjustable iron core
14. Ammeter for cathode filament
15. Primary of cathode filament transformer
16. Secondary of cathode filament transformer
17. X-ray tube
18. Milliammeter in high-voltage circuit

of milliamperes and seconds whose product is 20 MAS. MAS, then, is the proper way of designating exposure for a film.

Kilovoltage

The higher the kilovoltage applied to the tube, the faster the electrons are accelerated to the anode; the greater the speed with which they strike the target, the shorter are the wavelengths of the roentgen rays produced; and the shorter the wavelengths, the more penetrating are the rays. Kilovoltage, then, is not only a measure of electron speed but also of the penetrating power of the roentgen rays.[4]

X-RAY BEAM

When the electrons strike the target, roentgen rays are given off in all directions from the face of the target. These are called primary rays. Many are ab-

sorbed by the metal casing of the protective tube housing. Those that pass out through the aperture over the anode form the useful beam of primary rays. This useful beam, starting from a small spot on the target called the focal spot, fans out in a cone shape as it travels from the tube. Thus at a distance from the tube the rays in the beam are spread out over a larger area and are therefore less concentrated or less intense. The intensity of the beam follows the inverse square law (Fig. 13-6), which states that intensity varies inversely as the square of the distance. Thus at distance *D* the beam in the diagram covers four blocks, while at twice the distance, *2D*, it covers not twice the area but four times, or sixteen blocks. Conversely, a film placed at *D* would require only one fourth the exposure time as the same film placed at *2D*. Exposure time, then, varies *directly* as the square of the

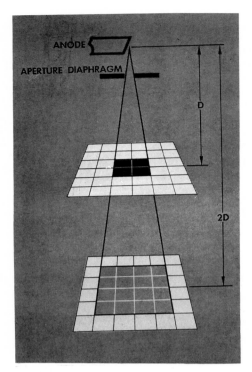

Fig. 13-6. X-ray beam. (From The fundamentals of radiography, ed. 9, Eastman Kodak Co., Rochester, N. Y.)

distance and may be computed from the following formula:

$$\frac{E_1}{E_s} = \left(\frac{D_1}{D_s}\right)^2$$

where E_1 is exposure time at the longer distance
E_s is exposure time at the shorter distance
D_1 is the longer source-to-film distance
D_s is the shorter source-to-film distance

Example: If a film is properly exposed in 3 seconds at an 8-inch source-to-film distance, what is the proper exposure time for the same film at a 16-inch source-to-film distance? The following formula demonstrates the substitution of values in order to solve for the number of seconds.

$$\frac{E_1}{3} = \left(\frac{16}{8}\right)^2; \ E_1 = 3 \times 4; \ E_1 = 12 \text{ seconds}$$

SPECIFIC ASPECTS OF DENTAL RADIATION

It has been stated that primary radiation consists of the rays coming off the target and that the useful beam of primary rays is a cone-shaped bundle coming out of the tube housing to the patient. When this useful beam strikes any object (up to the density of lead), that object will give off rays called secondary rays, which scatter in all directions. The useful beam travels in one general direction and is quite penetrating; secondary rays scatter in all directions and are less penetrating. When the useful beam enters the patient's head, some of the rays pass through and emerge from the opposite side in attenuated form, but most are absorbed in the patient's tissues. These tissues in turn give off secondary, or scattered, rays. (If roentgen rays were visible, the patient's head would glow like an electric light bulb!) Some of these secondary rays scatter onto the film, fogging it; some scatter into the room, creating a potential hazard to the operator; and some scatter to the patient's reproductive cells.

Effects of primary rays

Effects upon the patient. The effects of the useful beam directed at a localized area vary with the dose given. With small doses there is no detectable change; larger doses may produce a loss of hair (usually temporary), called alopecia; still larger doses can produce a reddening of the skin, called erythema; massive doses, such as those used to treat cancer, actually burn and kill the tissue. In dental roentgenography, of course, the dose of radiation does not even approach an erythema dose. In certain cases where a number of films in one area are necessary, the operator must know the limit of radiation that can be administered. Although the amount required to produce erythema (about 400 R) varies from one individual to another, the limit of exposure at an 8-inch source-to-film distance is 1,200 MAS (for example, 120 seconds at 10 mA) or 4,800 MAS at a 16-inch source-to-film distance. This limit is half of the average amount needed to produce an erythema.

Effects upon the operator. The operator should never expose herself to any of the primary rays. This means that the operator must *never*, under any circumstances, *hold a film in the patient's mouth.* In the past this careless habit has resulted in dermatoses of the hand and fingers, radiation ulcers, burns, loss of fingers, cancer, and loss of life. The effects of roentgen rays are cumulative; that is, a cell damaged today remains damaged and radiation tomorrow or next week adds damage upon damage. While it may take many years for the damage to become evident from just holding a film "every now and then," it is then too late to remedy it.

It has been stated that the metal casing of the tube housing absorbs the primary rays coming off the face of the anode. In some machines, however, the metal is not thick enough to stop all rays, and some get through, called leakage radiation. Therefore, the operator must never hold the tube housing during exposure,[5] for this would endanger her hand.

Effects of secondary rays

Effects upon the patient. The chief concern in respect to the patient is the scattering of secondary rays from his jaws to his reproductive cells. The effect upon these cells has been discussed previously, and it has been pointed out that the scatter of 0.0005 R from a full-mouth examination is extremely small as compared with natural background radiation or the 10 R limit recommended for persons in the procreative age group. Protection for persons in the procreative age group (birth to 30 years, including pregnant women) can be provided by lead-impregnated, flexible vinyl aprons or cloth-covered lead sheeting,

which has a lead equivalent of 0.25 to 0.5 mm.

Effects upon the operator. Should the operator be careless enough to stand close to the patient during exposure, a large portion of her body could be exposed to secondary rays. This could produce a dermatitis over the body, exposure of the reproductive cells, and/or damage to the blood-forming organs (bone marrow), resulting in lowered blood count or even in leukemia. The operator therefore must protect herself from the scattering. The ideal protection is afforded by a lead screen with a leaded-glass window. If this is not available, she must stand far enough away from the patient so that the rays do not reach her. A long cord on the timer is essential to accomplish this.

The National Bureau of Standards' Handbook 60[5] recommends that the operator in constant daily contact with roentgen rays receive no more than 0.3 R (300 mR) per week. Handbook 76 (1961) modifies this limitation by stating that the maximum permissible dose (MPD) to the operator's body from secondary radiation should be 0.3 R in any 1 week; 3 R in a 13-week period (one fourth of a year); and a total of 5 R per year.

A dental x-ray machine, equipped to function with 10 mA, total filtration equivalent to 2.25 mm. of aluminum, and a useful beam measuring 2.75 inches in diameter at the end of the short cone, could be operated for the number of seconds per day shown in Table 13-1, depending on the voltage and distances involved, before the operator would receive the maximum permissible exposure of 0.1 R per week.

If no lead diaphragm were used to limit the diameter of the x-ray beam to 2.75 inches and the total filtration were only equivalent to 0.5 mm. of aluminum, the permissible daily work loads would be one fourth of the values listed in Table 13-1 (Richards[6]).

Table 13-1. Permissible work load for operator's safety*

Distance between patient and operator (feet)	Permissible daily work load with 65 kVp (seconds)	Permissible daily work load with 90 kVp (seconds)
2	60	25
3	140	60
4	240	105
5	380	165
6	540	240
8	960	424
10	1,500	665

*From Richards, A. G., and others: X-ray protection in the dental office, J.A.D.A. **56:**514-521, 1958.

A number of different recommendations has been made over the years regarding a safe position for the operator when an exposure is made. Among the recommendations are standing at right angles to the path of the primary beam or behind the head of the x-ray unit, and, in either case, standing at least 5 feet from the patient. Basically, any position in which the operator is not in the path of the primary beam and is at least 5 feet from the patient may be considered safe. With any conceivable work load the operator's exposure to secondary radiation would not exceed the recommended limit of 0.1 R per week.

Although a number of positions can be considered safe, certain positions offer more relative safety than others for a particular projection. Richards[7] found that when the central incisors are examined, because of the symmetry of the patient's head, there are two positions of greatest safety for the operator. They are located on each side of the patient's head at an angle of 45 to 90 degrees to the central ray. For other projections the position of greatest safety is located at 45 to 90 degrees to the central ray, but the operator must stand behind the patient's head.

Determination of exposure to secondary radiation can be made by taping a coin over a dental film packet and carrying it in the pocket. If an image of the coin appears when the film is processed, it indicates exposure. This, however, does not tell how much exposure has been received. An accurate and practical means of quantitative determination is the radiation film badge (Fig. 13-7). This consists of a frame containing a film packet the same size as a dental film. The badge is clipped to the clothing and worn for 1 month. Then it is mailed to the company supplying the service. The film is processed and compared in a photodensitometer with films exposed to known amounts of radiation. A report, stating the number of milliroentgens recorded, is sent to the subscriber.

Size of useful beam

Since the useful beam of primary radiation is cone shaped, the area of the beam as it strikes the patient's face is determined by the size of the aperture through which the rays leave the tube housing. This aperture should be just large enough to permit the beam to cover the film completely; an area larger than the film gives the patient unnecessary radiation. Furthermore, the more tissues irradiated by the primary rays, the more secondary rays produced. It is sometimes necessary to change the size of the aperture by inserting a lead diaphragm (Fig. 13-8) at the base of the cone. This is a lead disk with a hole in the center, which reduces the size of the primary beam to a diameter of 2.75 inches at the end of the cone. By reducing the diameter of the primary beam from 3.5 to 2.75 inches with a lead diaphragm, the patient receives 38% less primary radiation, and the smaller area of irradiated tissue gives off fewer secondary rays, which reduces scattering to the patient's reproductive cells by 30%, to the film (less fogging), and to the operator (less hazard).[5]

There is one type of film holder (Fig. 13-9) that, in addition to holding the film and providing a guide for the alignment

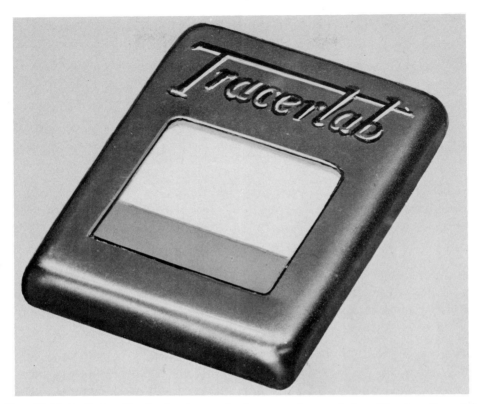

Fig. 13-7. Radiation film badge for monitoring secondary radiation. (Courtesy Tracerlab, Inc., Waltham, Mass.)

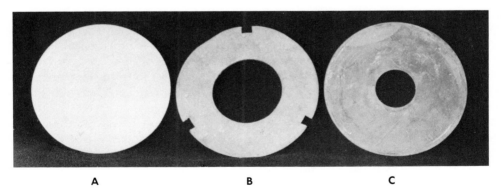

Fig. 13-8. A, Aluminum filter; **B,** lead diaphragm used to limit beam diameter to 2.75 inches at end of short cone; **C,** lead diaphragm used to limit x-ray beam diameter to 2.75 inches at end of long cone.

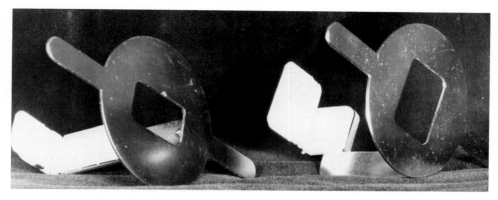

Fig. 13-9. Film-holding instruments that provide for alignment of x-ray beam and reduction of beam size to conform to the size and shape of the film. (Courtesy Precision X-ray Company, Nashville, Tenn.)

of the x-ray beam, also limits the size and shape of the beam to conform to the size and shape of the film. A substantial reduction in the radiation exposure of the patient is effected when an instrument of this type is used.

Wavelength

The useful beam is never made up of rays of a single wavelength but always contains some short and some long waves. The shorter waves are the ones that penetrate the tissues of the patient and register the image on the film. The longer waves do not have this penetrating power but are absorbed in the cheek and set up scattered radiation. They do not contribute to the image but rather detract from it by fogging the film and obscuring the image. Furthermore, they subject the patient to unnecessary radiation. For this reason they have been referred to as "burning" or "nuisance" rays.

Certain materials placed in the path of the useful beam have the ability to remove or filter the longer waves, thereby preventing them from reaching the patient. Aluminum is the filter most commonly used in the dental machine, and the National Bureau of Standards[5] recommends a thick-

ness of 1.5 mm., while Radiation Regulation 433 of Pennsylvania[8] requires 2.5 mm. This disk is placed inside the cone, covering the opening in the diaphragm (Fig. 13-8). The short waves have no difficulty penetrating the aluminum. They go on to enter the patient and produce the image on the film. The long waves, however, are absorbed in the aluminum and never reach the patient, thus reducing primary radiation to the patient and the secondary radiation it would produce.

With a slow, relatively less sensitive film, it is unnecessary to increase exposure time when the filter is added. A faster, more sensitive film, however, may require some additional time; even so, the patient still receives less radiation. The following measurements, made on an average dental machine, will illustrate the point. With no filtration the machine put out 1.8 R per second; 2.2 seconds were required for proper exposure of the film, and the exposure to the patient was 4 R. When 1.5 mm. of aluminum were added, the rate of delivery was reduced to 0.6 R per second, or one third of the unfiltered output; 3.3 seconds were then required to expose the film properly, but even with this increase in time the patient received 50% less facial exposure and 30% less gonadal exposure, and the secondary scatter to the operator was also reduced 30%.

Kilovoltage

As kilovoltage is increased, shorter wavelength and more penetrating rays are added to the useful beam. Kilovoltage is the primary factor that affects the contrast of the images on the film. Generally speaking the greatest degree of contrast is achieved by lower kilovoltage. Therefore the kilovoltage should not be increased or decreased without considering the effect such a change will have on the image quality.

Distance and time

As the source-to-film distance increases, the intensity decreases according to the inverse square law. Hence at a greater distance the patient will receive less radiation in a given time, but so will the film. Thus a fast film must be used when using a longer distance. Higher kilovoltage and milliamperage also will help to expose the film in less time. Film speed and distance must obviously be correlated for any given technic being employed.

Reduction of radiation exposure

The primary methods of keeping radiation exposure of the patient to a minimum may be summarized as follows.

Filtration. The total filtration of the primary beam should be equivalent to at least 2.0 mm. of aluminum. Some states require filtration equivalent to 2.5 mm. of aluminum.

Lead diaphragm. The lead diaphragm controls the size of the x-ray beam. The diameter of the beam should be no greater than 2.75 inches at the end of the cone, regardless of whether a short cone or long cone is used.

Film speed. The use of a "fast" film is the most effective single factor in minimizing the radiation exposure of the patient.

A medium-speed film requires approximately five times as much exposure as a fast film.

Processing. For conventional processing, if a film is properly exposed, it should require 5 minutes in developing solution at 68° F. If a shorter developing time is used, the film must be overexposed to achieve satisfactory film density. An additional benefit of minimal exposure and complete development is improved film quality.

The following methods, although less effective than the preceding ones, may be used for some additional reduction in the radiation exposure of the patient.

Cones. Open-end cones are preferred. The pointed cones produce some scattering of the x-ray beam. With open-end cones this source of scattered radiation is eliminated. An open-end cone that is lined with lead or stainless steel is called a shielded cone. The use of a shielded cone effects a modest further reduction in the scattered radiation exposure of the patient.

High kilovoltage. Recommendations for the use of high kilovoltage are usually based on the fact that the skin exposure is decreased when the kilovoltage is increased. However, the tissues beyond the film are exposed to more radiation and the rate of scatter is increased. The overall effect is probably a slight reduction in the total amount of absorbed radiation, but not to the extent that was once thought.

Lead apron. The lead apron can be used to decrease the amount of scattered radiation to the gonadal region. If the x-ray unit is properly controlled, however, the exposure to the gonadal region is extremely small. Therefore the lead apron can serve only to reduce this extremely small exposure to virtually zero.

DENTAL FILMS

A film is made of a clear cellulose acetate base coated with a photographic emulsion, which is a layer of gelatin in which silver bromide salts are suspended. If only one side of the film base is coated with emulsion, it is known as a single-coated film; if both sides are coated, it is called a double-coated film. Single-coated films are usually called *slow* or *regular* films. They contain more and finer grains of silver and therefore require a longer exposure time. Double-coated films require less exposure time and, depending upon the emulsion characteristics, are known as either *intermediate* or *fast* films. Film manufacturers are continually attempting to improve the emulsions, and they change the emulsion speeds quite frequently; hence, it is always advisable to read the recommended exposure time on the printed slip of paper included in the box of films.

Two kinds of films are used in dental roentgenography: intraoral films, which are placed within the mouth to be exposed, and extraoral films, which are held next to the face.

Intraoral films

There are three types of intraoral films: periapical, bite-wing, and occlusal, each designed to accomplish a specific objective. They all come in a light-proof, moisture-resistant assembly known as the film packet. It consists of an outer wrapping sealed against light and moisture, an inner fold of black paper, the film (if one film, called a single-film packet; if two, a double-film packet), and a backing sheet of lead foil. The lead foil in the back of the packet is to absorb the rays after they have registered on the film, preventing them from passing on into the tissues behind the packet and setting up scatter rays that would fog the film from the rear. Obviously, the packet must be placed in the mouth with the lead foil side away from the tube; otherwise the rays would be stopped by the foil before striking the film, and a blank or very faint image would result.

Periapical film. The objective of the periapical film, as the name suggests, is to show the apex of the tooth and the surrounding bone. The entire tooth shows on the film, but unless a sufficient amount of bone beyond the apex can be seen, the film has not fulfilled its objective, no matter how nicely the tooth itself is shown. A film half as large as the ordinary periapical film is available for small children and is known as the Type 0 size.

Bite-wing film. The bite-wing packet has a wing, or tab, on the side on which the patient bites. The posterior bite-wing film shows the crowns of the maxillary and mandibular bicuspids and molars and their alveolar crests. The adult, or Type 3, posterior bite-wing film is longer and narrower than the periapical film. The Type 2, is a periapical-sized film with a tab attached and is used for 6- to 12-year-old children; when used for adults, two films on each side of the arch are usually necessary. A bite-wing film for a small child may be made by attaching a tab to the front of a Type 0 periapical film packet.

Occlusal film. The occlusal film is considerably larger than the periapical film and is so named because the patient bites upon the entire film. The objective of the occlusal film is to show the entire maxillary or mandibular arch, large segments of the arches, or the floor of the mouth. It is employed to visualize the tissues above and beyond the area shown in a periapical film.

Extraoral films

Extraoral films are large—5 by 7 inches, 8 by 10 inches, and 10 by 12 inches. They are used to examine an entire side of the jaw, the skull, the temporomandibular joint, and so on. They do not come in packets but are marketed in boxes containing twenty-five or seventy-five sheets of unwrapped film. The sheet of film must be placed in a rigid, light-proof exposure holder in the darkroom. There are two types of extraoral films, no-screen film and screen film, and a specific type of exposure holder for each.

No-screen film. No-screen film is a fine-grained, double-coated film. It is used in a rigid cardboard exposure holder that has a lead-foil backing. Being a fine-grained film, it produces sharp detail but also requires longer exposure time. It is an excellent film for relatively thin structures, such as the mandible, but is contraindicated for heavy structures, such as the skull, because the exposure time would be too long.

Screen film. To reduce the time of exposure, intensifying screens are employed. These are two rigid sheets of cardboard coated with calcium tungstate (fluorescent salts that give off visible light when struck by roentgen rays). They are mounted in a rigid aluminum or plastic case called a cassette. In the darkroom the sheet of screen film is inserted between the two screens and the cassette clamped shut. Thus the film is sandwiched between the two screens, and, when roentgen rays strike the cassette, the screens glow and expose the film from both sides in a shorter time than roentgen rays alone could expose it. Actually 95% of the blackening of the film comes from the visible light given off by the screens.

There are three speeds of screens: slow or high definition, intermediate or par speed, and fast. The last is seldom used in dental roentgenography.

PERIAPICAL RADIOGRAPHIC EXAMINATION

The purpose of a periapical radiographic examination is to show the entire tooth or teeth, including the root ends and the associated supporting structures. A periapical film must show at least ⅛ inch, preferably ¼ inch, of the supporting bone adjacent to the root apices.

There are two basic methods of periapical radiographic examination—the Bisecting technic and the Paralleling technic.

The bisecting technic is based upon the geometrical theorem that states that two triangles are equal when they have two equal angles and a common side. In performing a periapical x-ray examination, the bisecting principle is applied as follows. The film is placed in contact with the crowns of the teeth and is inclined into the palate or the floor of the mouth. The resulting angle, one side formed by the long axis of the tooth and the other side by the film, is bisected and the center of the x-ray beam is directed through the apex of the tooth perpendicular to the bisecting line. If these procedures are performed correctly, the length of the tooth image on the film will be the same as the length of the tooth itself.

The paralleling technic is a method of periapical examination in which the films are placed parallel with the long axes of the teeth. It is sometimes called the "long cone" technic, which refers to the long extension cone that is required for the conventional dental x-ray unit to increase the distance from the x-ray tube to the film. The name "right angle" technic is sometimes used, too; this derives from the fact that the x-ray beam is directed at right angles toward the teeth and film.

Each technic has advantages and disadvantages and neither is perfect. Advantages most frequently claimed for the paralleling technic are: improved visualization of the periodontal structures, particularly the alveolar crest; projection of the shadow of the zygomatic process of the maxilla and the zygomatic bone above the apices of the maxillary molar teeth; and improved detail resulting from the increased source-to-object distance provided by the "long cone." One of the primary disadvantages is that for most patients anatomical conditions are such that it is impossible to achieve parallel placement of films to examine all regions of the mouth. When parallel placement is impossible it is necessary to use the bisecting technic or some modification of the paralleling technic.

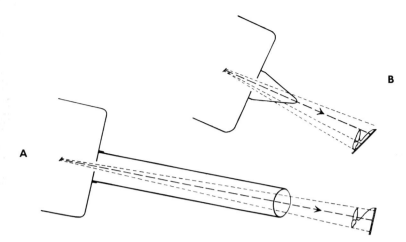

Fig. 13-10. A, Paralleling principle. **B,** Bisecting principle.

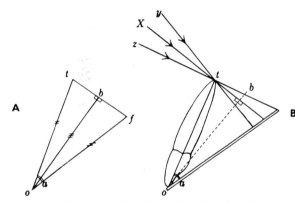

Fig. 13-11. A, Bisecting principle. Angle *a* is bisected by line *ob*; line *tf* is perpendicular to *ob*; therefore triangle *tob* equals triangle *fob*, since each has right angles at *b*, equal angles at *a*, and a common side, *ob*. Thus *to* equals *fo*. **B,** Cieszynski's law of isometry. Angle between tooth *to* and film *fo*, or angle *a*, is visually bisected by line *ob*. Central ray, *X*, is directed perpendicular to the bisection, *ob*. Thus two equal triangles are formed, as in **A,** and side *to* (length of tooth) of *tob* equals side *fo* (length of image) of *fob*.

Some advantages of the bisecting technic are: it may be used for examining essentially all regions of all patients' mouths; and, except for multirooted maxillary molars, x-ray images that are the same length as the teeth can be recorded. The primary disadvantages are distortion of the height of the alveolar crest, and, in the maxillary molar region, the superimposition of the zygomatic process of the maxilla and the zygomatic bone on the apical regions of the molar teeth.

We believe that the best results can be obtained by an operator who is thoroughly proficient with both technics. Then for each region of the mouth the operator may select the technic that will produce the best results. As a general guide, it is recommended that the paralleling technic be used for regions in which it is possible to place the film parallel with the teeth and far enough apically to record the periapical structures. When anatomical conditions make parallel placement impossible, the bisecting technic should be used.

In order to place a film parallel with the teeth, anatomical conditions usually require that the film be placed away from the teeth near the center of the mouth. Therefore, it is necessary to use a film-holding instrument. Many different instruments have been devised for this purpose. Most require visual alignment of the x-ray beam to direct it toward the film. The

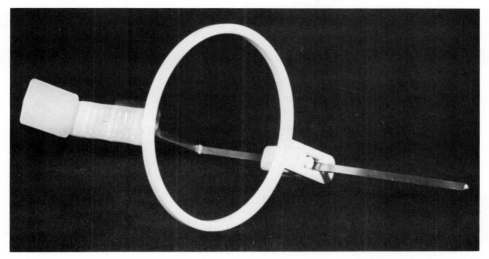

Fig. 13-12. Rinn XCP instrument used for periapical examination of anterior regions.

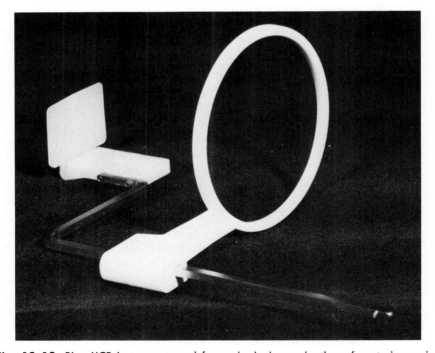

Fig. 13-13. Rinn XCP instrument used for periapical examination of posterior regions.

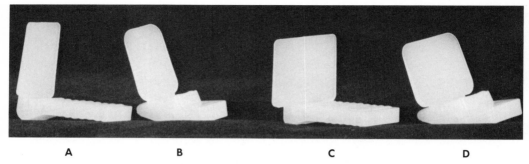

Fig. 13-14. Bite-blocks for Rinn XCP and bisecting angle film-holding instrument. **A,** Anterior bite-block for parallel technic; **B,** anterior bite-block for bisecting angle technic; **C,** posterior bite-block for parallel technic; **D,** posterior bite-block for bisecting angle technic.

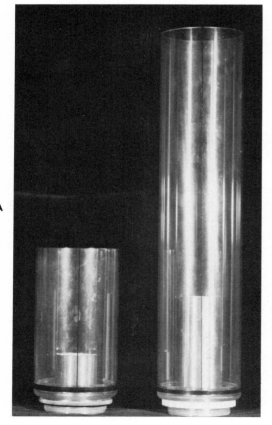

Fig. 13-15. A, Short open-end cone for use with bisecting technic; **B,** long cone for use with paralleling technic. (It may also be used with the bisecting technic.)

Rinn XCP instrument consists of a bite-block type of film holder plus an external guide ring for proper direction of the x-ray beam. The following description of the paralleling technic is based on the use of the Rinn XCP instrument. The instrument may be converted for use with the bisecting technic by removing the paralleling bite-block and replacing it with a bisecting bite-block. It is this conversion feature that makes it feasible to perform a periapical examination using the paralleling technic for some regions and the bisecting technic for other regions.

When the paralleling technic is used, a conventional x-ray unit must have a "long cone" to provide a 16-inch distance from the x-ray tube to the film. The "long cone" may also be used with the bisecting technic, although a short cone is permissible when only the bisecting technic is used.

The narrow Type 1 periapical film is recommended for use in examining the anterior regions of the maxilla and mandible. (It is also possible to use Type 0 pedodontic film for these regions.) The wider Type 2 periapical film may be used for the examination of the anterior regions when the bisecting technic is used. However, the narrow film is preferred when

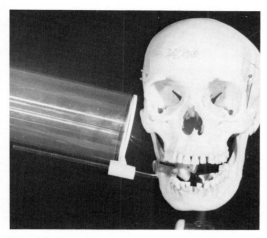

Fig. 13-16. Rinn XCP instrument as used to hold film in place for periapical examination of maxillary molar region. Also note the alignment of the extension cone to the guide ring for proper direction of the x-ray beam. (Photograph by David Sullivan, University of Pennsylvania, School of Dental Medicine, Philadelphia.)

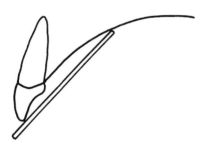

Fig. 13-17. Film placement for bisecting technic. The film is placed against the crowns of the teeth and the apical portion is inclined into the palate (or into the floor of the mouth)

parallel placement is desired, and it is also satisfactory for use with the bisecting technic. Five films are commonly used in the maxillary anterior region; three are recommended for the mandibular anterior region.

The Rinn film-holding instrument is called the XCP (X-tension Cone Paralleling) instrument when the bite-block for

parallel film placement is used. When the bisecting angle bite-block is used it is called the bisecting angle instrument. For either technic the x-ray beam is directed toward the film by the alignment of the end of the cone to the external guide ring of the instrument. The procedure is similar for the examination of all periapical regions of the mouth.

The basic procedure for the examination of any one of the periapical regions is as follows. Select the proper (anterior or posterior) film-holding instrument. Attach the appropriate bite-block (bisecting or paralleling, narrow for anterior, wide for posterior). Insert the film into the slot of the bite-block. Place the bite-block portion of the film holder in the patient's mouth and place the film to the correct position. The bite-block should be placed in contact with the incisal edges or occlusal surfaces of the teeth being examined. Instruct the patient to close firmly on the bite-block to retain the instrument and film in place. A cotton roll may be inserted between the opposing teeth and the block for improved stability. Slide the guide ring on the rod toward the patient's face until it is close to the skin surface. Align the cone of the x-ray unit to direct the x-ray beam through the guide ring. Set the timer and make the exposure.

Film placement for maxillary central incisor region

The narrow Type 1 film packet is placed vertically in the slot of the bite-block.

For parallel placement, place the bite-block well back into the mouth so that the incisal edges of the maxillary central incisors contact it near the end. Rotate the film upward into the midpalatal region. Instruct the patient to close firmly against the bite-block to retain the film in position. A cotton roll may be placed between the mandibular incisors and the bite-block to improve stability.

For bisecting placement, place the film

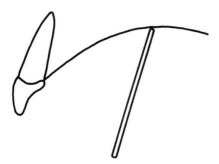

Fig. 13-18. Film placement for paralleling technic. The film is placed near the center of the mouth and parallel with the teeth.

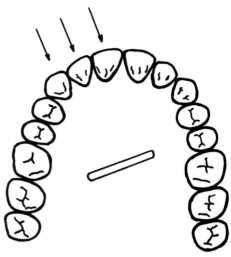

Fig. 13-21. Film placement and beam direction for maxillary lateral incisor, paralleling technic.

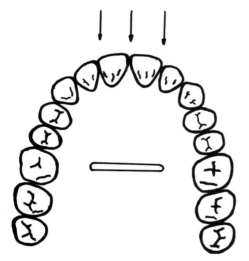

Fig. 13-19. Film placement and beam direction for maxillary central incisor, paralleling technic.

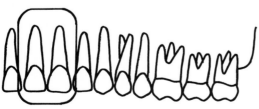

Fig. 13-20. Film placement for maxillary central incisor, paralleling and bisecting technics.

directly behind the central incisors so that it contacts the crowns of the incisors and the palatal tissues. The incisal edges of the teeth should contact the bite-block near the film slot. Instruct the patient to close firmly against the bite-block to retain the film in position. A cotton roll may be placed between the mandibular incisors and the bite-block to improve stability.

Note: The closing to retain the film in position is similar for all periapical regions. Therefore, the preceding detailed description of the procedure will not be repeated for the other regions that follow.

Film placement for maxillary lateral incisor region

The Type 1 film packet is placed vertically in the slot of the bite-block.

For parallel placement, place the bite-block well back into the mouth so that the incisal edge of the lateral incisor contacts it near the end. Rotate the film upward into the midpalatal region. Instruct the patient to close.

For the bisecting placement, place the center of the film directly behind the

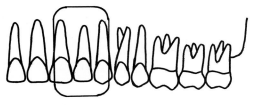

Fig. 13-22. Film placement for maxillary lateral incisor, paralleling and bisecting technics.

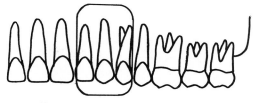

Fig. 13-24. Film placement for maxillary cuspid, paralleling and bisecting technics.

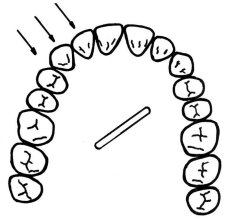

Fig. 13-23. Film placement and beam direction for maxillary cuspid, paralleling technic.

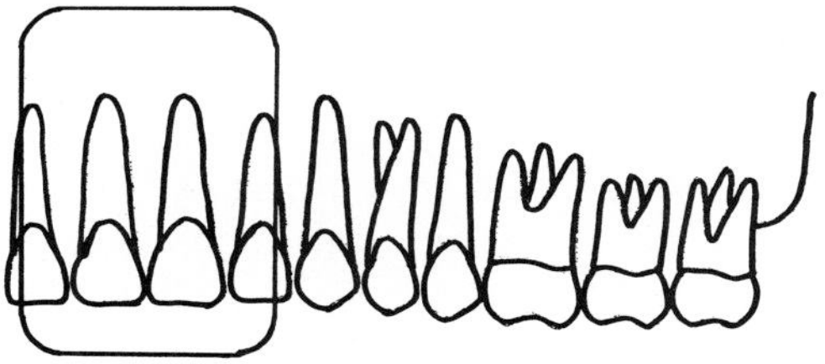

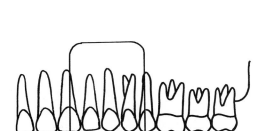

Fig. 13-25. Type 2 film placement for maxillary incisor, bisecting technic.

lateral incisor so that it contacts the crown of the tooth and the palatal tissues. The incisal edge of the tooth should contact the bite-block near the film slot. Instruct the patient to close.

Film placement for maxillary cuspid region

The Type 1 film packet is placed vertically in the slot of the bite-block.

For parallel placement, place the bite-block well back into the mouth so that the incisal edge of the cuspid contacts it near the end. Rotate the film upward into the midpalatal region. Instruct the patient to close.

For bisecting placement, place the center of the film directly behind the cuspid

Fig. 13-26. Type 2 film placement for maxillary cuspid, bisecting technic.

crown so that it contacts the crown of the tooth and the palatal tissues. The incisal edge of the tooth should contact the bite-block near the film slot. Instruct the patient to close.

Note: Type 2 film packets may be used in place of Type 1 when the bisecting technic is used. With Type 2 films only one incisor film plus cuspid films of the right and left sides are required for the anterior region.

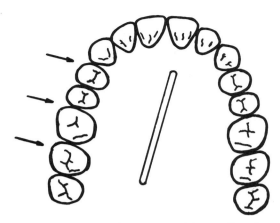

Fig. 13-27. Film placement and beam direction for maxillary bicuspid, paralleling technic.

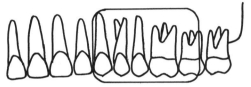

Fig. 13-28. Film placement for maxillary bicuspid, paralleling and bisecting technics.

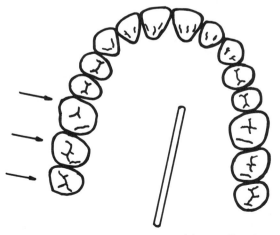

Fig. 13-29. Film placement and beam direction for maxillary molar, paralleling technic.

Film placement for maxillary bicuspid region

The Type 2 film is placed horizontally in the slot of the bite-block.

For parallel placement, place the upper edge of the packet in the midpalatal region behind the bicuspids. Keep the film well forward to be sure that the first bicuspid and at least one-half of the cuspid will be shown. Place the bite-block against the occlusal surfaces of the bicuspids. Instruct the patient to close.

For bisecting placement, place the lower part of the packet against the lingual surfaces of the bicuspids and first molar teeth. Keep the packet well forward so that the front edge covers at least one half of the cuspid. Tilt the upper portion of the packet upward to the palatal tissues. The occlusal surfaces of the bicuspids should contact the bite-block near the film slot. Instruct the patient to close.

Film placement for maxillary molar region

The Type 2 film is placed horizontally in the slot of the bite-block.

For parallel placement, place the upper edge of the packet in the midpalatal region behind the molars. Keep the film well back to be sure that the third molar region and tuberosity will be shown. If the front edge of the film is no farther forward than the mesial surface of the first molar, it will usually give adequate coverage of the third molar and tuberosity. Place the bite-block against the occlusal surfaces of the molars. Instruct the patient to close.

For bisecting placement, place the lower part of the packet against the lingual surfaces of the molar teeth. Keep the packet well back to be sure that the third molar and tuberosity will be shown. Usually, if the front edge of the film is no farther forward than the mesial surface of the first molar, the third molar and tuberosity will be covered adequately. Tilt the upper por-

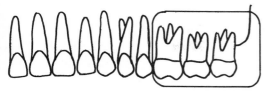

Fig. 13-30. Film placement for maxillary molar, paralleling and bisecting technics.

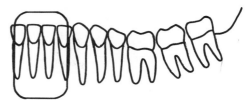

Fig. 13-32. Film placement for mandibular incisor, paralleling and bisecting technics.

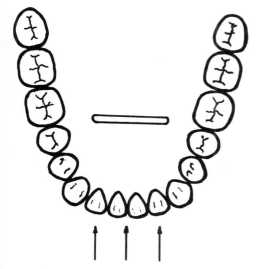

Fig. 13-31. Film placement and beam direction for mandibular incisor, paralleling technic.

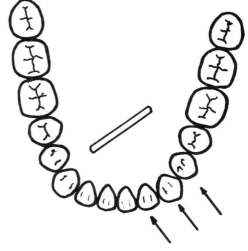

Fig. 13-33. Film placement and beam direction for mandibular cuspid, paralleling technic.

tion of the packet upward to the palatal tissues. The occlusal surfaces of the molars should contact the bite-block near the film slot. Instruct the patient to close.

Film placement for mandibular incisor region

The Type 1 film packet is placed vertically in the slot of the bite-block.

For parallel placement, place the lower edge of the packet into the floor of the mouth, under the tongue, about 1 inch behind the incisors. (The tongue should be relaxed during the placement of all mandibular films.) Tilt the film as re-

quired to place it parallel with the long axes of the incisors. The incisal edges of the incisors should contact the bite-block near the end. Instruct the patient to close.

For bisecting placement, place the lower edge of the packet into the floor of the mouth, under the tongue, about 1 inch behind the incisors. Tilt the upper portion of the packet forward until it touches the lingual surfaces of the incisors. The incisal edges of the incisors should contact the bite-block near the film slot. Gently rotate the lower portion of the packet as far forward as the soft tissues will permit. Instruct the patient to close.

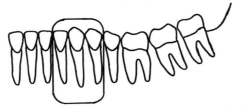

Fig. 13-34. Film placement for mandibular cuspid, paralleling and bisecting technics.

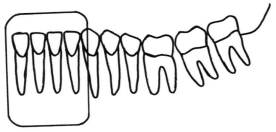

Fig. 13-35. Type 2 film placement for mandibular incisor, bisecting technic.

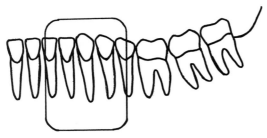

Fig. 13-36. Type 2 film placement for mandibular cuspid, bisecting technic.

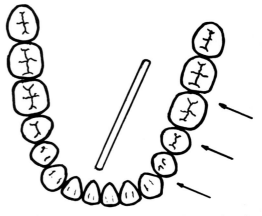

Fig. 13-37. Film placement and beam direction for mandibular bicuspid, paralleling technic.

Film placement for mandibular cuspid region

The Type 1 film packet is placed vertically in the slot of the bite-block.

For parallel placement, place the lower edge of the packet into the floor of the mouth, under the tongue, about 1 inch behind the cuspid. Tilt the film as required to place it parallel with the long axis of the cuspid. The incisal edge of the cuspid should contact the bite-block near the end. Instruct the patient to close.

For bisecting placement, place the lower edge of the packet into the floor of the mouth, under the tongue, about 1 inch behind the cuspid. Tilt the upper portion of the packet until it touches the lingual surface of the cuspid. The incisal edge of the cuspid should contact the bite-block near the film slot. Gently rotate the lower portion of the packet as far toward the cuspid as the soft tissues will permit. Instruct the patient to close.

Note: Type 2 film packets may be used for examining the mandibular incisor and cuspid regions when the bisecting technic is used.

Film placement for mandibular bicuspid region

The Type 2 film packet is placed horizontally in the slot of the bite-block.

For parallel placement, place the lower edge of the packet into the floor of the mouth, between the tongue and the lingual surfaces of the bicuspids. Move the film toward the center of the mouth, displacing the tongue at the same time until it is approximately ½ inch from the teeth. Gently move the film downward into the

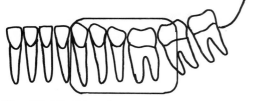

Fig. 13-38. Film placement for mandibular bicuspid, paralleling and bisecting technics.

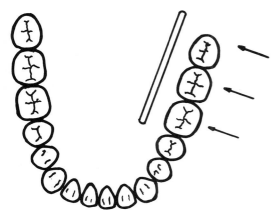

Fig. 13-39. Film placement and beam direction for mandibular molar, paralleling technic.

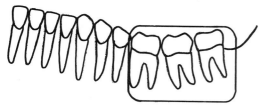

Fig. 13-40. Film placement for mandibular molar, paralleling and bisecting technics.

floor of the mouth, keeping it well forward so that at least one half of the cuspid will be shown. Tilt the film as required to place it parallel with the long axes of the bicuspids. The bite-block should rest against the occlusal surfaces of the bicuspids. Instruct the patient to close.

For bisecting placement, place the lower edge of the packet into the floor of the mouth, between the tongue and the lingual

surfaces of the bicuspids. While keeping the upper part of the packet in contact with the teeth, tilt the lower part toward the midline. Gently move the packet downward into the floor of the mouth, keeping it well forward so that at least one half of the cuspid will be shown. The occlusal surfaces of the bicuspids should contact the bite-block near the film slot. Gently rotate the lower portion of the packet as far toward the bicuspids as the soft tissues will permit.

Film placement for mandibular molar region

The Type 2 film packet is placed horizontally in the slot of the bite-block.

For parallel placement, the lower edge of the packet is placed into the floor of the mouth between the tongue and the lingual surfaces of the molars. In some patients it may be moved directly downward, with gentle pressure, to the necessary depth. If resistance is encountered in getting the film down to the required depth, move the film toward the midline, displacing the tongue until it can be placed to the proper depth. Keep the film well back to be sure that the third molar region will be shown. If the front edge of the film is no farther forward than the mesial surface of the first molar, it will usually give adequate coverage of the third molar region. Tilt the film as needed to place it parallel with the long axes of the teeth. The bite-block should rest against the occlusal surfaces of the molars. Instruct the patient to close.

For bisecting placement, the procedure is essentially the same as for parallel placement. The only difference is that the upper portion of the packet is placed in contact with the molar crowns rather than being tilted slightly away from the teeth to achieve parallel placement.

Bite-wing technic

Except for edentulous patients, a bite-wing examination of the posterior teeth is

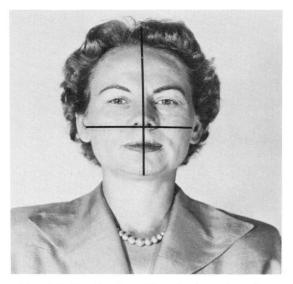

Fig. 13-41. Head position for bite-wing films showing midsagittal plane perpendicular to the floor and occlusal plane parallel with the floor. The occlusal plane is parallel with a line from the ala of the nose to the tragus of the ear. Therefore, placing the ala-tragus line parallel with the floor will establish the correct position of the occlusal plane.

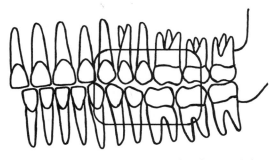

Fig. 13-42. Film placement for bicuspid–first molar bite-wing.

usually a standard part of a full-mouth x-ray examination. Also, bite-wing examinations are frequently done without a full-mouth periapical examination at the time of patients' periodic recall appointments.

The primary purpose of the bite-wing examination is to reveal carious lesions involving the mesial or distal surfaces of the teeth and to show a portion of the supporting bone between the teeth. The film packets used for bite-wing examinations are similar to periapical packets except for a tab that is attached to the packet. The purpose of the tab is to retain the packet in position in the mouth. The patient "bites" on the tab to retain the packet, hence the name "bite-wing."

One posterior bite-wing film on each side is usually all that is required for children under 12 years of age. Two films of the Type 2 size for each side are recommended for the adult patient. A Type 3 film, which is somewhat longer and slightly narrower than the Type 2, may also be used. Only one film is required for each side when Type 3 is used.

Bicuspid–first molar bite-wing technic. Position the patient's head so that the occlusal plane of the maxillary arch is parallel with the floor and the midsagittal plane is perpendicular to the floor. The Type 2 bite-wing film is "relieved" by bending the lower anterior corner of the packet over the index finger so that when it is placed in the mouth that corner will curve gently toward the midline.

If the film is to be placed on the patient's right side, grasp the tab with the left thumb and index finger; if it is to be placed on the patient's left side, use the right thumb and index finger. Place the lower half of the packet down between the tongue and the lingual surfaces of the bicuspids and first molar. The front edge of the packet should be adjacent to the middle of the cuspid crown. (It is deceptive to check this while standing in front of the patient. The film appears to be farther forward than is actually the case. Observe the film position while standing at the side of the patient to determine whether or not the front edge is at the middle of the cuspid crown.) Hold the tab firmly against the occlusal surfaces of the teeth with one index finger; use the

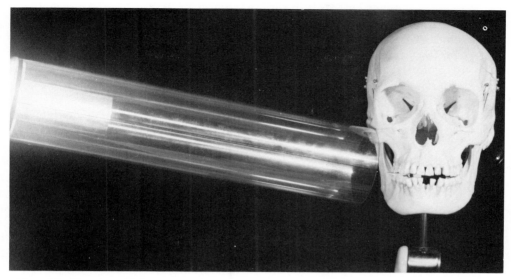

Fig. 13-43. Bicuspid–first molar bite-wing technic. Long cone is shown; however, short cone may also be used.

other index finger to tilt the upper portion of the packet toward the midline. Instruct the patient to "close slowly on your back teeth." When the upper teeth touch the finger holding the tab, rotate the finger outward and downward so that the tab is held firmly against the buccal surfaces of the teeth. As the patient continues to close the mouth, keep the upper portion of the packet tilted toward the midline until the teeth touch the finger. Then remove the finger and have the patient continue to close until he is biting firmly on the tab. The index finger holding the tab may then be removed.

Check patient's head position; readjust occlusal and midsagittal planes if necessary. A standard vertical angulation of +10 degrees is used. (The cone is directed 10 degrees downward.)

The horizontal angulation of the x-ray beam is adjusted to direct the beam through the interproximal spaces of the bicuspid region. For most patients, when the horizontal angulation is correct the x-ray beam will be directed toward the midsagittal plane at an angle of approximately 80 degrees.

The center of the x-ray beam, the central ray, is directed to a point on the cheek ½ to ¾ inch from the corner of the mouth and level with the lip line. The central ray is thereby directed through the occlusal plane in the second bicuspid region. Set time and make exposure.

For children the bite-wing technic is the same as for the adult bicuspid–first molar technic. The Type 2 film can usually be used for children 6 to 12 years of age. Younger children, up to approximately 6 years of age, usually require the smaller Type 0 film. Frequently the relief of the film packet must be more pronounced in order to accommodate it to the child's smaller arches.

Molar bite-wing technic. For the molar bite-wing, follow the procedure for the bicuspid–first molar bite-wing, with the following exceptions:

Film placement. The front edge of the film is placed adjacent to the mesial portion of the mandibular first molar crown.

Horizontal angulation. The x-ray beam is directed through the interproximal spaces of the molar region. For most patients, when the horizontal angulation is correct, the x-ray beam will be directed toward the midsagittal plane at an angle of approximately 85 degrees.

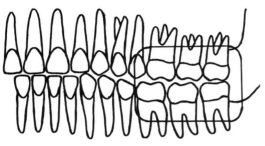

Fig. 13-44. Film placement for molar bite-wing.

Point of entry. The center of the x-ray beam is directed to a point on the cheek 1¼ inches from the corner of the mouth and level with the lip line. The central ray is thereby directed through the occlusal plane in the second molar region.

A patient who has some posterior teeth missing may not be able to bite on the tab to retain the film in position. A cotton roll may be placed in the area where the teeth are missing; this makes it possible for the patient to bite and hold the tab between the teeth and the cotton roll. Cotton rolls of various lengths and diameters should be readily available for such use.

An alternate method of performing the posterior bite-wing examination utilizes a film-holding instrument similar to the Rinn XCP and Bisecting Angle instruments. An

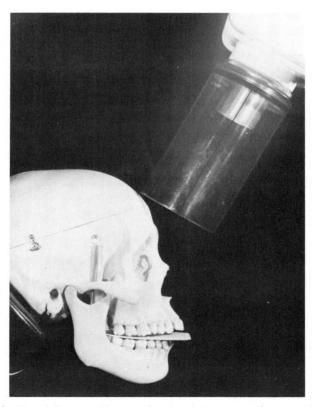

Fig. 13-45. Midline maxillary occlusal technic as seen from a side view.

external guide ring indicates the vertical angulation, horizontal angulation, and point of entry. Periapical films may be used, since the bite-block eliminates the need for bite-wing tabs. However, we prefer the preceding technic, which does not utilize the film-holding instrument, because we believe it gives better results.

Occlusal film technic

Occlusal films are the largest of the intraoral films. They are called occlusal films because they are placed in the occlusal plane; the patient bites on the packet to retain it in position. For edentulous patients it is sometimes necessary to place the patient's index finger against the front edge of the packet to prevent it from slipping forward.

An occlusal examination may be performed using either a long or a short cone. However, in some cases it is difficult to achieve correct alignment with a long cone because of the limits in the range of movement of the x-ray tube head. If it is difficult or impossible to align the long cone properly, the short cone should be used.

Film placement is similar for all the basic occlusal technics. With the patient's mouth opened approximately ½ inch, the packet is centered in the midline and carried well back into the mouth. Then the patient is asked to bite to retain it. The exposure side of the packet must be up for maxillary films and down for mandibular films.

Maxillary midline occlusal technic. Position the patient's head so that the occlusal plane is parallel with the floor and the midsagittal plane is perpendicular to the floor. A standard vertical angulation of +65 degrees is used. The horizontal angulation is adjusted to direct the x-ray beam parallel with the midsagittal plane, and the center of the x-ray beam is directed through the bridge of the nose.

This technic is also useful for taking

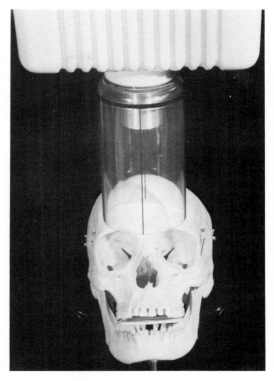

Fig. 13-46. Midline maxillary occlusal technic as seen from a frontal view.

anterior periapical films of patients who have extremely narrow arches. It is also useful for examining the anterior regions of small children; the Type 2 periapical film is usually used for this technic.

Mandibular symphysis occlusal technic. Position the patient's head so that the occlusal plane is at an angle of 45 degrees to the floor and the midsagittal plane is perpendicular to the floor. A standard vertical angulation of −20 degrees is used. The horizontal angulation is adjusted to direct the x-ray beam parallel with the midsagittal plane, and the center of the x-ray beam is directed through the midline at the tip of the chin.

This technic is also useful for examining the anterior regions of small children; the Type 2 periapical film is usually used.

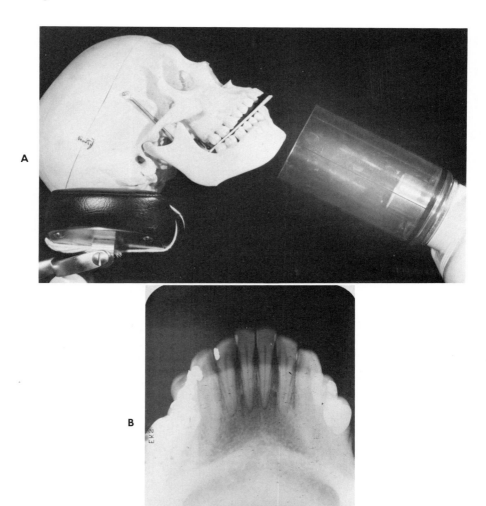

Fig. 13-47. A, Mandibular symphysis occlusal technic and **B,** film.

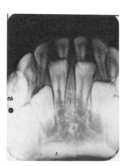

Fig. 13-48. Mandibular symphysis occlusal film for a child, using periapical film.

Mandibular floor-of-the-mouth occlusal technic. Position the patient's head so that both the midsagittal and the occlusal planes are perpendicular to the floor. A standard vertical angulation of 0 degrees is used. The horizontal angulation is adjusted to direct the x-ray beam parallel with the midsagittal plane, and the center of the x-ray beam is directed through the midline, 1 inch below the mandibular symphysis.

Panoramic radiography

During the past decade, panoramic radiography has become a routine procedure in many dental offices. At present,

three panoramic x-ray units are available—Panorex, Orthopantomograph, and G.E. 3000. A panoramic radiograph shows the entire dentition and the supporting structures on one extraoral film.

The panoramic radiograph does not eliminate the need for periapical and bite-wing radiographs. When maximum detail is required—for example, to show small carious lesions—periapical and bite-wing radiographs are indispensable. The panoramic radiograph is satisfactory, however, for many examinations that do not require maximum detail. The examination of a child to determine the progress of the developing permanent teeth is one example

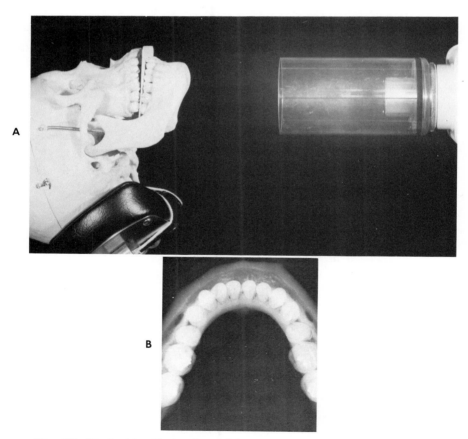

Fig. 13-49. A, Mandibular floor-of-the-mouth occlusal technic and **B,** film.

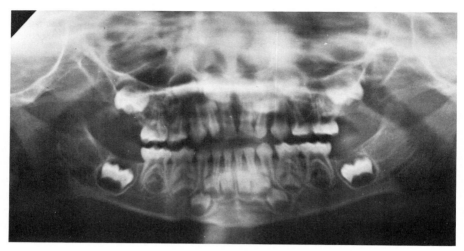

Fig. 13-50. Panoramic radiograph of a 3-year-old child.

of an examination that does not require maximum detail.

A panoramic x-ray unit is rather complex from a mechanical standpoint but its operation is comparatively simple. Almost anyone can learn the necessary basic procedure in 30 minutes. Accurate positioning of the patient's head is probably the most important single factor in producing good panoramic radiographs. If the patient is not positioned correctly, portions of the radiograph will have a blurred or "out of focus" appearance.

Some additional advantages of the panoramic examination are:

1. It shows portions of the jaws that extend beyond the range of periapical films. This is especially desirable when large lesions are present.
2. Certain "difficult" patients, such as those with physical and/or mental handicaps, extreme "gaggers," and young children can be examined more satisfactorily with panoramic procedures than with intraoral procedures.
3. The examination requires only a short time, approximately 3 minutes per patient.

4. The radiation exposure of the patient is less than required for a full-mouth periapical examination.

A panoramic radiograph, when supplemented by a bite-wing examination, is a satisfactory x-ray examination for many patients.

The film used for panoramic radiography is of the "screen" type, which means that the film is placed in a cassette, between intensifying screens, prior to being exposed. It is necessary to have a darkroom safelight equipped with a Wratten Series 6-B filter to provide the proper illumination when films of this type are processed.

FILM PROCESSING

When roentgen rays strike the light-sensitive silver salts (silver bromide, AgBr) in the film emulsion, the energy is stored in the form of a latent image. When the film is immersed in certain chemical solutions, a change takes place in which particles of metallic silver are deposited and the latent image becomes visible. These aggregations of silver constitute the black and gray shadows seen when the

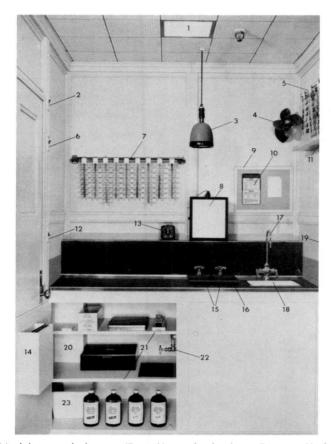

Fig. 13-51. Model x-ray darkroom. (From X-rays in dentistry, Eastman Kodak Co., Rochester, N. Y.)

1. Ceiling light
2. Master switch for all processing-room lights and outlets
3. Darkroom lamp with safelight filter, Wratten Series 6B
4. Electric fan
5. Bar for holding hangers when drying radiographs
6. Switch for ceiling light
7. Bar for holding hangers when not in use
8. Utility safelight lamp, Model C, for viewing wet radiographs
9. Bulletin board
10. Exposure and processing chart for dental x-ray films
11. Drip pan
12. Switch for safelight lamp
13. Timer
14. Open-end box for sheet-film hangers
15. Valves controlling hot and cold water to processing tank
16. Dental processing tank, 8 x 10 inches
17. Blending faucet with high gooseneck spout
18. Sink
19. Switch for electric fan
20. Chute connecting opening in bench with wastebasket
21. Storage shelves
22. Valve for draining processing tank
23. Wastebasket

film is held in front of light. The term for the several operations that collectively produce the visible, permanent images is *processing*. These operations consist of developing, rinsing, fixing, washing, and drying and are carried out in a darkroom.

The darkroom

The old adage, "A place for everything and everything in its place," never applied more aptly than to the darkroom. Since the processing operations are carried out in near-total darkness, every piece of equipment must be in its specific place. Fig. 13-51 shows a well-planned and well-equipped darkroom. The first requisite is the exclusion of all external light. Dental film emulsions are extremely sensitive to visible light, and any light leaking around a door or window or through a window curtain will fog and spoil the films. Aside from processing tanks, loading benches, storage cabinets, sink, and ventilation, other requisites are film hangers, a floating thermometer to check solution temperatures, an accurate interval time clock, enameled or plastic buckets for mixing solutions, a plastic stirring paddle, a plastic apron to protect clothing, an abundant supply of towels, and a proper safelight. The safelight should contain a 10-watt bulb and should be mounted 4 feet above the level of the bench and tanks. The Wratten Series 6-B safelight filter may be used for all x-ray films. Some film manufacturers are now marketing intraoral films that are less sensitive to visible light. With such films an increased level of illumination may be used in the darkroom. Kodak, for example, recommends a Type ML-2 safelight filter for use with their Morlite dental x-ray film, and they state that it provides up to sixty times more safelight illumination in the darkroom. When extraoral films are to be processed, however, it is necessary to use only the illumination provided by the Wratten Series 6-B filter.

Equally as important as proper facilities is the care of the darkroom. It should be considered a chemical laboratory and the same meticulous care given to it. It should be kept as free of dust as possible, and any drippings of solution should be wiped up with clear water immediately. The solutions should be covered when not in use, and the tanks should be scrubbed clean every time solutions are changed. To remove the deposits that often form on the walls of the developer tank the following solution is helpful:

Commercial hydrochloric acid	1.5 oz.
Cold water	16 oz.
Lukewarm water, to make	1 gallon

This formula is for a 1-gallon tank. Drain the old developer and wipe the walls of the tank with clear water. Mix the cleaning solution in the tank, let it soak for 30 minutes, and then drain and rinse thoroughly with fresh water. The addition of tablets to the developer to control algae is recommended.

Chemistry of processing

Processing involves chemical reactions that, like all chemical reactions, are critical, and meticulous attention to detail must be practiced. The sequence of the processing procedure is as follows:

Development → Rinse → Fixation → Wash → Dry

Development. When silver bromide salts that have received x-ray energy are acted upon by chemical developers, they are reduced or split into metallic silver particles, which are precipitated in the gelatin of the emulsion, and bromide, which goes into solution.

$$2 \text{ AgBr (in light)} \rightleftharpoons 2 \text{ Ag} + \text{Br}_2$$

Chemicals. The following chemicals are used in developing films.

DEVELOPING AGENTS, OR REDUCERS: There are two chemicals in the developing solution that act to reduce, or split, the silver bromide salt into metallic silver and bromine. These are hydroquinone and Elon, each reducing in a different manner. Elon is important in producing detail in the image and hydroquinone in giving contrast.

PRESERVATIVE: Hydroquinone and Elon have a great affinity for oxygen and, when oxidized, become inactive. A substance with a greater affinity for oxygen (sodium sulfite) is added as a preservative.

ACTIVATOR: Hydroquinone and Elon work best in an alkaline medium. To activate these agents, then, sodium carbonate is added to create the alkaline medium.

RESTRAINER: If only the chemicals just described were to act upon the film, the development would take place too rapidly, producing a chemical fog. To retard the reaction potassium bromide is added as a restrainer.

VEHICLE: The developer chemicals are dissolved in distilled water for proper dilution.

Rinsing. A brief rinsing in running water prevents the developer on the surface of the film from being carried into the fixer.

Fixing. Silver bromide salts that were not struck by roentgen rays are not acted upon (split) in the developer but remain as silver bromide salts. The fixing solution dissolves these remaining salts, leaving in the emulsion only the metallic silver particles precipitated by the developer.

Chemicals. The following chemicals are used for fixation.

"HYPO": Hyposulfite of soda (sodium thiosulfate) is the chemical that has the ability to dissolve undeveloped silver bromide salts, removing them from the emulsion.

ACID: While in the developer, the emulsion becomes swollen, soaking up the alkaline developer much like a sponge. Rinsing removes the developer from the surface, but the emulsion carries much of the developer with it into the fixer. Acetic acid is added to the fixing solution to neutralize this alkali, stopping further de-

velopment and permitting the "hypo" to take over its function.

PRESERVATIVE: As in the developing solution, sodium sulfite is added to prevent deterioration of the "hypo" by oxidation.

HARDENER: To shrink and harden the soft, swollen emulsion an alum compound is added.

VEHICLE: The chemicals are mixed in distilled water as the vehicle.

Washing. Since the gelatin of the emulsion soaks up the processing chemicals, prolonged washing in fresh running water is necessary to remove them completely. If not completely removed, a brown stain will appear weeks or months later, which spoils the film. After 2 minutes of washing, one half of the chemicals in the emulsion will have been removed. After another 2 minutes, one half of the remaining chemicals will have been removed, and so on. Thus, after 20 minutes only about 1/1,000 of the original chemicals would remain in the emulsion, at which point it can be considered thoroughly cleansed.

Drying. Drying of the films should take place in a clean, dry, well-ventilated area. Lint, dust, or dirt particles will stick to a wet film and cannot be removed without tearing the emulsion.

Time and temperature. All chemical reactions take place at an optimum temperature in an optimum time, and the same applies to film processing. The optimum temperature for developing and fixing is 68° F. (20° C.). If the temperature is higher, the developer acts more quickly; if it is too high, it will produce a chemical fog. If it is lower, the reaction takes place more slowly; if it is too low, the hydroquinone will not act at all, resulting in a thin (faint) image. In the absence of a refrigerated tank that maintains a constant temperature of 68° F., the solutions may be cooled by putting cracked ice in a rubber glove, tying it at the wrist, and floating it on the surface of the solutions. Never add ice directly to the solutions since it will dilute them and reduce their efficiency. The temperature of the rinse and wash water need not be exactly 68° F. but should not be much above or below. If the wash water is too warm, the emulsion will expand, and as it contracts during drying, it will cause cracks called "reticulation."

The optimum times are 5 minutes in the developer, 30 seconds in the rinse, 5 minutes in the fixer, and 20 minutes in the wash. Certain developing solutions require 4½ minutes' development; it is therefore always advisable to check the manufacturer's specifications on the package. No-screen film should be developed for 8 minutes and fixed for 10 minutes. Screen film should be developed for 5 minutes and fixed for 10 minutes.

Mixing solutions. Processing solutions are available either in the powdered form for "do-it-yourself" mixing or in liquid, ready-mixed solutions requiring only the addition of water. While the latter may be prepared more quickly, they have a shorter life and are, therefore, less economical than solutions prepared from powder. With either type the mixing instructions recommended by the manufacturer on the label of the container must be strictly adhered to.

The proper level of the developing and fixing solutions may be maintained by replenishing each day. When the developer starts to become exhausted, the films will come out light or show a thin image. Hypo exhaustion is evident when the film has not cleared (the milky coating has not disappeared) in 2 minutes of fixation. Rather than risk spoiling films by waiting until the signs of exhaustion appear, it is better to drain and clean the tanks and add fresh solution every 2 to 3 weeks routinely. In the average office the developer and fixer deteriorate more rapidly from oxidation than from actual use. To prolong the life of the solutions a floating cover is recommended. Cut a piece of ½ inch

thick cork to the exact size of the tank opening, dip it in hot paraffin so it will not soak up solution, and float the cover on the solution. Since the cover is in direct contact with the solution, oxidation will be greatly retarded when the solutions are not in use.

Wetting agents. Several chemical preparations are on the market that reduce surface tension. When they are added to the developer, the film will be developed more evenly and uniformly. After the 20-minute washing in running water the film should be immersed for a minute or two in a bucket of water containing the wetting agent. It will then dry much more rapidly and without streaking.

Cutting reducers. Whereas chemical reducers (hydroquinone and Elon) are used in the developer to split silver bromide salts, cutting reducers dissolve the metallic silver deposits in the completely processed film layer by layer. If a processed film is slightly too dark, it may be immersed in the cutting reducer to lighten it. This is not a panacea for careless exposure or developing technic, for the grays as well as the blacks on the film will be lightened as the layers of silver are removed; the black areas may end up as gray, but the grays may be completely removed. The cutting reducer should be used for films just slightly too dark.

Farmer's Reducer may be prepared as follows:

Dissolve 1 ounce of potassium ferricyanide in 16 ounces of water. Store in a brown bottle, labeled Solution A.

Dissolve 1 ounce of hypo crystals (not fixing solution) in 16 ounces of water. Store in a separate brown bottle, labeled Solution B.

The film may be reduced immediately after fixing, with the light on. If the film has dried, soak it in water for several minutes. Mix only as much as is needed of equal parts of Solutions A and B, dip the film for a few seconds, rinse in water, and examine it. Repeat until the desired density is attained, wash for 20 minutes in running water, and dry.

Automatic film processing

Automatic processing units are a recent innovation in dental film processing. One of the primary advantages of automatic processing is that a film may be developed, fixed, washed, and dried in less than 5 minutes, compared to approximately 1 hour for conventional processing. Some obvious advantages of this are: less personnel time is required for processing, and the diagnosis and treatment for a patient may be expedited by having the radiographs available in such a short time.

Most automatic processing units utilize a roller transport system; the films are passed progressively from one pair of rollers to the next and are thereby carried through the solutions. In some units the solutions are automatically replenished to maintain them at constant strength. For each film fed into the unit, small amounts of fresh developing and fixing solutions are automatically pumped into the corresponding tanks.

The conventional developing and fixing solutions are not suitable for automatic processing units. The solutions specified by the manufacturer must be used. Also, the processing is done at higher temperatures; 80° to 85° F. is the usual developer temperature.

The routine daily maintenance required for starting, stopping, and cleaning takes only a few minutes. Cleanliness and proper maintenance is extremely important, however, in keeping the unit functioning properly.

FAULTY ROENTGENOGRAMS

Shadows on the film caused by "unnatural" objects (not within the tissues) or by manipulation are called "artifacts." Some of the imperfections on films and their causes are as follows:

1. Reticulation ("fish-net" or "orange-peel" crinkled lines)
   CAUSE: Washing water too warm, causing shrinking and crackling of emulsion when film is dried
2. Blotchy, fogged film
   CAUSE: Outdated film; check manufacturer's expiration date stamped on film package
3. Splash marks, darker than rest of film
   CAUSE: Film splashed with developer before being immersed in developer, causing overdevelopment in splashed areas
4. Splash marks, lighter than rest of film
   CAUSE: Film splashed with fixer before being immersed in developer; fixer removes silver bromide salts in these areas so that no silver remains to be precipitated by developer
5. Splash marks, same density as rest of film
   CAUSE: Film splashed with water after being processed and dried; wash again for 20 minutes in running water and dry
6. Black lines
   CAUSE: Creasing of film packet
7. Black marks, elliptical
   CAUSE: Pressing fingernail or thumbnail against film; usually occurs when unwrapping packet in darkroom—*handle with care!*
8. Outline of another film, light
   CAUSE: Contact with another film in developer, preventing complete development in contacting area—*never crowd the tank!*
9. Outline of another film, dark
   CAUSE: Contact with another film in fixer, preventing dissolution of the silver bromide salts in contacting area—*never crowd the tank!*
10. White streaks

CAUSE: Dirty film hanger; if film hanger is not thoroughly washed after use, hypo will dry on it in powder form; when film is clipped to it later, dried hypo powder will dissolve upon entering developer, run across film, and remove silver bromide salts before they have had opportunity to be developed

11. White spot(s)
    CAUSE: (a) Dust, dirt, or particles of chemical powder on surface of film in developer, preventing developer from reaching emulsion; keep darkroom clean; use wetting agent in developer. (b) Foreign body in pointer cone, blocking roentgen rays before they strike film; remove cone and clean at frequent intervals

12. Partial image
    CAUSE: "Cone-cutting"; roentgen ray beam does not cover entire film; check film placement and point of entry

13. "Stretched" image
    CAUSE: Bending of film packet in mouth

14. Thin image
    CAUSE: Insufficient exposure to roentgen rays, exhausted developer, cold developer, insufficient time in developer, packet placed in mouth backward, or failure to stir developer before using

15. Dense image
    CAUSE: Overexposure to roentgen rays, overdevelopment, or developer too warm

16. Fogging
    CAUSE: Unsafe storage of films, before and/or after exposure at chair, outdated film, lack of filtration (with aluminum filter) of useful beam, diaphragm opening for useful beam too large, light leak in darkroom, or unsafe safelight in darkroom

IDENTIFICATION OF FILMS
Right or left side of mouth

All intraoral films now being manufactured are double coated; that is, there is a coating of emulsion on both sides of the plastic film base. Along one border of the film is an embossed dot. The depressed, or concave, side of the dot denotes the side of the film that was toward the tongue during exposure. The raised, or convex, side of the dot indicates the side of the film that was toward the teeth or toward the x-ray tube during exposure. If the viewer looks at the film from the depressed, or concave, side, it is as though she were looking out through the tissues from a position within the mouth. Conversely, if she views the raised, or convex, side, it is as though she were looking through the tissues from a position outside the mouth. The dot, therefore, enables the viewer to determine whether a given film was exposed on the patient's right or left side. Fig. 13-52 shows a dental hygiene student viewing the films after they have been dried.

Extraoral films are double coated and do not have the embossed dot. They must be marked at the time of exposure by placing a lead letter R or L on the tube side of the cardboard exposure holder or cassette.

Tooth area

The particular tooth area that the film shows is readily recognized by identifying the teeth; this, of course, presupposes a thorough knowledge of dental anatomy. In an edentulous area, however, certain anatomical landmarks must be identified in order to determine the area. Fig. 13-53 shows a dental hygiene student inserting films into a film mount.

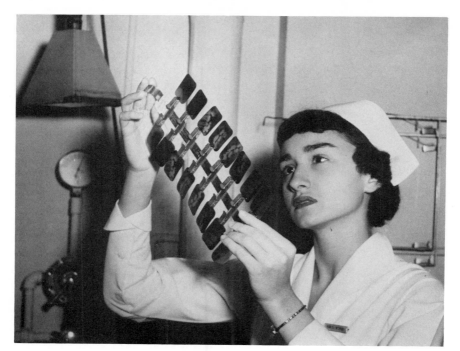

Fig. 13-52. Dental hygiene student viewing films in holder after they have been dried.

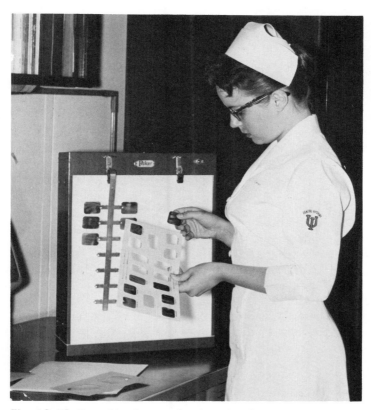

Fig. 13-53. Dental hygiene student inserting films into film mount.

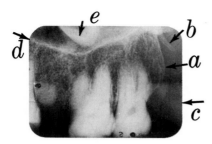

Fig. 13-54. Maxillary molar area. *a,* Posterior wall of tuberosity (of maxilla); *b,* hamular process (of pterygoid plate of sphenoid bone); *c,* coronoid process (of mandible); *d,* inferior wall of maxillary sinus; *e,* malar process.

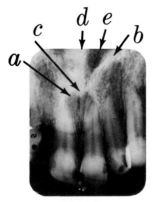

Fig. 13-55. Maxillary incisor area. *a,* Incisive foramen; *b,* anterior wall of nose; *c,* anterior nasal spine; *d,* median septum of nose; *e,* nasal fossa.

Light shadows on a film are produced by the passage of roentgen rays through relatively dense structures that absorb the rays and prevent all or part of them from reaching the film. These are known as roentgenopaque (radiopaque) shadows and include metallic restorations, cement, enamel, dentin, lamina dura, and cortical bone. Darker shadows are produced when roentgen rays pass through less dense structures, which permit more rays to reach the film to darken it. These are known as roentgenolucent (radiolucent)

shadows and are caused by pulp chamber and canal, periodontal membrane space, medullary (marrow) spaces in spongy bones, sinuses, canals, foramina, and plastic restorations.

Landmarks

Maxillary molar area. See Fig. 13-54 for the following landmarks: *a,* posterior wall of the maxillary tuberosity curving upward behind the third molar area; *b,* hamular process—a spur of bone extending down behind the posterior wall of the maxillary tuberosity; *c,* coronoid process of the mandible—a rounded triangular shadow of bone that may be seen behind, below, or over the maxillary tuberosity; *d,* maxillary sinus—a roentgenolucent shadow with a roentgenopaque outline (the cortical-bone wall of the sinus) in the area of the molar roots; in size and configuration the sinus has many normal variations; *e,* malar process—this roentgenopaque shadow of the zygomatic bone is often superimposed over the shadow of the sinus; the anterior part is usually a U- or V-shaped roentgenopaque shadow, with a roentgenopaque band (the shadow of the zygomatic bone) extending backward off the edge of the film.

Maxillary bicuspid area. The shadow of the maxillary sinus often appears in this area. A roentgenopaque line running across the upper portion of the sinus shadow is the floor of the nose and above it the roentgenolucent shadow of the nasal fossa.

Maxillary incisor area. See Fig. 13-55 for the following landmarks: *a,* incisive foramen—a rounded roentgenolucent shadow in the midline, above and between the roots of the first incisors; this is the oral end of the nasopalatine canal; *b,* anterior walls of the nose—roentgenopaque shadows curving in from either side, above the roots of the incisors, and joining at the anterior nasal spine; these shadows are formed by the ridges of cortical bone under each of the nares (nostrils); *c,*

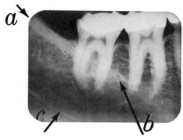

Fig. 13-56. Mandibular molar area. a, External oblique line; b, mylohyoid ridge; c, inferior border of mandibular canal.

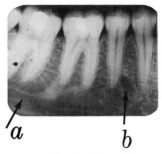

Fig. 13-57. Mandibular bicuspid area. a, Mandibular canal; b, mental foramen.

anterior nasal spine—a roentgenopaque, pointed shadow in the midline above or superimposed upon the shadow of the incisive foramen; it is a sharp, bony spine and can be palpated under the cartilaginous septum of the nose; d, median septum of the nose—a roentgenopaque shadow running from the anterior nasal spine to the top of the film; this is the bony septum of the nose; e, nasal fossae—two roentgenolucent shadows on either side of the median septum of the nose; they often contain a rounded, slightly roentgenopaque shadow, which is the shadow of the turbinate bones on the lateral walls of the nasal fossae, and are more often seen in occlusal films.

Mandibular molar area. See Fig. 13-56 for the following landmarks: a, external

oblique line—a roentgenopaque line running from the crest of the alveolar ridge behind the third molar to the middle of the roots of the first molar; this is continuous with the cortical bone of the anterior crest of the ramus and runs along the buccal aspect of the alveolar bone covering the molar teeth; b, mylohyoid ridge—another roentgenopaque line, lying below the external oblique line, which starts at the third molar area and runs anteriorly to the first molar or bicuspid area; it is the ridge of bone on the lingual surface of the mandible that gives attachment to the mylohyoid muscle in the floor of the mouth; c, mandibular canal—a roentgenolucent shadow, with roentgenopaque upper and lower borders, running anteriorly from the back of the film; it is the canal, lined with cortical bone, that carries the inferior dental nerve and vessels from the mandibular foramen in the ramus to the front of the mandible.

Films placed sufficiently deep will show the roentgenopaque shadow of the lower border of the mandible, usually a relatively thick shadow.

Mandibular bicuspid area. See Fig. 13-57 for the following landmarks: a, mylohyoid ridge—this shadow sometimes appears in this area; mandibular canal—the shadow of the canal may be seen running up to a round roentgenolucent shadow, the mental foramen; b, the mental foramen may be seen as a roentgenolucent shadow lying below and between the root apices of the bicuspids.

Mandibular cuspid area. The shadow of the mental foramen often appears on the back portion of the cuspid film.

Mandibular incisor area. See Fig. 13-58 for the following landmarks: a, mental ridge—a roentgenopaque line just above the lower border of the mandible, sweeping in from either side of the film and meeting at a point in the midline; this is the shadow of a ridge of bone on the labial aspect of the mandibular symphysis; it does

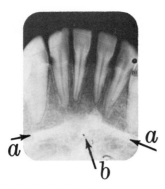

Fig. 13-58. Mandibular incisor area. *a*, Mental ridges; *b*, lingual foramen.

not always show in the film; *b*, lingual foramen—a small roentgenolucent dot in the midline, well below the roots of the teeth; this also is not always seen in incisor films; it is the shadow of a foramen on the lingual surface of the mandible that transmits a branch of the lingual artery to supply the anterior mandible; it is located between and slightly above the genial tubercles.

The genial tubercles are roentgenopaque spurs of bone, usually two or more in number, jutting lingually from the inner surface of the lower border of the mandible, giving attachment to the geniohyoid muscles of the floor of the mouth.

USING ROENTGENOGRAMS

A thorough understanding of the roentgenographic technics and processing procedures, which are described in the preceding pages, is indispensable for the production of high-quality roentgenograms. The ultimate purpose of the roentgenographic examination is to provide diagnostic information for the dentist. *Roentgenographic interpretation* is the term applied to the extraction of diagnostic information from roentgenograms.

The information obtained from the roentgenograms is utilized by the dentist; he correlates it with the information ob-

tained from other diagnostic aids to make a diagnosis. Although the hygienist does not use the roentgenograms for diagnosis, she should have a knowledge of interpretation that will enable her to determine whether or not a roentgenogram is of the best possible quality. A knowledge of the physical factors that affect film quality and the ability to recognize the effects of various factors is essential for the hygienist who desires to produce high-quality roentgenograms. An understanding of the physical factors that affect film quality, as presented here, along with the knowledge of roentgenographic technics and processing procedures of the preceding pages, will enable the hygienist to make competent evaluations of the quality of roentgenograms.

Factors affecting film quality

The diagnostic quality of the image seen in the roentgenogram is affected by the factors known as sharpness, density, contrast, and amount of distortion of the roentgenographic image. Sharpness, or detail, refers to the clear definition of the images of objects and the recording of fine details of objects. Density refers to the overall darkness of the film. Contrast refers to the differences in darkness of areas of the film, which are caused by differences in the density of the objects under examination. Distortion is the change in shape or size of the image as compared to the object.

Factors affecting image detail, or sharpness

Geometrical factors. Geometrical factors control the amount of fuzziness of an image. It is most evident at the image borders, where it is known as the penumbra.

SIZE OF FOCAL AREA: The focal area is that portion of the anode that is bombarded by electrons to produce roentgen rays. Ideally, the roentgen rays should

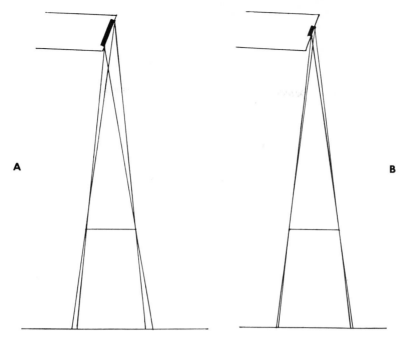

Fig. 13-59. A, Large focal area produces a relatively wide band of fuzziness (penumbra) at image borders. **B,** Small focal area produces a relatively narrow band of fuzziness at image boders. Therefore, image sharpness is improved.

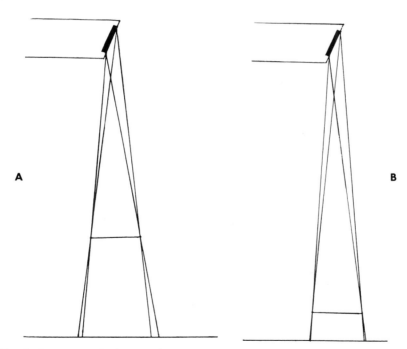

Fig. 13-60. A, Increased object-to-film distance produces a relatively wide band of fuzziness (penumbra) at image borders. **B,** Decreased object-to-film distance produces a sharper image.

emanate from a point, or extremely small area, for maximum sharpness (Fig. 13-59). However, the electron bombardment also produces heat, which requires that it be spread over a sufficiently large area to avoid damage to the x-ray tube. Most dental x-ray units have effective focal areas of 1 to 1.5 mm. square. The size of the focal area is determined by the manufacturer and cannot be changed by the operator. It is one factor that should be considered during the selection of an x-ray unit.

OBJECT-TO-FILM DISTANCE: Object-to-film distance refers to the distance between the object being examined (the teeth) and the film. Maximum sharpness results when the film is placed as close to the teeth as possible. Placing the film close to the teeth decreases the width of the penumbra, or fuzzy area, at the image borders. The placement of films parallel with the teeth, as in the paralleling technic, usually re-quires that the object-to-film distance be increased. The increased distance is, in itself, undesirable, but the undesirable effects are minimized by increasing the source-to-film distance, which is discussed next. An increase in the object-to-film distance also results in greater magnification of the image (Fig. 13-60).

SOURCE-TO-FILM DISTANCE: The source-to-film distance is the distance between the focal area of the x-ray tube, where the roentgen rays are produced, and the film. maximum sharpness results when the longest practical source-to-film distance is utilized (Fig. 13-61). As seen before, the intensity of the x-ray beam varies in accordance with the inverse square law; also, an increased target-to-film distance requires wider excursions of the tube head. These two factors limit the amount of increase in the source-to-film distance that is clinically practicable. For intraoral films relatively

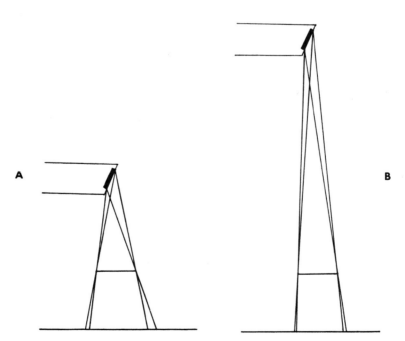

Fig. 13-61. A, Short source-to-film distance produces a relatively wide band of fuzziness. **B,** Increased source-to-film distance decreases width of penumbra and results in improved image sharpness.

little increase in sharpness is gained by using a source-to-film distance greater than 16 inches.

Motion. Movement of the x-ray tube, the patient, or the film during the exposure results in a blurring or fuzziness of the images on the film. The operator should make sure that the patient's head is positioned firmly against the headrest, that he retains the film firmly and with the hand properly braced, and that the x-ray tube head is steadied if necessary to stop oscillations before making the exposure. The tube head must not be held during the exposure.

Film. The size of the silver particles that constitute the image affects the image detail. Small grain size is necessary for maximum sharpness. Films having large grain size are said to appear grainy. Films having the smallest grain size require the greatest exposure, however, while larger grains produce a faster film that requires less exposure. The grainy appearance of fast films was formerly objectionable. Some manufacturers have improved their fast films in recent years to the extent that recent research indicates that in clinical practice the fast films cannot be distinguished from the slower films, which require greater exposure. The thickness of the emulsion and whether the emulsion is coated on one or both sides of the film base also affect detail, but a discussion of these factors is beyond the scope of this chapter.

Fog. Fog is an overall darkening of the film that tends to obscure detail. It is impossible to avoid all fogging of roentgenograms; however, it can be kept to a minimum by eliminating as many causes as possible.

When roentgen rays strike an object, some of them are scattered in all directions. Some of the scattered rays reach the film. This radiation produces an overall exposure of the film that is superimposed on the useful image. Fog from this source can be minimized by using the smallest practical beam size and proper filtration. These factors decrease the amount of radiation exposure of the patient's tissues, which in turn decreases the amount of scattered radiation and its potential for fogging the film. The lead foil in the back of the film packet helps to prevent fogging of the film by absorbing the scattered and secondary rays from the tongue and other tissues beyond the film. For extraoral films a grid may be used to absorb the scattered rays before they reach the film, but this method is not applicable to intraoral films.

Some other causes of fogging are as follows:

1. Unsafe storage of films. If films are exposed to secondary or scattered radiation before or after exposure, such exposure causes fogging.
2. Old film. An expiration date is placed on each box of film by the manufacturer. The film accumulates fog slowly from the time it is manufactured. The expiration date is that time, on the average, when the film has become fogged to the extent that makes it unsuitable for use.
3. Unsafe safelight in the darkroom. A safelight filter that is damaged or unsuitable will allow light rays to expose and fog the film.
4. Light leak in the darkroom. White light leaking into the darkroom around the door or other opening produces fogging of the film. To test for light leaks enter the darkroom and close the door. Keep the room dark for 5 minutes until the eyes become adapted. Then look for any leakage of light around the door, walls, floor, and ceiling. If none is observed, the darkroom is satisfactory.
5. Chemical fog. This type of fogging may be produced by the developer temperature being too warm or by

leaving the film in the developer for too long a time.

Factors affecting film density or darkening

Amount of radiation. The primary factor that determines the density is the amount of radiation delivered to the film. The quantity of roentgen rays produced is determined by the milliamperage supplied to the x-ray tube and the length of time the tube is energized. Exposure, therefore, is expressed in terms of milliampere-seconds (MAS).

Kilovoltage. A secondary factor that affects the density is the kilovoltage. Since the kilovoltage affects the wavelength and, therefore, the penetrating power of the roentgen rays, it naturally has some effect on density. The rays must be able to penetrate the tissues and reach the film in order to blacken it.

Fog. As was pointed out in the preceding section, fog contributes to the overall density of the film. It is an undesirable form of darkening in that it tends to obscure fine detail.

Factors affecting film contrast. Contrast refers to the differences in darkness of areas on the film, which result from differences in the density of the objects under examination.

Kilovoltage. The primary factor that affects contrast is the kilovoltage, which determines the penetrating power of the roentgen rays. The optimum kilovoltage for a given object under examination is that which is selectively absorbed by the object in such a manner that the fine details of the object may be readily visualized on the film. The greater the penetrating power of the roentgen rays, the smaller the area-to-area variations in the absorptions within the subject. Therefore increasing the kilovoltage reduces contrast; decreasing kilovoltage increases contrast.

Milliamperage. A secondary factor that does not affect the contrast directly but that does affect visualization of the structures shown on the film is the milliampere-seconds of exposure. If the film is extremely light or extremely dark the visibility of the recorded images is adversely affected.

Fog. Fog has a deleterious effect on contrast in that it smothers the film with dull gray shadows.

Factors affecting image distortion

Distortion. Distortion is a variation in shape or size of the roentgenographic image as compared with the object under examination. It is impossible to obtain an image that is not distorted to some degree. Distortion may be of two types: magnified and irregular.

OBJECT-TO-FILM-DISTANCE: Placement of the film close to the object under examination decreases the amount of magnification of the image.

SOURCE-TO-OBJECT DISTANCE: An increase in the distance from the source to the object will decrease the amount of magnification of the image.

FILM NOT PARALLEL WITH OBJECT: Irregular distortion of the image occurs when the film is not parallel with the object and when the radiation does not strike the object and film at right angles.

BENDING: Bending of a film packet produces irregular distortion of at least a part of the image. Obviously the film packet should be kept as flat as possible to minimize distortion.

When these factors are considered it becomes obvious that some distortion of the image occurs regardless of which basic technic is used. The bisecting technic, when properly effected, results in a tooth image that is exactly the length of the object. But magnification of the mesiodistal dimension of the tooth is unavoidable, and irregular distortion results from the film being placed at an angle to the tooth. The paralleling technic, on the other hand, results in a regular magnification of the entire tooth image.

When the factors that affect film quality

are considered as a whole, it is evident that some incompatibilities arise in an attempt to combine all of the optimum features into a single perfect technic. For example, the desirable parallel placement of films in the mouth requires than an undesirable increase in the object-to-film distance be tolerated. Therefore, no single combination can be given that is best in all instances.

Interpretation of roentgenograms

A roentgenogram is, essentially, a two-dimensional shadow picture of a three-dimensional object. In view of the many factors that affect the image on the film, as described in the preceding section, it is evident that a comprehensive knowledge of these factors is necessary for accurate interpretation of the images recorded on the film. Also, the dentist must have a thorough knowledge of the many normal anatomical variations and their roentgenographic appearances, plus a knowledge of the roentgenographic changes produced by pathological processes, in order to be able to extract the maximum diagnostic information from the film.

Roentgenographic changes that may be observed are of three basic types: a change in density, a change in structure, and a change in form or shape. A change in density would be revealed by a darker (roentgenolucent) image or a lighter (roentgenopaque) image. A change in the structure would be revealed by a change in the fine detail of an object; a change in the trabecular pattern of bone would be a change in structure. A change in form would be observed as a change in the normal outline; expansion of the cortical plates by a cyst and a break in continuity observed in cases of fractures are changes in form.

The dentist must correlate the information obtained from the interpretation of roentgenograms with the history, signs and symptoms, clinical examination, and any other necessary diagnostic aids in

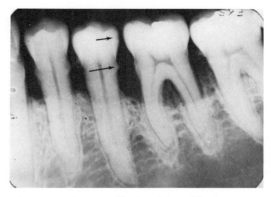

Fig. 13-62. Mandibular bicuspid roentgenogram. Calculus deposits are present just below the enamel caps of the teeth. Lower arrow indicates one calculus deposit. Can you find the others? Upper arrow indicates a dark zone in the enamel that is suggestive of caries. Also observe the height of the bone between the teeth. It is lower than normal. This is indicative of horizontal bone resorption.

order to make a diagnosis. Since the diagnosis depends on many factors, it is important that the hygienist avoid discussing the roentgenographic findings with the patient.

A systematic procedure is required for best results in the interpretation of roentgenograms. The following procedure is recommended. The first step is to determine the area shown by the film. A knowledge of the anatomy of the teeth is necessary to identify the area shown by the film. In Fig. 13-62, for example, the two bicuspids with single roots and the molar with two roots give sufficient information to identify the area shown as the mandibular bicuspid region. The second step is to determine whether or not the film shows the region adequately. Are the apices of the teeth shown? Are the images distorted? Was the film processed satisfactorily? Are the contrast, detail, and density satisfactory? The hygienist should become fully competent in identifying the area shown; this knowledge is necessary for mounting

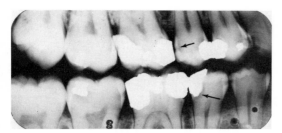

Fig. 13-63. Bite-wing roentgenogram. Upper arrow indicates a carious lesion in the distal surface of the maxillary second biscupid. Lower arrow indicates recurrent caries beneath the restoration in the distal surface of the mandibular second bicuspid. Can you find other areas of caries and recurrent caries? A temporary restoration is present in the distal surface of the maxillary first molar; observe the slight difference in density of the temporary restoration and the metallic restoration in the mesial surface of the same tooth. The alveolar bone level is normal; compare with Fig. 13-62.

films. She should also be able to make a competent determination of whether or not a film is technically adequate.

The interpretation of roentgenographic changes produced by pathological processes are normally performed by the dentist. However, the hygienist can learn to interpret common findings such as calculus deposits on the teeth and interproximal caries. This information is useful when scaling a patient's teeth and when charting the mouth. Figs. 13-62 and 13-63 show the typical radiographic appearance of calculus and caries.

The hygienist is in a position to render a most valuable service to the dentist and to the patient by producing roentgenograms of the highest possible quality.

REFERENCES

1. Glasser, O.: Dr. W. C. Röntgen, Springfield, Ill., 1945, Charles C Thomas, Publisher.
2. National Academy of Sciences: The biologic effects of atomic radiation—a report to the public, Washington, D. C., 1960, U. S. Government Printing Office.
3. Richards, A. G.: Roentgen-ray doses in dental roentgenography, J.A.D.A. **56**:351-368, 1958.
4. Wuehrmann, A. H., and Curby, W. A.: Radiopacity of oral structures as a basis for selecting optimum kilovoltage for intra-oral roentgenograms, J. Dent. Res. **31**:27-32, 1952.
5. X-ray protection, National Bureau of Standards' Handbook 60, Washington, D. C., 1955, U. S. Government Printing Office.
6. Richards, A. G., and others: X-ray protection in the dental office, J.A.D.A. **56**:514-521, 1958.
7. Richards, A. G.: Sources of x-radiation in the dental office, Dent. Radiogr. Photogr. **37** (3):67-68, 1964.
8. Radiation protection, Regulation 433, Commonwealth of Pennsylvania, Department of Health, Bureau of Environmental Health, Harrisburg, Pa., 1936.
9. Fitzgerald, G. M.: Dental roentgenography: Part I. An investigation in adumbration, or the factors that control geometric unsharpness, J.A.D.A. **34**:1-20, 1947.
10. Fitzgerald, G. M.: Dental roentgenography: Part II. Vertical angulation, film placement and increased object-film distance, J.A.D.A. **34**:160-170, 1947.
11. McCormack, D. W.: Mechanical aids for obtaining accuracy in dental roentgenology, J.A.D.A. **40**:144-153, 1950.
12. Waggener, D. T.: Principles of extension cone technique, J. Missouri Dent. Assoc. **30**:204-207, 1950.
13. Updegrave, W. J.: Paralleling extension-cone technique in intraoral dental radiography, Oral Surg. **4**:1250-1261, 1951.
14. Richards, A. G.: Roentgenographic technics made to order, J.A.D.A. **39**:396-402, 1949.
15. Richards, A. G.: Control of gagging in dental radiography, Dent. Radiogr. Photogr. **23**:37-38, 1950.
16. Berry, H. M., Jr.: Radiopaque materials in the roentgenographic interpretation of periodontal lesions; a preliminary report, J.A.D.A. **43**:278-284, 1951.

SUGGESTED READINGS

Berry, H. M., Jr.: The role of roentgenology in oral diagnosis, Dent. Clin. N. Amer., March, 1963, pp. 55-66.
Eastman Kodak Company: X-rays in dentistry, Rochester, N. Y., 1964.
Ellinger, F.: Medical radiation biology, Springfield, Ill., 1957, Charles C Thomas, Publisher.
Ennis, L. M., Berry, H. M.,, Jr., and Phillips, J. E.: Dental roentgenology, ed. 6, Philadelphia, 1967, Lea & Febiger.

McCall, J. O., and Wald, S. S.: Clinical dental roentgenology, Philadelphia, 1957, W. B. Saunders Co.

Peterson, S.: The dentist and his assistant, ed. 3, St. Louis, 1972, The C. V. Mosby Co.

Shawkat, A. H.: A quantitative study of scattered radiation fog on low- and high-speed dental roentgenograms, Oral. Surg. **20:**42-55, 1965.

REVIEW QUESTIONS

1. When, by whom, and how were roentgen-rays discovered?
2. By means of a sketch show the relation of roentgen rays to other radiations in the electromagnetic spectrum.
3. Name three properties of roentgen rays and tell how they are utilized in the medical sciences.
4. Briefly discuss ionizing radiations and genetics.
5. What is meant by natural background radiation? Fallout? Radioactive waste disposal?
6. With a modern x-ray machine, whose beam is properly filtered and collimated, how much radiation would scatter to the reproductive cells of an adult male during a full-mouth series of sixteen films? More or less to female gonads?
7. State the recommendation of the National Research Council regarding the limit of radiation to the reproductive cells.
8. How are roentgen rays produced?
9. What is thermionic emission?
10. What are the components of a modern x-ray tube?
11. Why is tungsten used as the material for the target?
12. What is the function of the autotransformer? The high-tension transformer? The low-tension transformer?
13. Discuss milliamperage, kilovoltage, MAS, and the inverse square law as they apply to the intensity of the x-ray beam.
14. If a film is properly exposed in 2 seconds at an 8-inch source-to-film distance, what would be the proper exposure time at a 16-inch distance?
15. What is primary radiation? Secondary radiation?
16. Define erythema dose. What is the average erythema dose in roentgens?
17. What is the danger to the operator from holding films in patients' mouths?
18. How can the operator protect herself from secondary rays? What is the limit of secondary radiation that the operator can receive per week?
19. How can the operator determine whether she is being exposed to secondary radiation?
20. What is the recommended diameter of the x-ray beam at the cone tip? How can this be altered?
21. What is the function of an aluminum filter? How does a filter affect the patient? The film? The exposure time? The operator?
22. What is a film emulsion? A single-coated film? A double-coated film?
23. What are the intraoral films, and what is the objective of each?
24. What are extraoral films? What film is used in a cardboard exposure holder? What film is used with a cassette?
25. What is a cassette? What are intensifying screens, and how do they act?
26. Discuss the principles upon which the paralleling and bisecting technics are based.
27. State the rule for the patient's head position for maxillary and mandibular periapical films; for bite-wing films; for occlusal films.
28. Describe the placement of the fourteen periapical films.
29. Describe bite-wing film placement.
30. What are the tube angulations for the occlusal films?
31. What are the steps in film processing?
32. What are the essentials for a dental x-ray darkroom?
33. What is the function of the developer? What are its components and their functions?
34. What is the function of the fixer? What are its components and their functions?
35. Why is it necessary to wash films for 20 minutes?
36. Name several artifacts and their causes.
37. How may gagging be minimized?
38. Name the roentgenopaque landmarks of the maxilla and the mandible.
39. Name the roentgenolucent landmarks of the maxilla and the mandible.
40. Define sharpness as it applies to film quality.
41. Diagram and describe the three geometrical factors affecting image detail, or sharpness.
42. Compare the bisecting and paralleling technics in regard to the geometrical factors affecting film quality.
43. What are some causes of fogged films?
44. What is the primary factor affecting film density?
45. What is the effect of fog on film density?
46. What is the primary factor affecting film contrast?
47. What are some factors that cause image distortion?

48. Describe the distortion produced when the bisecting technic is used.
49. Describe the distortion produced when the paralleling technic is used.
50. Why should the hygienist refrain from discussing roentgenographic findings with the patient?

chapter 14

STERILIZATION AND SANITATION

Milton Siskin, B.A., D.D.S.

First impressions are easy to create and very difficult to dispel. Consequently every effort should be made by the dentist and his ancillary personnel to provide as favorable an initial impression for the patient as is possible. One of the vehicles essential to the accomplishment of this objective is that of cleanliness. In the dental office, cleanliness not only implies the absence of filth but also freedom from disease-producing germs. Methods that may be utilized in the dental office to control and destroy microorganisms will be discussed in detail in subsequent portions of this chapter. At this point the discussion is concerned with and directed toward physical surroundings and personnel. Most patients do not have basic or detailed information relative to the pathogenicity of microorganisms or a comprehension of methods by which disease-producing organisms are transmitted. However, almost everyone is familiar with the "germ theory of disease" and the fact that microorganisms may be harbored on dirty or contaminated fomites or objects containing excreta and waste. When a patient walks into a dental office and is greeted by personnel who are neat, tidy, and clean in appearance and when sterilizing equipment is prominently displayed and the surroundings have an "aseptic" look and odor, he is given the impression that this

is an office concerned with his welfare. A feeling of confidence that can be engendered in no other way is imparted to the patient. This confidence, and the tranquility of mind that goes with it, will be conveyed to all other experiences related to the dental practice. At this first exposure the patient is made aware that his dental problems are to be disposed of in a precise and professional manner and that simultaneously every precaution is taken to protect his health.

It is the responsibility of the dental hygienist, along with every other member of the office team, to assure the patient that his health and welfare are of prime consideration and to reinforce this concept and impression. In the light of present knowledge cleanliness is just good common sense and a sound practice. Negatively it should be emphasized that carelessness and laxity can be responsible for the transmission of a communicable disease, and this in turn could have serious professional and legal consequences.

PERSONAL HYGIENE

It is axiomatic that members of the dental health team must be neat in appearance and should follow all of the rules conducive to good personal hygiene. In addition there are a few specific rules relative to personal cleanliness and grooming that must be observed with special care. Obviously the uniform and shoes must be clean. Since the hygienist will be handling instruments and supplies that will be used in the patient's mouth, care of the hands is of paramount importance. The following rules concerning care of the hands must be followed:

1. The sink to be used for washing the hands should be in a prominent place; the fixture must be spotless and clean, unstained towels always available.
2. The hands must be thoroughly scrubbed before each patient is treated. It is desirable to perform this act in front of the patient. After the hands are washed the hygienist must not touch instruments or equipment that have not been sterilized.
3. Detergents that have a good hexachlorophene content will greatly minimize the number of organisms to be found on the skin. When such detergents are used repeatedly it has been demonstrated that the hexachlorophene will produce a water-insoluble film that will remain adherent to the hands, and thus a continued and long-acting bacteriostatic effect is achieved.
4. In the event that it becomes necessary for the hygienist to leave the operatory to attend to other office duties, the hands must be washed before again contacting the patient or before handling instruments to be used in the patient's mouth.
5. Fingernails must be kept short and clean.
6. When nailpolish is worn, it should be clear or of a conservative shade.
7. If or when the hygienist has a sore or a wound on one of her fingers, she must not perform duties for the patient or handle instruments unless a finger cot is used.
8. Great care should be exercised to wash the hands in front of the patient whenever the dental hygienist has touched her face or hair or any object that might be construed as less than sterile.

TERMINOLOGY

In all areas of human endeavor precise methods of communication are extremely important. This is particularly true in fields of the healing arts. One's comprehension of terms related to one's field of interest is essential, and knowledge of the meaning of these words is mandatory if communication is to take place. Semantically speaking one should be able to say what one means and mean what one says. There is a group of terms that are an integral part of the lexicon related to cleanliness and sterilization, and those in most frequent usage are listed here.

aerobe (aerobian) A microorganism that can live and grow only in the presence of adequate quantities of oxygen.

aerobiosis The act of living or the existence of life in an atmosphere that contains oxygen.

anaerobe A microorganism that lives best or that may live only when in an environment free of oxygen.

anaerobiosis The existence of life in an atmosphere that is free of oxygen.

antisepsis The destruction of germs that cause disease, fermentation, or putrefaction.

antiseptic A substance or agent that has the capacity to inhibit bacterial growth and reproduction.

asepsis A condition or state in which living pathogenic organisms are absent.

aseptic Characterized by a state of asepsis.

aseptic technic The utilization of those procedures and precautions that will prevent the access of viable microorganisms.

asepticize To render aseptic or sterile.

bactericide An agent that will cause the death of bacteria.

bacteriostatic An agent or drug that will arrest the growth of bacteria. This term has essentially the same meaning as *antiseptic* and is used in its stead.

disinfectant An element or chemical compound capable cf destroying organisms that cause disease, fermentation, and putrefaction.

facultative anaerobe A microorganism that has the

ability to carry on all of the attributes of life in an environment that may or may not contain oxygen.

fumigation Exposure to the fumes of sulfur or to the action of a disinfectant gas. (This method of sanitation of premises is presently believed to be ineffective.)

fungicide An element or compound capable of inducing the destruction of fungi.

germicide Essentially a synonym for disinfectant; any agent capable of destroying germs or microbes.

in vivo Refers to vital processes occurring in the living being.

ionization Dissociation into ions, which occurs when an electrolyte is dissolved.

iontophoresis The introduction of ions by means of a direct current into tissues or cells. When the ions have medicinal or therapeutic value, the process is known as ionic medication. When the ions are germicidal the process may be used to accomplish sterilization.

obligatory anaerobe A microorganism that must be in an oxygen-free environment in order to carry on essential metabolic activities.

pasteurization A process for destroying living bacteria in liquids without appreciably affecting the flavor or the bouquet of the liquid. The process consists of heating the liquid in question at 140° to 155° F. for 30 minutes, then cooling immediately to 50° F. or lower. Spores usually are unaffected by the temperature but are kept from developing by the sudden cooling. This process is used to destroy pathogenic bacteria in milk, wines, beer, fruit juices, and other liquids.

sterile The state of being free of living organisms.

sterility The condition of being sterile.

sterilization The process by which all forms of life are completely destroyed in a given circumscribed area.

sterilization temperature That temperature at which microorganisms will be destroyed.

sterilizer Any apparatus used to produce a sterile state.

RECOGNITION OF RESPONSIBILITY

It is the practice in most dental offices to delegate the responsibility of carrying out sterilizing procedures. This may or may not be included among the duties of the hygienist, but in any event it is mandatory that she be familiar with all aspects of the process. This is a confidence that must be recognized, accepted, ap-

preciated, and never violated. The dental hygienist should be thoroughly familiar with methods of sterilization used in the practice of dentistry. She needs to be aware of the operation and operating procedures for all sterilizing equipment. A knowledge of the particular method by which each item requiring sterilization can be best rendered sterile is essential. Since disease can be transmitted from patient to patient by instruments or other fomites that are unsterile, sterilizing procedures or the supervision of sterilizing procedures is among the hygienist's most important duties.

STERILIZING ROOM OR ALCOVE

Every dental office should have a site set aside and designated for the purpose of carrying out sterilizing procedures. This room or alcove needs to be centrally located in the floor plan and easily accessible from all parts of the office. The area should be well lighted, easy to keep clean, and conveniently arranged. It should contain a spacious sink equipped with hot and cold water. There must be ample facilities for the storage of supplies, instruments, and equipment after sterilization. The sterilizing area should be equipped with a sonic or ultrasonic cleaner, a pair of transfer forceps, a container for chemical or cold sterilization, hot water sterilizer, and autoclave; a hot air or dry heat sterilizer is optional.

Every instrument and dressing or any other item to be placed in the mouth must be sterilized. Considerable time may be conserved and the sterilizing procedure disposed of with dispatch if a definite routine is established and followed empirically. Each item used in caring for the patient should be assigned a specific method for sterilization. Storage methods must be devised and utilized to maintain sterility of supplies, instruments, and equipment until they are needed.

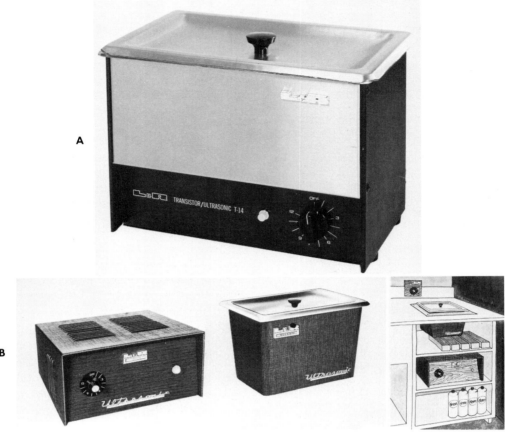

Fig. 14-1. Transistorized ultrasonic cleaning machines. **A,** Table-top model; **B,** with solid state circuitry. (Courtesy L & R Manufacturing Co., Kearny, N. J.)

ULTRASONIC CLEANER

All instruments must be carefully and thoroughly cleansed before any method of sterilization is employed. It is possible to accomplish this by manual scrubbing with a stiff brush. However, this method is relatively time consuming and somewhat ineffective as compared to other technics. The old method of scrubbing cannot in any way compare with the efficiency and thoroughness of the ultrasonic cleaner (Fig. 14-1). The ultrasonic cleaner is a relative newcomer to the dental armamentarium, but it is a piece of equipment that should be commonplace in every den-

tal office. If instruments are to be rendered completely sterile, they must be free of extraneous material prior to sterilization. The ultrasonic cleaner accomplishes this thoroughly, effectively, and consistently, and the process requires a minimum of effort.

The ultrasonic cleaner is composed of an electronic generator and a bath solution. When the generator is in operation, it places the liquid of the bath in a state of high-frequency vibration. While in this state the solution undergoes cavitation of an order that will produce myriads of submicroscopic bubbles, which are formed and will collapse almost instantaneously. The formation and collapse of the bubbles produce intense pressure changes resulting in a mechanical scrubbing action. Instruments are placed in a basket and then immersed in the cleaning solution. Vibrations set up in the solution will initiate the cleaning action and thus free the solid objects of extraneous material and leave them clean and free of surface contaminants. The cleaning cycle is automatically controlled, and the process requires a time interval of 2 to 10 minutes. The value of this instrument has been conclusively demonstrated.

METHODS OF STERILIZATION

Methods of sterilization can be categorized under one of the following processes or combination of processes: physical, chemical, or mechanical. The most significant and important procedure for sterilization is the application of heat, which is a physical process. Chemicals must be regarded as disinfectants. It is only in special instances that complete sterilization is accomplished by this means. An example of a mechanical method of sterilization is filtration. This process is used primarily for the purpose of removing microorganisms from liquids or solutions.

Chemical method or cold sterilization

In comparison with the several methods of sterilization available in the dental office, the chemical method is the least effective. It is a very unreliable procedure for destroying organisms with spores and has several other disadvantages that surely limit the effectiveness of this type of sterilization. In most instances the use of cold sterilization should be limited to instruments that do not lend themselves to other methods of sterilization and to instruments that have sharp cutting surfaces that must be maintained. Disinfectant solutions never should be used in an attempt to sterilize needles.

When a chemical disinfectant is to be used for sterilization, it is necessary to follow a rigid regimen. The solution should be placed in a dry, clean container that has a well-fitted top (Fig. 14-2). The lid should be kept closed at all times except for the placement and removal of instruments. Forceps should be used for the transfer of instruments to and from the solution (Figs. 14-3 and 14-4). Since the effectiveness of the solution may be altered by airborne organisms or by those contained upon the hands, the foregoing precautions should be followed without exception. Keeping the container sealed has the added advantage of minimizing evaporation from the solution. The solution should be changed at frequent and regular intervals, since the concentration may be altered and the effectiveness diminished by evaporation or dilution. Before placing instruments into a chemical solution they should be carefully cleansed or scrubbed, then rinsed and dried. Should foreign material be left upon instruments, it may act as a protective shield and prevent the disinfectant from coming in contact with the organisms that lie between the instrument and the encrusted matter. The instruments to be sterilized must be dry in order to obviate an alteration in the concentration of the solution. Once the sterilizing cycle has begun, the instruments should be left in the solution for 20 to 30 minutes. If additional instruments are placed in the sterilizer after a cycle has begun, the timing must be restarted.

There are many compounds that are marketed as chemical disinfectants. To list them all or even those in common usage is impractical. However, most of those in frequent use are either quaternary ammonium compounds, aldehydes, chlorine compounds, phenols, mercurials, or alcohols. Since all chemical disinfectants do not have the same capacity for destroying organisms, their germ-killing potential is usually compared to a known quantity.

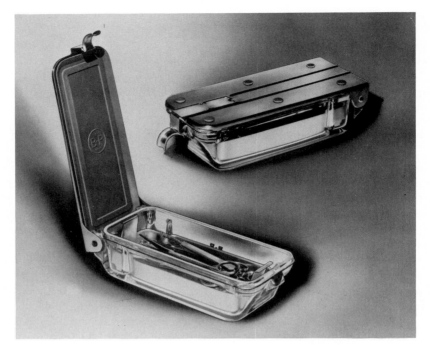

Fig. 14-2. Bard-Parker sterilizing container. (Courtesy American Hospital Supply Corp., Evanston, Ill.)

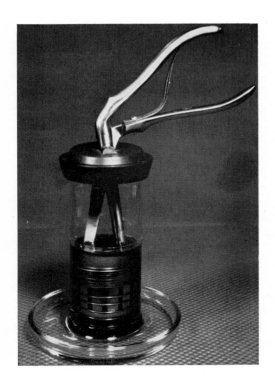

Fig. 14-3. Bard-Parker transfer forceps. (From Peterson, S., editor: The dentist and his assistant, ed. 3, St. Louis, 1972, The C. V. Mosby Co.)

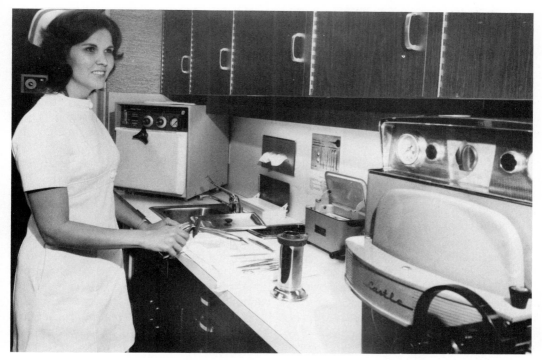

Fig. 14-4. The use of sterilized transfer forceps for moving sterile instruments.

The standard was developed by Rideal and Walker and is known as the "phenol coefficient." The phenol coefficient is an index or a measurement of the ability of a solution to destroy living organisms. Thus by being aware of the coefficient one is able to determine the effectiveness of various solutions and the dilutions that are used as chemical disinfectants. It should be remembered that most chemical disinfectants are effective against the vast majority of vegetative forms of bacteria if allowed to remain in contact with the organism for 30 minutes; 14 to 15 hours are required for spores, and most are unreliable against the various species of *Mycobacterium*.

Instruments ordinarily cared for by the chemical or disinfecting procedures are as follows:

1. Mirrors
2. Explorers
3. Cotton pliers
4. Plastic instruments
5. Suction tips (except surgical tips)
6. Orthodontic pliers
7. Impression trays
8. Instruments for cavity preparation
9. Amalgam instruments
10. Water syringe tips
11. Air syringe tips
12. Burs (except surgical burs)

There are items of equipment that do not lend themselves to the various methods of sterilization in common usage, but these items are likely to come in contact with the patient, with instruments to be used in the mouth of the patient, or with the hands of the operator. These pieces of equipment would include the water and air syringes, bracket table, and light handles. They should be carefully wiped or swabbed down with an alcohol sponge prior to seating the patient.

Heat sterilization

Microorganisms, generally, are extremely responsive to temperature. It is a well-established point that metabolic activity in bacteria is at a minimum at 0° C. Reproduction of organisms at this temperature undergoes complete cessation. The optimum temperature for microbial metabolism and reproduction is near body temperature. The range of temperatures for reproduction may be from 15° to 38° C. As a general rule, the more pathogenic the organism, the more specific the optimum temperature requirements, and the closer that temperature approaches 37.5° C. Temperatures of 60° C. or greater are totally destructive to bacteria. The most efficient method of utilizing heat for the destruction of microbial organisms is in the form of moist heat.

All organisms do not manifest the same degree of susceptibility to destruction by heat. Bacteria that are nonsporeformers and the vegetative forms of the sporulating organisms are least resistant to elevations in temperature. These organisms may be destroyed by moist heat at temperatures ranging from 55° to 65° C. applied for periods of 10 to 60 minutes. All organisms except spores can be killed by moist heat in 60 minutes at 80° C. Spores are extremely resistant to heat. When attempting to eliminate bacterial spores, it should be noted that dry heat is less effective than moist heat. There are some spores that can resist boiling for 3 hours. Because of this, one should not rely on boiling alone to accomplish the purpose. The most effective method for killing spores is by using steam under pressure. This can be effected in 30 minutes at a temperature of 121.5° C. It is interesting to note that only the bacilli produce spores and that there are approximately 150 species with this potential.

The manner by which death of microorganisms is accomplished when using heat for sterilization is dependent upon the application. When moist heat is used, the proteins of the protoplasm of the bacteria will undergo denaturation and coagulation. Death of bacteria produced by dry heat is attributable to dehydration and the resulting oxidation. One should know that dry heat will bring about a drying out of a spore and initially will increase its resistance to the sterilizing process. This does not occur with the use of moist heat. Thus when dry heat is being used and spores are likely to be present, it is well to use a hold time that is longer than that considered to be optimum.

It is essential to note that when heat is utilized to produce a sterile state, there are two factors that are of paramount importance: time and temperature. The lethal effect of this mode of sterilization is equated with the intensity and the time that the heat is applied. For sterilization the requirement of each is inversely proportional to one another. The greater the amount of time used in the sterilizing process, the lower the temperature requirement. The higher the temperature used in sterilization, the shorter the amount of time needed to complete the process.

Moist heat sterilization

Boiling water. Of all the methods available for sterilization, boiling water is probably the most commonly used agent for sterilizing instruments in the dental office. Boiling water is also one of the most efficient, effective, and satisfactory methods of disinfecting instruments (Fig. 14-5). This process requires no elaborate equipment, it is inexpensive, and it is most effective except in instances where spores are involved. As has been mentioned, some spores may be resistant to boiling for up to 3 hours. The bactericidal action of boiling water can be enhanced by the addition of an alkali (3% saponated cresol solution or 5% phenol) to the water. Alkalies and boiling water are not only effective against all vegetative organisms but against viruses as well. This is of particular importance in guarding against the spread of infectious hepatitis.

Sterilization by boiling does have limita-

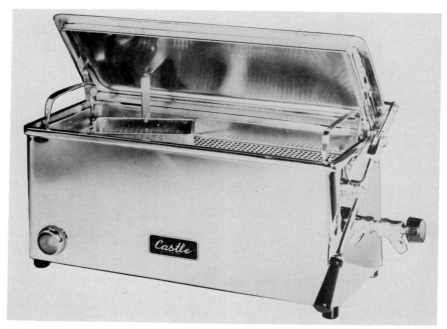

Fig. 14-5. Castle instrument boiler. (Courtesy Ritter Co., Inc., Rochester, N. Y.)

tions, since it tends to dull sharp instruments and to rust some metals. Boiling should not be used for those instruments that are expensive or adversely affected. In most instances the deleterious effects of boiling can be minimized by the addition of antirust preparations, the use of distilled or mineral-free water, the addition of alkalies, the elimination of scale from the boiler, and the removal and drying of instruments at the completion of the boiling cycle.

Instruments to be sterilized by boiling must be freed of debris prior to placing them in the water bath. Should needles be included, a stylet must be passed through the lumen to dislodge any trapped material. The water must be boiling before the instruments are inserted into the tank. If the placement of the instruments lowers the temperature of the water below the boiling point, the timing of the sterilizing cycle cannot begin until the water returns to a vigorous boil. The instruments must

be completely submerged in the boiling water. The cycle should not be broken by the addition of more instruments. The most commonly accepted duration for the sterilizing cycle by boiling is 20 minutes. Since this interval is not long enough to be effective against spores, as was previously thought, 10 minutes may be long enough to accomplish disinfection, exclusive of spores.

After sterilization, instruments are to be removed from the water immediately. The transfer is accomplished by the use of sterile forceps, and the instruments are placed between a sterile towel and then thoroughly dried. At this point instruments with moving parts may be lubricated with sterile oil. The lubricant can be applied with a sterile cotton applicator or toothpick. Storage of the instruments in such a manner as to prevent recontamination should be effected. It is essential that sterilized instruments not be touched with the hands.

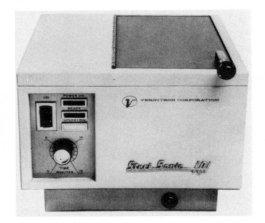

Fig. 14-6. Steri-Sonic 101C (gross and frontal view) designed to clean, disinfect, and sterilize ultrasonically. (Courtesy Vernitron Medical Products, Inc., Carlstadt, N. J.)

The instruments that lend themselves to sterilization by boiling are as follows:

1. Syringes
2. Hand instruments without sharp cutting surfaces
3. Surgical instruments
4. Needles
5. Impression trays
6. Glass slabs
7. Scalers and other periodontal instruments
8. Suction tips

Thermal and ultrasonic wave sterilization (Fig. 14-6). Thermal and acoustical shock wave sterilization is accomplished by the use of a unique electronic device with the trade name Steri-Sonic 101C. The equipment is designed to perform several functions: cleaning, disinfecting, and sterilizing. The unit contains a tank that is filled with 3 quarts of distilled or demineralized water to which is added ½ oz. of Vernitron's Hematergent, a blood solvent. The solution is preheated to 180° F. and at this point the cleaner/sterilizer is ready for operation. The items to be placed in the tank for cleaning and sterilization are carefully rinsed. After placing them in the tank the timer is set for 5 to 15 minutes and the power switch is then pressed into the "on" position.

The functions of the unit are performed by producing a high-frequency, high-intensity cavitation in hot water containing Hematergent. The high-frequency, 400,000 cps (Hz.) affects the transmission of compression waves through the hot chemical solution. In turn this action will produce cavitation. The bubbles resulting from the 400,000 Hz. per second are 100 times smaller than those produced by equipment capable of generating only 25,000 to 70,000 cps. Thus there is significant increase in the penetration and the effectiveness of the cleansing action. It is presumed that the cavitation bubbles, with the dimensions made possible by this equipment, not only enhance thoroughness and efficiency but facilitate penetration into cavities and recesses previously inaccessible.

Studies have been done on the time and kill rate on mixed cultures and mixed molds as related to the sterilization efficiency of the Steri-Sonic 101C. It has been demonstrated that complete sterilization, including the destruction of *Clostridium sporogenes* and *Bacillus subtilis,* can be accomplished after 4 hours of continuous processing with this equipment. The manufacturer, as well as a private test laboratory, maintains that disinfection is achieved within 5 to 15 minutes.

Steam under pressure (autoclave). There are several methods of sterilization available to the dentist; however, the most effective and efficient is steam under pressure. The apparatus that provides for this method of sterilization is known as an autoclave. Steam under pressure can be raised to temperatures higher than that of free-flowing steam or boiling water. It is the heat that sterilizes (Figs. 14-7 to 14-11). This method of providing heat has several advantages:

1. The desired temperature can be attained with ease and in a short period of time.
2. Anything that is not adversely af-

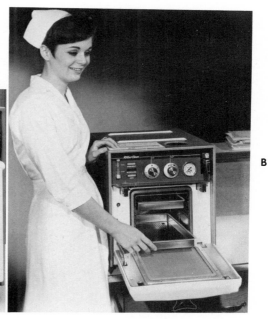

Fig. 14-7. A, Ritter autoclave, Ritter-Clave. This is a general purpose autoclave and one designed for use in a dental office. **B,** Interior design and construction of the chamber of this general purpose autoclave. (Courtesy Ritter Co., Rochester, N. Y.)

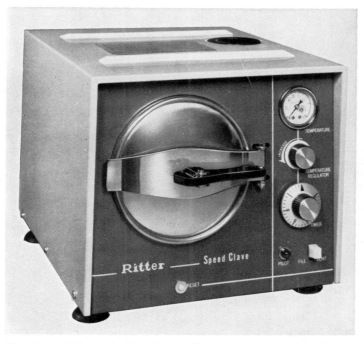

Fig. 14-8. Ritter Speed Clave; designed to sterilize instruments and small packages. (Courtesy Ritter Co., Inc., Rochester, N. Y.)

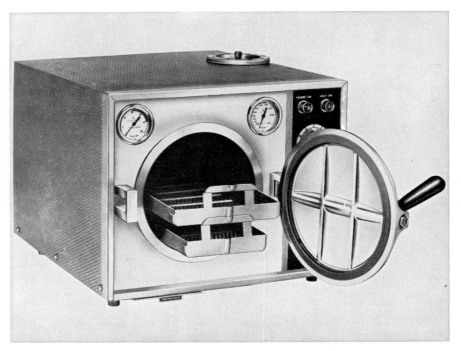

Fig. 14-9. Omniclave may be used for both autoclaving and dry heat sterilization. (Courtesy Pelton & Crane, Charlotte, N. C.)

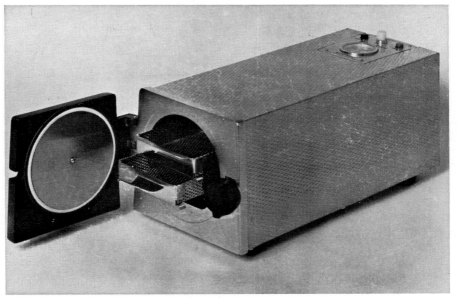

Fig. 14-10. Instru-Clave. A compact autoclave used to sterilize dental instruments. (Courtesy Pelton & Crane, Charlotte, N. C.)

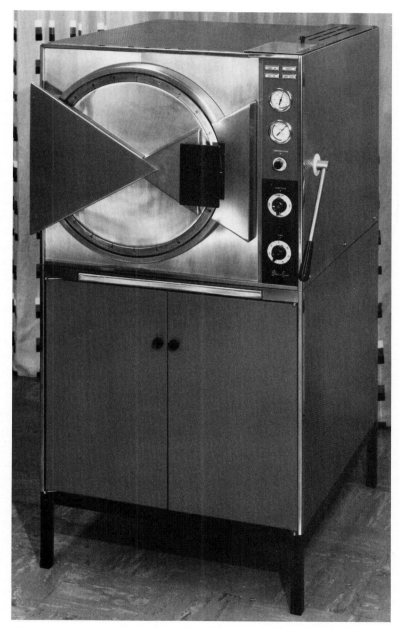

Fig. 14-11. Magna-Clave, a large general purpose autoclave. (Courtesy Pelton & Crane, Charlotte, N. C.)

fected by heat can be sterilized in an autoclave.

3. The damage to instruments is minimal.
4. Sterilization is effective and complete.
5. Spores are destroyed in a relatively short period of time.
6. Dissipation of heat into the room is minimal.

Sterilization in an autoclave is routinely accomplished at 250° F. (121° C.). This temperature is attained when the steam is under 15 pounds of pressure per square inch. The duration of the sterilizing cycle is 15 to 20 minutes at this temperature. However, the cycle can be shortened by elevating the temperature, and this may have some practical value when emergencies arise.

When using an autoclave, there are several essential steps that must be observed:

1. Heat the apparatus until steam is generated.
2. Insert the material to be sterilized.
3. Seal the door tightly.
4. Evacuate air.
5. Elevate the temperature within the chamber to the desired level. Allow enough at this point for all objects that were placed in the autoclave to reach the temperature of the chamber (lag time or preheating time).
6. Provide adequate exposure time to the sterilizing temperature (holding time).
7. Release the steam.
8. Allow for drying time.

There are several aspects relative to sterilization by the use of the autoclave that are deserving of special attention. Before placing instruments into the autoclave they must be cleansed meticulously. Since the temperature of the autoclave is evenly distributed by the penetration of the steam, the apparatus never should be packed too tightly. If the materials are packaged prior to sterilizing, they should be wrapped in a towel, paper, or cloth. If tubes or metal containers are used for packaging, they never must be sealed tightly and should be placed on their side to prevent the accumulation of moisture. Metal objects do have a tendency to undergo corrosion when exposed to the action of steam. This should be taken into account and necessary precautions taken. One method available for the protection of metal instruments is the use of Proclave. This regimen utilizes two solutions, one a detergent and the other an emulsion. The instruments are first placed in the detergent, which helps to cleanse and lower the surface tension. They are then submerged in the emulsion, which coats them with a layer that acts as a lubricant and then protective film. Another method of protecting metal products to be autoclaved and of enhancing their longevity is by use of an additive to the water that is placed in the autoclave tank. Such a product is Credo-Clave. This solution can be properly referred to as an additive. It does not enhance but it has no adverse effect upon the sterilizing equipment or efficiency and reliability of the sterilizing process. It has been adequately demonstrated that via the use of Credo-Clave undesirable changes in anything containing metal can be decreased or negated without inconvenience and at a minimal or inconsequential expense.

When needles or objects with long thin lumina are to be sterilized in an autoclave, they should not be covered by a cotton roll, since the cotton will prevent the steam from gaining access to the lumen and thus prevent adequate sterilization. It is permissible to sterilize the needle and the cotton roll independently and then to cover the needle by inserting it into the cotton roll before completely removing it from the autoclave.

Instruments and objects to be autoclaved may be placed loose into the apparatus. Upon completion of the sterilization cycles they can be removed with sterile forceps and placed into a sterile

Table 14-1. Temperature, exposure time, and load arrangement for steam pressure sterilization*

Article	Arrangement of load	Temperature	Exposure time (min.)
Instruments	Layer of muslin placed in bottom of tray; instruments arranged so do not contact one another; covered with second layer of muslin	250° F.	15
Instruments (alternate method)	Layer of muslin placed in bottom of tray; instruments arranged so do not contact one another; covered with second layer of muslin	270° F.	3
Surgical dressings, small packs, other textiles	Flat compact packages wrapped with double-thickness muslin; packages placed in tray on end, never tightly packed together	250° F.	20
Rubber gloves, rubber-dam material	Flat compact packages wrapped with double-thickness muslin; packages placed in tray on end, never tightly packed together; dusting powder sprinkled between two layers of rubber	250° F.	15
Empty glassware and utensils	Wrapped in muslin and inverted or placed on side	250° F.	15
Solutions	Sealed in 50-ml. Pyrex flasks or test tubes up to 100 mm. long	250° F.	15
	Sealed in 125- to 200-ml. Pyrex flasks	250° F.	20

*From Kanterman, C. B.: Autoclave sterilization, W. Virginia Dent. J. **29:**154-155, 1955.

container. However, the most advantageous method is to prepackage instruments in groupings as they are routinely to be used. Care needs to be taken to use a wrap that can be effectively penetrated by steam. Once packaged, sterilization is effected. When instruments are packaged, they may be stored for relatively long periods of time without fear of breaking the sterility. A label with a thermochromatic indicator may be affixed to each package. This serves two purposes; one to identify the content and the other to indicate that the package has been sterilized.

Hot oil sterilization. Hot oil sterilization (Fig. 14-12) is used primarily for the sterilization of conventional handpieces, contra-angles, burs, and instruments that are hinged or jointed. The apparatus closely resembles a miniature hot water sterilizer. Instead of using water as the bath, oil is used. Mineral oil, silicones, and the other synthetic oils are used in the disinfection process. All objects must be cleansed thoroughly before being completely submerged in the oil. The cycles most frequently used are 150° C. (300° F.) for 10 minutes or 121° C. (250° F.) for 15 minutes. This time-temperature ratio will kill all organisms except spore formers. However, oil can be an effective sterilizing agent at a temperature of 150° C. (300° F.) and with an exposure time of 1½ hours.

There is no one oil with all the properties desirable for use in hot oil sterilization. Ideally the oil used should be non-irritating, chemically inert, and clear; have a high flash point; and be a good lubricant. The hydrocarbon oils are good lubricants but, when heated to the desired temperature, they break down and give off an offensive odor. They cannot be heated above 250° C. because of their flash point.

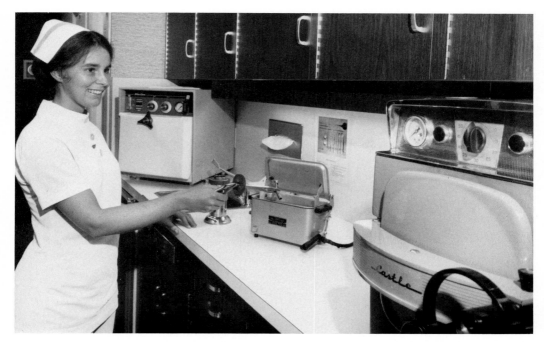

Fig. 14-12. Hot oil sterilization of a dental handpiece. The transfer forceps are used to remove the handpiece upon completion of sterilization.

A

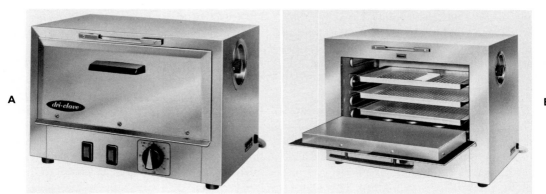

B

Fig. 14-13. A, Dri-Clave, a dry heat sterilizer. **B,** Interior design and construction of a dry heat sterilizer. (Courtesy Dri-Clave Corporation, Westbury, N. Y.)

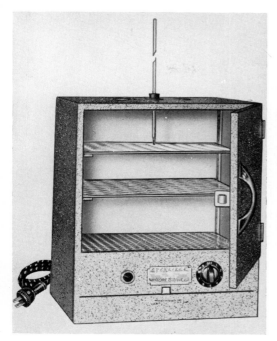

Fig. 14-14. Adjustable dry heat sterilizer. (Courtesy Union Broach Co., Inc., Long Island City, N. Y.)

Silicones are more stable but are relatively poor lubricating agents. In spite of the inherent disadvantages and limitations, this method is recommended for disinfecting handpieces.

Dry heat sterilization (Figs. 14-9, 14-13, and 14-14). Dry heat sterilization is an effective method of sterilization, and the end results compare favorably with those achieved by the use of the autoclave. However, there are two distinct disadvantages present when using this method of sterilization. A longer sterilizing time is needed to achieve sterilization, and materials that are adversely affected by dry heat cannot be sterilized by this procedure. Dry heat sterilization is usually reserved for objects that do not lend themselves to moist heat and to those that rust readily. Root canal instruments, injection and surgical needles, and instruments with sharp cutting surfaces are fre-

quently sterilized with dry heat. When a minimum load is placed in the oven of the dry heat sterilizer, the sterilizing cycle is 1 hour at 160° C. (320° F.). However, should the oven be loaded to near capacity, the time interval must be increased to 2 hours. Timing of the cycle or holding time can begin only when the sterilizing temperature is achieved. In most instances the high temperature that is required for this method of sterilization is injurious to fabrics. Towels and sponges can be sterilized by this technic, but the temperature is critical; 160° C. must be maintained for sterilization, while anything over this amount of heat will usually produce charring.

The dry heat method of sterilization, even where it may be used, is not always practical for the dental office because of the time factor and the need for sterilizing some instruments several times during the course of a single day. Dry heat, in addition to being used for metal objects with sharp edges, is frequently utilized in scientific laboratories and for sterilizing objects where maintaining complete dryness is mandatory.

Flaming or direct flame sterilization. Flaming sterilization is accomplished by dipping an object in 95% alcohol and then exposing the object to the direct heat of a flame. In some instances the alcohol dip is omitted. This method is effective in destroying vegetative forms of organisms but is not completely efficient for all spores. It should be emphasized that direct flame sterilization includes more than just passing an object through a flame. The temperature of the object must be elevated to a minimum of 60° C. Because of the effect that heat has on metals, at this temperature it is not a routinely useful method of sterilization. The only real advantage of flaming is that it affords sterilization of metal objects in a very short period of time.

Glass bead, salt, or molten metal steri-

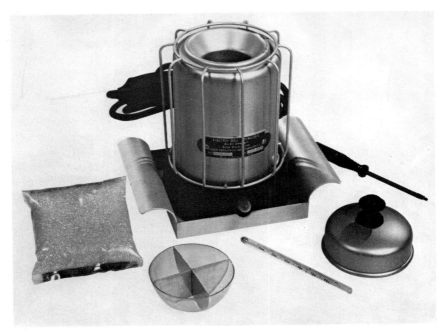

Fig. 14-15. Electric glass bead sterilizer. The accessories shown in the illustration, from left to right, are a package of glass beads, divider for glass dish, and a thermometer. (Courtesy Union Broach Co., Inc., Long Island City, N. Y.)

lizer. The glass bead, salt, or molten metal sterilizer consists of an apparatus containing a small pot in which the temperature can be maintained at 204° C. to 280° C. (400° to 536° F.). These sterilizers are generally of two types: one is electrical (Fig. 14-15); the other requires gas heat (Fig. 14-16). Molten metal, glass beads, or salt is placed in the pot, and the temperature within the container is elevated to the desired level. Small objects can be inserted into the contents of the pot and left for the desired period of time, usually from 5 to 10 seconds. This method of sterilization will destroy vegetative organisms, but there is some question concerning the reliability of the device to kill spores within a reasonable length of time. Since the reliability of this form of sterilization is in question and it can only be used for very small objects, it is recommended that other forms of sterilization be utilized.

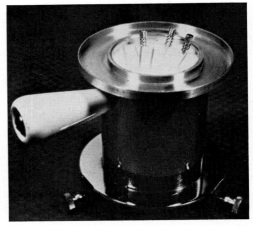

Fig. 14-16. Glass bead or salt sterilizer. This particular type is attached to the Bunsen burner on the dental unit and a gas flame is used. Sterilizers of this type are primarily used in endodontics. Files and paper points are inserted between the hot beads in this illustration. (From Peterson, S., editor: The dentist and his assistant, ed. 3, St. Louis, 1972, The C. V. Mosby Co.)

This piece of equipment is used primarily in the field of endodontics to sterilize the working end of small metal instruments, paper points, and cotton pellets. Molten metal has the tendency to adhere to the surface of objects placed in it and, as a result of this disadvantage, has been discarded in favor of salt or glass beads.

Ultraviolet light sterilization

Ultraviolet light or radiation will destroy airborne organisms and organisms found upon exposed surfaces. It has no penetrating ability, consequently the application of this form of sterilization is limited. Ultraviolet light is used successfully to reduce the bacterial count in a room, to sterilize drawers or cabinets, and to render sterile exposed surfaces of objects that cannot be sterilized by any other means.

Ultraviolet light is irritating to the eyes and skin. Unless it is being used in a closed or shielded place, it should not be in use while the operator is in the room.

Gaseous sterilization

Gases have been utilized for sterilization for a number of years, and among those that have been used are sulfur dioxide and formaldehyde. However, the gas that is of primary interest in this discussion is ethylene oxide because of its penetrating potential and ability to destroy spores. This gas is being used to sterilize many drugs, including antibiotics, biologicals, and enzyme preparations. It is also used to render sterile plastics, surgical material, processing equipment, and other pieces of apparatus. In short, ethylene oxide usually can be used to sterilize almost any object that will be adversely affected by heat or moisture. One of the several applications of ethylene oxide sterilization in dentistry is the sterilization of disposable needles and plastic syringes.

Ethylene oxide, a cyclic ether having the formula $(CH_2)_2O$, is a colorless gas at room temperature. It is inflammable and, when mixed with air, is explosive. In order that the hazard of explosion may be reduced, the gas (10% to 20%) is mixed with carbon dioxide and this mixture used for sterilization. Special autoclaves are used for this type of sterilization. When the temperature and pressure conditions are ideal, the penetration of this gaseous mixture is extremely efficient and effective. The sterilization time varies from 4 to 8 hours.

Bacterial filtration

The bacterial filtration form of sterilization is useful in removing organisms from thermolabile solutions. This solution is passed through special types of filters, which are capable of retaining microorganisms, spores, and many types of viruses. There is some question as to the complete effectiveness of this method of cold sterilization against all viruses. However, bacterial filtration is extremely useful in sterilizing solutions when other methods are impractical or unavailable.

HEPATITIS

There are two virus diseases, both of which primarily involve the liver, that are known as "hepatitis." Because of the possibility of spreading these diseases from one patient to another in the dental office by the use of contaminated instruments, it is well to have some familiarity with them.

Infectious hepatitis is one of the most common of all infectious diseases and is transmitted by direct contact or by contact with contaminated fomites or food and water. Serum hepatitis is spread by contact with blood or plasma that contains the virus. In view of the manner by which these diseases are spread, sterilization of instruments and objects that may come in contact with the patient is essential. Particular care must be taken of instruments that come in contact with blood or of those that are used to penetrate the skin or mucous membranes. Autoclaving is the most reliable method available in the dental office for destroying viruses and thus preventing the transmission of these diseases via contaminated instruments.

SPECIAL CONSIDERATIONS

Storage of instruments after sterilization. After sterilization, instruments must be kept sterile until used. This may be accomplished in several ways. In order to maintain sterility of instruments the following precautions must be taken:

1. Instruments that have been autoclaved or sterilized in boiling water must be removed from the sterilizer only with sterile instrument forceps; they never must be touched by the hands.
2. The instruments are then placed in designated drawers or cabinets between towels that have been sterilized previously in the autoclave. Instruments that have been wrapped for autoclaving should be left in the package until placed on the instrument tray.
3. Instruments must not be removed from the storage cabinet or container with the fingers but only with sterile forceps.

Instruments disinfected by chemical means are usually stored in the dental cabinet after they are rinsed and then dried with a sterile towel.

Preparation of anesthetic syringe. Because it is so very important that injections be made under sterile conditions, special consideration must be given to sterilizing the syringe and preparing it for use.

After use the anesthetic carpule is removed from the syringe and discarded. The contents of the carpule never must be saved, even though only a portion of it was used. If a disposable needle is used, it also is removed from the syringe and discarded. The syringe itself is then scrubbed with a stiff brush in warm soapy water, rinsed thoroughly, placed in the ultrasonic vibra-

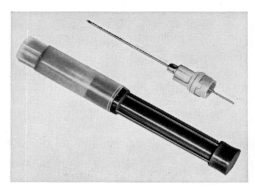

Fig. 14-17. Presterilized disposable dental needle. (Courtesy Sherwood Medical Industries, Inc., St. Louis, Mo.)

tor, and sterilized by boiling or by autoclaving. After the syringe is sterilized it is removed from the sterilizer with sterile instrument forceps and placed in a sterile storage area.

When needed, the syringe is removed from its sterile container, and the needle and hub are assembled if they were sterilized separately. In this case the hub and needle are picked up with sterile forceps, since the needle must not be touched by the hands. Many offices are now using presterilized, disposable needles (Fig. 14-17). When the manufacturer's instructions concerning assembly of the syringe are followed, the disposable needle can be placed on the syringe with no danger of contamination. With the needle assembly in place the anesthetic carpule is removed from a germicidal solution and inserted in the syringe. The syringe is now ready for use, but the assistant must be extremely careful that the needle does not touch any nonsterile object before injection. Should the disposable syringe be used, the same degree of safety can be expected and the the same precautions must be exercised (Fig. 14-18). If a tray is used, it should be covered with a towel that has been autoclaved.

Tray preparation. A sterile tray setup

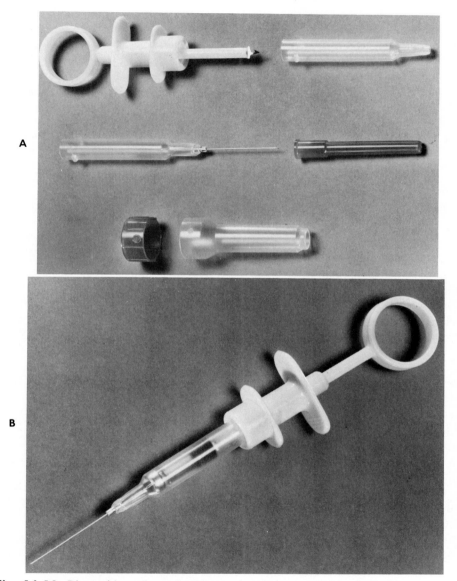

Fig. 14-18. Disposable syringe. **A,** Disassembled disposable syringe displaying the components. **B,** An assembled disposable syringe with anesthetic carpule in place and ready for use. (Courtesy Sherwood Medical Industries, Inc., St. Louis, Mo.)

should be used whenever practical. A container of autoclaved towels should be kept next to the sterilizer, and towels should be removed only with the instrument forceps. The tray is first covered with a sterile towel, and sterile forceps are then used to place the required instruments and supplies in proper order on the tray. If instruments have been autoclaved in individual paper containers, they should be removed and placed on the tray without being touched by the hands. A sterile towel is then placed over the instrument arrangement, and the tray is ready for use. Offices that routinely use the tray system usually will have a number of trays that have been completely outfitted and autoclaved in advance. These, of course, are available for immediate use.

SUMMARY OF STERILIZATION PROCEDURES

Upon completion of each appointment a definite routine should be followed for the care and sterilization of instruments and equipment. In general this routine should be as follows:

1. All instruments are removed from the bracket table or tray, scrubbed thoroughly with a stiff brush in warm soapy water, rinsed in clear water, and then cycled in the ultrasonic vibrator.
2. Air and water syringe tips and oral evacuator tips are removed and scrubbed thoroughly, as in the case of operating instruments.
3. The instruments, syringe tips, and oral evacuator tips are then sterilized by autoclaving, boiling water, or chemical means. All surgical instruments must be autoclaved or boiled. Instruments used in examination, cavity preparation, and restorative procedures may be placed in the chemical solution.
4. Cement slabs and spatulas are scrubbed, rinsed, dried, and replaced in the proper storage place.

5. Conventional handpieces, contra-angles, and prophylaxis handpieces are removed from the dental unit and placed in the hot oil sterilizer. Handpieces that cannot be sterilized by this method are wiped carefully with an alcoholic sponge.
6. The bracket table or tray cover is removed and discarded (if made of paper) or placed in a laundry receptacle.
7. The rim of the bracket table and the air and water syringes are wiped carefully with an alcohol sponge.

SUGGESTED READINGS

Addison, B. A., and others: Sterilization of surgical sutures; comparison of heat and irradiation, Amer. Surg. 31:242, 1965.
Antonovich, E. I.: The dry air sterilizer SS-1, Med. Promyshl. SSSR 18:52, 1964.
Avis, K. E.: What to watch for in sterilization technic, Mod. Hosp. 100:98-104, 1963.
Avis, K. E.: How effective are your sterilization procedures? Hosp. Pharmacy 1:34-40, 1966.
Beeby, M. M., and others: A bacterial spore test piece for the control of ethylene oxide sterilization, J. Appl. Bact. 28:349-360, 1965.
Buchbinder, M.: Sterilization of cotton points and gutta percha points; description of technique, New York J. Dent. 36:200-201, 1966.
Burrows, W.: Textbook of microbiology, ed. 19, Philadelphia, 1968, W. B. Saunders Co.
Burton, W. E.: Changing requirements for sterilization, J. Prosth. Dent. 14:127, 1964.
Central sterile supply, Nurs. Times 61:1795, 1965.
Central sterile supply principles and practices, London, 1963, Oxford University Press.
Cheatle, E. L., and others: An evaluation of some disinfectants, Amer. J. Clin. Path. 45:412-414, 1966.
Christensen, E. A.: Recent sterilization methods, Ugeskr. Laeg. 126:330, 1964.
Christensen, E. A., and others: Inactivation of dried bacteria and bacterial spores by means of ionizing radiation, Acta Path. Microbiol. Scand. 58:225, 1964.
Cleary, D. J.: Residual effects of ethylene oxide sterilization, Bull. Parenteral Drug Assoc. 23:233, 1969.
Colombo, B. M.: Sterilization on an industrial scale with ethylene oxide, Boll. Chimicofarm. 103:554, 1964.
Conte, E. A.: How to sterilize with ethylene oxide gas, Mod. Hosp. 102:122, 1964.

Coughlin, J. W., and others: Comparison of dry heat, autoclave and vapor sterilizers, J. Ontario Dent. Assoc. **45**:137, 1968.

Crawford, J. J., and others: Practical methods of office sterilization and disinfection, J. Oral Med. **22**:133, 1967.

Crowley, M. C.: Obtaining and maintaining surgical cleanliness, Dent. Clin. N. Amer., Nov., 1957, pp. 835-844.

Custer, F., and Hamilton, L.: Evaluation of an autoclave make-up water additive, Dent. Dig. **73**:260-263, 1967.

Custer, F., and others: Physical changes of instruments during sterilization, J. Periodont. **36**:382-386, 1965.

Custer, F., and others: Instrument changes during sterilization, J. Dent. Res. **49**:487, 1970.

Darmady, E. M.: The cleaning of instruments and syringes, J. Clin. Path. **18**:6-12, 1965.

Dittmer, H. H.: Sterilization of local anesthetics, Pharm. Prax. **2**:197, 1963.

Dyer, E. D., and others: Bacteriologic study of muslin and parchment wrapped sterile supplies, Nurs. Res. **15**:79-80, 1966.

Ehrlen, I. R.: Advances in sterilization techniques, Pharm. Weekbl. **99**:1430, 1964.

Ehrlen, I. R.: Advances in sterilization techniques, Svensk. Farm. T. **68**:818, 1964.

Eshleman, J. R.: Methods used for sterilization or disinfection of instruments, J. Dent. Educ. **32**:330, 1968.

Fajers, C., and others: On steam corrosion and steam corrosion inhibition; autoclave corrosion experiments on carbon steel test samples enclosed in nylon foils; preliminary report, Odont. Rev. (Malmo) **17**:40-43, 1966.

Fallon, R. J.: Sterilization of air filters for high pre-vacuum autoclaves, J. Clin. Path. **16**:259, 1963.

Finsterbusch, W.: Experiments with cold sterilization using ethylene oxide under increased tension during one year of clinical use, Wien. Klin. Wschr. **76**:255, 1964.

Gasthalter, F. M.: Importance of sterilization in dental practice (a review of the literature), W. Virginia Dent. Assoc. **36**:154, 1962.

Gillette, W. B.: Ethylene oxide sterilization in dentistry, J. Oral Ther. **2**:440, 1966.

Gimborn, H. von: Sterilization technic, Pharm. Prax. **9**:197, 1963.

Ginsberg, F.: Ethylene oxide is boon to hospital asepsis, Mod. Hosp. **102**:118, 1964.

Gould, D.: Sterilization of medical instruments with gamma rays, Elektromedizin **9**:38, 1964.

Grabar, P.: Biological effects of ultrasonic waves, Advances Biol. Med. Phys. **3**:191-246, 1953.

Gunther, D. A.: Balanced pressure sterilization with ethylene oxide—a new technique, Bull. Parenteral Drug Assoc. **24**:193, 1970.

Haberman, S.: Some comparative studies between a chemical vapor sterilizer and a conventional steam autoclave on various bacteria and viruses, J. S. Calif. Dent. Assoc. **30**:163, 1962.

Harding, H. B.: A sterility control program for the central supply service, Hosp. Top. **43**:81, 1965.

Hepatitis, Washington, D. C., 1955, Health Information Series No. 82, U. S. Department of Health, Education and Welfare.

Hesselgren, S. G., and others: A new method of sterilizing handpieces and contra-angles, J. Oral Ther. **3**:340, 1967.

Hok, R., and others: Ultrasonic tonometer sterilization, Amer. J. Ophthal. **58**:676, 1964.

Holmlund, L. G.: Standardization, by means of ultrasonic treatment, of test samples for laboratory steam-corrosion tests, Acta Odont. Scand. **21**:321, 1963.

Hot enough for long enough, Nurs. Times **62**:406-407, 1966.

Hunter, H. A., and Madlener, E. M.: Disinfection of dental instruments, Int. Dent. J. **11**:312, 1961.

Johnsen, G. N.: Our experience with a high-vacuum sterilizer, Hospitals **37**:77, 1963.

Jossel, N.: Instrument sterilization in dental practice; some limited observations, J. Soc. Dent. Res. **13**:10, 1964.

Kelsey, J. C.: Sterilization and disinfection techniques and equipment, J. Med. Lab. Techn. **22**:209-215, 1965.

Kürer, J.: Immediate root-canal sterilization, Dent. Pract. (Bristol) **16**:404-407, 1966.

Lane, C. R., and others: High-temperature sterilization for surgical instruments, Lancet **1**:358, 1964.

Larato, D. C.: Sterilization of the high speed dental handpiece, Dent. Dig. **72**:107-109, 1966.

Lawrence, C. A., and Block, S. S.: Disinfection, sterilization and preservation, Philadelphia, 1968, Lea & Febiger.

Lubianitskii, G. D.: Ultrasonic device type UM2-2 for cleaning of medical instruments, Med. Promyshl. SSSR **18**:49, 1964.

McCulloch, E. C.: Disinfection and sterilization, ed. 3, Philadelphia, 1945, Lea & Febiger.

McLundle, A. C., and others: Sterilization in general dental practice, Brit. Dent. J. **124**:214, 1968.

Mercer, J. F.: The challenge of sterilization in the dental office, Dent. Assist. **38**:10, 1969.

Olander, J. W.: New facilities and equipment for radiation sterilization, Bull. Parenteral Drug Assoc. **17**:14, 1963.

Opfell, J. B., and others: Penetration by gases

to sterilize interior surfaces of confined spaces, Appl. Microbiol. **12:**27, 1964.

Opfell, J. B., and others: Cold sterilization techniques, Advances Appl. Microbiol. **7:**81-102, 1965.

Perkins, J. J.: Principles and methods of sterilization, ed. 2, Springfield, Ill., 1969, Charles C Thomas, Publisher.

Perkulis, B., and others: Ultrasonics and benzalkonium chloride as a method of sterilizing dental instruments, J. Dent. Child. **37:**69, 1970.

Rittenbury, M. S., and Hench, M. E.: Preliminary evaluation of an activated glutaraldehyde solution for cold sterilization, Ann. Surg. **161:**127, 1965.

Rubbo, S. D., and Gardner, J. F.: A review of sterilization and disinfection as applied to medical, industrial, and laboratory practice, Chicago, 1965, Year Book Medical Publishers, Inc.

Shaner, E. O.: Acoustical-chemical parameters for the ultrasonic sterilization of instruments: a status report, J. Oral Ther. **3:**417, 1967.

Sheahan, J.: Methods of sterilization and disinfection; a survey of current practice in 50 hospitals in England and Wales, Nurs. Times **62:**795-798, 1966.

Sterilization of surgical material; a symposium, London, 1961, The Pharmaceutical Press.

Stratford, B. C.: An ultra-violet water-sterilizing unit, Med. J. Aust. **1**(1):11, 1963.

Sykes, G.: Disinfection and sterilization, ed. 2, Philadelphia, 1965, J. B. Lippincott Co.

Taguchi, J. T., and others: Serious limitations of a portable ethylene oxide sterilizer, Amer. J. Med. Sci. **245:**299, 1963.

Thexton, R.: Supply of sterile instruments and dressings; a central sterilisation system applied to the dental department of a district general hospital, Brit. Dent. J. **119:**344-346, 1965.

Trexler, P. C.: Microbic contamination control, Bull. Parenteral Drug Assoc. **18:**8, 1964.

Walker, G. G.: Basic principles of sterilization and pre-packing of dressings and instruments, Trans. Assoc. Industr. Med. Officers **15:**72-74, 1965.

Walker, R. O., and others: The sterilisation of syringes; a survey of current methods and recommendations, Brit. Dent. J. **118:**151, 1965.

Watson, D. D., and others: Sterilizing techniques with ethylene oxide, Hospitals **37:**81, 1963.

West, E. I., and others: Color coding to control rotation of sterile supplies, Hosp. Top. **45:**111-112, 1965.

Winchell, S. W., and others: Sterilization and care of equipment, Clin. Anesth. **1:**337-348, 1965.

Winge-Heden, K.: Ethylene oxide sterilization without special equipment, Acta Path. Microbiol. Scand. **58:**225, 1963.

chapter 15

DENTAL MATERIALS

Ralph W. Phillips, B.S., M.S., D.Sc.

In many dental offices the hygienist seldom will be required to assist the dentist at the chair or to carry out laboratory procedures. However, it is imperative that she be adequately prepared to handle such assignments if necessary. This chapter will acquaint the student with the more commonly used clinical materials and with the essential manipulative steps that must be controlled. It must be recognized that real proficiency can be attained only by further laboratory training. Fundamentals will be stressed, but many of the minor details associated with specific technics must of necessity be omitted.

A working knowledge of dental materials is also of great importance to the hygienist from the standpoint of her relationship to the patient, to the dentist, and to her profession. She must be cognizant of office routine and the responsibilities of the dentist in order to appreciate fully her own work and her obligations as a member of the dental team. Discussions of problems related to the use and clinical behavior of dental materials arise daily in the dental office, and lack of understanding can be embarrassing and a deterrent to personal progress. This is particularly true at the present time, for numerous new materials and technics are in use and are of keen and pertinent interest to both the patient and the dentist. If and

when the dental hygienist assumes additional professional responsibilities, her training in the field of dental materials science will be markedly expanded. It is with that concept that this chapter should be studied and assimilated.

BIOLOGICAL CONSIDERATIONS

The requirements that are placed upon all dental materials used in the oral cavity are heroic. The biting stresses on restorations amount to thousands of pounds per square inch. Sudden temperature changes with hot and cold foods may produce cracking or disintegration. The warm humid environment of the oral cavity is most conducive to corrosion, while widely varying pH changes contribute to disintegration. During the course of a meal, instantaneous temperature changes as great as 100° F. may occur. These temperature fluctuations from hot and cold foods and beverages may produce dimensional changes in restorative materials or craze or crack the surface.

One of the greatest deficiencies of all of the materials that have been used to restore the carious lesion is that none actually adheres to the adjoining tooth structure. The tooth is not well suited for the tenacious attachment of an adhesive. It is wet, nonhomogenous in composition, rough, covered with tenacious microscopic debris,

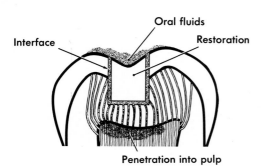

Fig. 15-1. Diagram of the microleakage phenomenon. Gross leakage, as illustrated here, can produce irritation to the pulp. (After Massler, M.: Adhesive retstorative materials, Spencer, Ind., 1961, Owen Litho Service, p. 56. From Phillips, R. W., Swartz, M. L., and Norman, R. D.: Materials for the practicing dentist, St. Louis, 1969, The C. V. Mosby Co.)

and relatively unreactive (low surface energy). All of these factors tend to prevent wetting of the surface by the adhesive. Thus leakage of microorganisms, acid, and debris can occur along the tooth-restoration *interface*, as diagrammed in Fig. 15-1. Such leakage patterns may on occasion result in secondary (recurrent) caries at the margins of restorations, corrosion and stain at the margins, and postoperative sensitivity resulting from the irritation produced to the pulp. Thus the dentist selects materials and technics designed to produce intimate adaptation of the material to the cavity preparation and thus reduce the possibility of deleterious effects from the phenomenon.

A great deal of research centers on the development of adhesive systems that would produce a chemical bond to enamel and/or dentin. One of the developments of particular interest to the dental hygienist is that concerned with sealants for pits and fissures, so-called prophylactic odontonomy. Fluorides are not as effective in inhibiting caries in those areas as they are when applied topically to smooth proximal surfaces. Several resins are now being evaluated as to their efficacy when used to fill in pits and fissures in child patients. Although long-term observations are needed, the early reports are encouraging.

The advent of adhesive dental materials opens other exciting avenues for changes in currently used dental therapies. For example, an adhesive cement would make it possible for the orthodontist to place appliances directly to the enamel surface with small brackets and thus eliminate the unsightly bands now required. It is not beyond the realm of possibility for adhesive films to be developed that, when applied to the tooth surface, could act as a barrier to the accumulation of the dental plaque and thereby act to prevent caries or periodontal disease.

Factors such as those and others require the use of highly specialized compositions and rigid manipulative technics in order to assure clinical success. It is for this reason that approximately one third of the current research effort in dentistry is devoted to improving the materials used by the dentist and his auxiliaries.

The basis for the science of dental materials is thus centered upon the biological and physical characteristics of materials and their interaction with the formidable oral environment.

AMERICAN DENTAL ASSOCIATION SPECIFICATIONS

The American Dental Association, through its fellowship at the National Bureau of Standards since 1928, has established specifications for most of the commonly used materials. These twenty-three specifications cover the pertinent physical and chemical properties and assure the dentist of a material intelligently designed to meet the rigid requirements of the oral environment. Therefore, the dentist is well advised to select only those materials that are on the approved list of certified American Dental Association products, since they are uniform and properly compounded.

At the present time most of the widely used materials are encompassed in the specification program, with a number of others soon to be added. Eventually all of the commonly employed materials used in the oral cavity or required in dental laboratory procedures will be covered by such specifications. An international specification program, sponsored by the Fédération Dentaire Internationale, is now in existence.

In spite of the excellent materials that are available today and the rigid control exerted by both the American Dental Association and the manufacturer, clinical failures are common with all types if materials. These failures may be caused by fracture, corrosion, excessive dimensional change, recurrent caries, gross disintegration in oral fluids, and the like. Seldom can such failures be attributed to use of inferior products but rather to improper manipulation of a basically well-designed material, adequate to meet the demands placed upon it. All dental materials, regardless of the brand, are extremely susceptible to manipulative variables. Every step involved in their preparation and use has a definite influence on the resultant chemical and physical properties. More important, these properties are reflected in the behavior of the material in the oral cavity. Routine success can be achieved only by a knowledge of these properties, an appreciation of the influence of the manipulative variables, and strict adherence to a scientifically sound and standardized procedure.

Obviously there is insufficient space in this book to prepare the student adequately in this field. However, this chapter should acquaint the student with most of the materials she will encounter daily and with the pertinent factors that influence their behavior. It is hoped that it will stimulate her interest to learn more in this highly important area of dentistry.

PLASTER AND STONE

Two of the most commonly used of all dental materials are plaster and stone. They serve as impression materials, are used in the construction of casts and models on which prosthetic appliances are fabricated, serve for study models in orthodontics, and are essential ingredients in many other products. Both plaster and dental stone, which is also often incorrectly referred to as hydrocal, are manufactured from gypsum ($CaSO_4 \cdot 2H_2O$). When mixed with water, both materials harden to reform gypsum. Plaster and stone have the same chemical formula ($(CaSO_4)_2 \cdot H_2O$), but the particles of stone are somewhat more regular in shape and less porous. Because of this physical difference, stone requires less water for making the original mix and is considerably harder and stronger. Thus stone is preferred wherever maximum strength, density, and resistance to abrasion are desired.

The setting time (the time required for the material to harden) of the materials, of course, is important. Obviously rapidity of set has a definite effect on many of the resultant physical properties. More important, though, is its relationship to the handling characteristics. If the plaster hardens too rapidly, there may be inadequate time to take an impression or to pour a model. Likewise prolonged setting will inconvenience both the patient and the dentist. Although the formulas are adjusted to regulate the setting time within proper limits, certain variables will influence the speed of the reaction. These variables are the water-powder ratio, the temperature of the gauging water, the speed of mixing, and the addition of chemical retarders or accelerators. The manufacturer actually adds carefully controlled amounts of retarders and accelerators in order to provide a proper setting time. Generally the most suitable manner of regulating setting time is by the use of

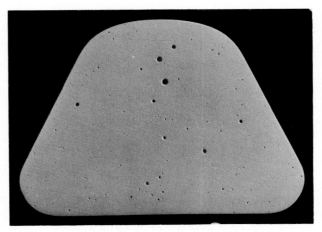

Fig. 15-2. Gross porosity, as seen in cross section of plaster model, that occurred when powder was merely dumped into water. (From Lindquist, J. I., Brennan, R. W., and Phillips, R. W.: J. Prosth. Dent. **3:**274, 1953.)

warm water to accelerate the set or cold water to retard it. It is important that the manufacturer's water-powder ratio be carefully followed. The strength and density are directly related to the amount of powder used; thus, the maximum amount possible should be employed.

The most important problem associated with the manipulation of these materials is minimizing air bubbles or voids. Lack of density may result in fracture, a poor surface on the model or cast, and inaccurate reproduction of essential detail. Porosity can usually be traced to these causes:

1. Air present in the original mass of powder
2. Air incorporated during the mixing procedure
3. Air trapped during pouring of the model

To minimize the air voids inherently present in the mass of plaster powder, the powder should be gently sifted into the water (Figs. 15-2 and 15-3) and vibrated aftermixing. Dumping large masses of plaster into the water carries large quantities of air present in the dry powder into the mix. In mixing, the plaster never should

be whipped but should be mixed by a swiping motion of the spatula against the bowl. The use of auxiliary equipment for mixing, such as vacuum or power-driven spatulators, is a valuable adjunct and definitely reduces the human variable. In pouring impressions the plaster or stone should be added a little at a time to the same area of the impression. A mechanical vibrator should be employed, using *mild* vibration during pouring. Excessive vibration can readily produce voids.

In recent years a still harder and stronger stone has been developed. These stones, technically referred to as Class II stones as compared to the previously discussed Class I stone, are widely used for working models in the fabrication of gold appliances. These stronger materials permit the laboratory technician to prepare and finish the wax pattern directly on the model without as great a danger of destroying or mutilating the surface of the stone. Another advantage of the Class II stones is that they have a lower setting expansion, 0.08%, as compared to the Class I stones, where setting expansions may be as high as 0.20%. Thus a more accurate reproduction of the original impression is

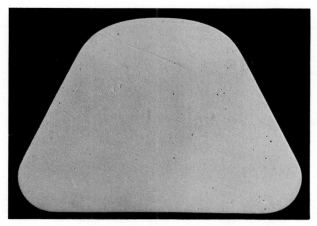

Fig. 15-3. Porosity is minimized when plaster is carefully sifted into water and when whipping is avoided during mixing. (From Lindquist, J. I., Brennan, R. W., and Phillips, R. W.: J. Prosth. Dent. **3**:274, 1953.)

attained. The improved properties are again accomplished by modification of particle size and shape. Although these materials are available in a wide variety of colors, all have essentially the same physical properties.

AMALGAM

The term *amalgam* refers to an alloy of two or more metals, one of which is mercury. Dental amalgam alloys generally contain silver, tin, copper, and often zinc. The dental amalgam restoration is made by mixing small particles of the alloy with mercury and then condensing this plastic mass into the cavity preparation. When the particles are mixed with mercury, a subsequent series of complex chemical and physical reactions ensues, which is accompanied by a hardening of the plastic mass.

The setting reaction may be summarized as follows:

$$Ag_3Sn + Hg \longrightarrow Ag_3Sn + Ag_2Hg_3 + Sn_8Hg$$
$$\text{(gamma)} \quad \text{(gamma-1)} \quad \text{(gamma-2)}$$

Thus the set amalgam is composed of particles of the original particles (gamma phase) surrounded by a crystalline matrix of silver-mercury and tin-mercury compounds. The weakest component in the final structure is the gamma-2 phase, while the strongest is the gamma phase.

The mixing process is referred to as *trituration* and is merely the mechanical combination of the mercury with the alloy. This trituration may be done either by hand with a mortar and pestle or by mechanical devices. During this process the slight oxide film on the alloy particles is abraded to permit the ready attack of the particles by the mercury.

Silver amalgam still remains the most commonly used restorative material, and approximately 80% of all restorations are amalgam. Although amalgam will eventually be replaced by a more esthetic material (such as the composite resins discussed later in this chapter), for the immediate future it will remain the material most commonly used for stress-bearing restorations. Because it remains the backbone of restorative dentistry, greater space will be devoted to amalgam than to the others. Arguments concerning the superiority of the amalgam restoration, as compared to an inlay or a gold foil, are unprofitable. As yet, no *ideal* restorative material has been developed—that is,

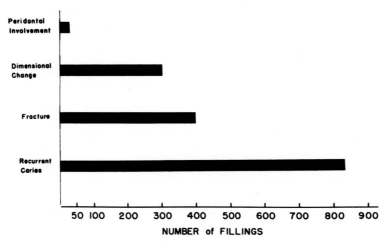

Fig. 15-4. Summary of types of failures observed in a clinical survey of 1,526 faulty amalgam restorations. (From Healey, H. J., and Phillips, R. W.: J. Dent. Res. **28:**439, 1949.)

one that would actually bond to the tooth and be esthetically and physically comparable to enamel and dentin.

Selection of any particular material must be governed by indications and contraindications, past experiences, and the proficiency of the operator in handling the material. For example, an inherent weakness in present amalgam alloys is their lack of ductility (brittleness). Thus, although this property can be controlled to a certain extent, some chipping and fracture at the margins of the restoration may be anticipated. On the other hand, amalgam is unique in that the leakage around the restoration tends to decrease with time in the oral cavity because of corrosion products filling in the area between the restoration and the cavity walls. Thus all restorative materials have certain inherent advantages and disadvantages, which the dentist must acknowledge and take into consideration upon selecting the proper material for that particular situation. Of greater concern in this discussion are the factors that contribute to a good or bad amalgam or to a good or bad inlay.

Surveys have shown, however, that the percentage of failures in amalgam restorations is lower than with any of the other restorative materials. Nevertheless, daily observations in the dental office do reveal large numbers of amalgam restorations that have failed. These failures occur in the form of recurrent caries, fracture, excessive dimensional change, and pulp or periodontal involvement (Fig. 15-4). The success of the amalgam restoration is dependent upon the control of and attention to many variables. Everything that is done from the time that the cavity is prepared until the final restoration is polished has a very definite effect upon the physical properties and thus directly on the success or failure of the restoration. An investigation has shown that improper cavity preparation is the causative factor in approximately 56% of all amalgam failures, while faulty manipulation of the alloy or its contamination at the time of insertion accounts for approximately 40% of all failures (Fig. 15-5). It is with this 40% that the hygienist and chairside assistant must be interested.

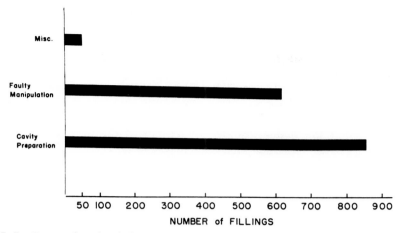

Fig. 15-5. Causes for the failures analyzed in Fig. 15-4 may usually be attributed to neglect or abuse. (From Healey, H. J., and Phillips, R. W.: J. Dent. Res. **28:**439, 1949.)

Pertinent physical properties

The three properties that especially influence the clinical behavior of amalgam are dimensional change, compressive strength, and flow. Proper control of all three of these properties is essential if failure is to be avoided. An understanding of these properties and their clinical significance is necessary in order to appreciate the importance of the various manipulative factors that will be discussed.

Dimensional change. Dimensional change in the restoration should, of course, be at a minimum. The American Dental Association's specification for amalgam states that 24 hours after its insertion the dimensional change shall be $0 \pm 20\mu$ per centimeter. Although slight deviations from these limits apparently are not clinically significant, changes of greater magnitude may lead to disastrous results. Obviously gross contraction could lead to leakage and recurrent caries at the margins, while excessive expansion could produce protrusion, possible postoperative pain because of the pressure upon the pulp from the expanding materials, and opening of the margins.

Compressive strength. There is no doubt that adequate strength is essential to the success of the amalgam restoration. Fracture, even of a small area, will hasten recurrence of decay and subsequent clinical failure. The conventional test for this property is compressive strength and is measured by gradually increasing compression stress until the specimen breaks. Approximately 26% of all failures of amalgam restorations may be attributed to fracture (Fig. 15-4). Although compressive strength has long been the principal strength property associated with such failures, it must be remembered that during mastication an amalgam restoration is subjected not only to compressive stress but also to shear and tensile stresses. However, generally those manipulative variables influencing one strength property will also alter the others accordingly.

Since amalgam is particularly susceptible to fracture during the period before it has completely hardened, the current A.D.A. Specification No. 1 includes an early strength test (a tensile type test). In addition to selecting only alloys that are certified to meet this strength requirement, the patient should be warned against biting on the restoration during the first few hours. Although the material may feel hard and strong, its 1-hour strength may be only one fourth of that which it will ultimately attain.

Gross fracture or severe marginal breakdown may usually be attributed to (1) improper cavity preparation design or (2) faulty manipulation of the material. The former is under the control of the dentist, but the latter may be the major responsibility of the chairside assistant. Three manipulative factors are especially important in controlling the strength—the original alloy-mercury ratio, the amount of trituration, and the pressure used in condensing the amalgam into the cavity preparation. The first two of these variables are generally under the care of the assistant. Thus an exacting manipulative procedure is essential if maximal strength in the restoration is to be attained.

Flow or creep. The strength of the amalgam is closely associated with another property called flow (also referred to as creep). Certain materials, but particularly amorphous ones, will deform or flow under a given load. Although this property is advantageous in many cases (for example, the flow of an impression material into the cavity preparation), it is deleterious to a restorative material. Marked flow under biting stress leads to deformation, loss of anatomical contour, and failure. In the flow test for amalgam the flow is measured as the shortening in length of a specimen subjected to a compressive load. Although the flow test makes use of a static load, it is generally believed that fillings with high flow are more likely to result in some type of distortion of the restoration, such as flattened contact points, overhanging margins, and in severe cases a slight protrusion from the cavity preparation. Recent clinical studies have shown that marginal breakdown may be more closely associated with the "dynamic creep" of the amalgam than any other one property. Dynamic creep is the flow occurring under the normal intermittent, not continuous, forces brought to bear on the restoration during mastication. Again it must be remembered that the flow of any acceptable alloy will vary within wide limits under the influence of the various factors in the manipulative procedure. For example, undertrituration may raise the flow value to as high as 8%, which is more than twice the maximum value permitted by the A.D.A. specification. Light condensation pressure, resulting in excess mercury left in the restoration, likewise increases flow. Thus any step in the technic that tends to reduce the strength will also increase the flow and will make the restoration more susceptible to change in shape during clinical service.

It cannot be overemphasized that a knowledge and appreciation of the importance of these three fundamental properties to the success of the amalgam restoration are necessary if routinely sound restorative dentistry is to be obtained. Failure to control dimensional change and to maintain adequate strength can result only in clinical failure. Probably in no other dental material are the clinical manifestations of even slightly deficient properties so vividly evident in daily practice.

Selection of the alloy

Most of the popular alloys now used have approximately the same chemical composition, the main difference being the size and shape of the grains. The principal exceptions are the recently introduced "dispersion" alloys. A dispersed filler (a silver-copper particle) is added to the conventional silver-tin alloy. It is claimed that such alloys have reduced creep properties and higher strength. However, more clinical data are needed to establish the advantage, if any, of such a composition.

Amalgams usually fall into three general types according to particle size. One type is composed of very small filings or shavings, which amalgamate readily in the mortar and pestle. Other alloys are composed of longer and thinner filings. These filings also amalgamate readily, since they break up into very small particles during trituration. The third type, now seldom seen, has large chunky grains that do not amalgamate well. Even after thorough trituration the mix from such an alloy is still quite coarse and granular. When restorations made from these large-grained alloys are carved, particles are pulled out, leaving a very rough surface that is more susceptible to tarnish and corrosion. It also has been shown that, with all other manufacturing variables controlled, smaller grain size provides greater strength.

Although there are objective reasons why some operators prefer a certain commercial brand of alloy because of color, setting time, ease of carving, or whatever, generally a smaller grained alloy or one whose filings readily break up into a small particle size is preferred. Trituration is probably more rapid with this type of alloy, the adaptation to the cavity walls is better, and the finished carved surface is smoother. For these reasons most of the popular alloys make use of a small-grained particle.

It is possible to manufacture the alloy in the form of small round balls or spheres, as shown in Fig. 15-6. Such an alloy is referred to as a spherical alloy. Several of these types have been introduced commercially. Although more research is required to establish their proper role in amalgam technology, it appears that such a particle shape may provide a slightly smoother carved surface, have higher early strength, and make condensation somewhat less exacting. As yet there is not clear evidence that the somewhat higher physical properties of spherical alloys lead to a superior restoration. It could well be that their principal merit is that they are not as susceptible to certain manipulative variables; in other words, they tend to be somewhat more "foolproof."

Filings or spherical alloys also may be supplied in the form of pellets. The alloy particles are lightly compressed to form a

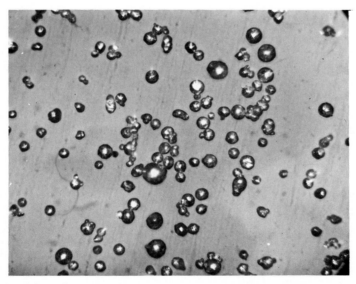

Fig. 15-6. Particles of a typical spherical amalgam alloy. (×170) (From Phillips, R. W., Swartz, M. L., and Norman, R. D.: Materials for the practicing dentist, St. Louis, 1969, The C. V. Mosby Co.)

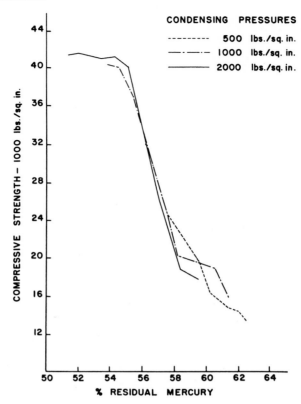

Fig. 15-7. The compressive strength, at various condensation pressures, plotted against residual mercury. Results indicate definite correlation and marked reduction in strength at values above 55%. (From Swartz, M. L., and Phillips, R. W.: J. Dent. Res. **35**:458, 1956.)

pellet or "pill." These pellets then break up readily into the individual filing particles during trituration. The pellet form of the alloy offers convenience and standardized weights of alloy.

Space does not permit a discussion of the manufacturing process. However, the final physical properties are dependent on critical control of composition, heat treatment of ingot and particles, cutting of the particles, and so on.

Effect of residual mercury

Probably the greatest single factor that controls the strength of the alloy, and thus its resistance to fracture, is the final mercury content in the restoration, which will be referred to as residual mercury. A def-

inite correlation has been established between the amount of mercury that remains and the compressive strength at the high mercury values that are often found in the amalgam restoration. It is not uncommon to find clinical restorations in which the residual mercury is well over 60%, even though the loss in compressive strength when the mercury exceeds 55% is dramatic (Fig. 15-7). Apparently the other strength properties of amalgam, such as tensile and transverse strength, are also controlled by the residual mercury content. An example of the clinical significance of a high residual mercury content in the restoration may be seen in the failure shown in Fig. 15-8.

What factors will govern the final per-

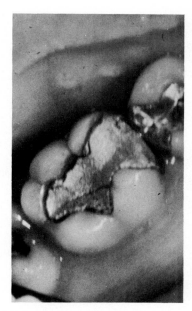

Fig. 15-8. Clinical failure of an amalgam restoration produced from excessive residual mercury content.

centage of mercury in the restoration and thus the ability of the restoration to resist biting stress? They are (1) the original mercury-alloy ratio, (2) trituration, and (3) condensation pressure and technic. Only the minimum amount of mercury needed to obtain a workable mass of material must be employed. Guessing at the ratio or adding mercury to amalgam that has partially set will inevitably lead to excess mercury in the final restoration regardless of the condensation technic. The greater the amount of mercury in the original mix, the greater is the mercury content in the final restoration. In the past it was common to use alloy-mercury ratios as high as 5:8 (5 parts of alloy by weight to 8 parts of mercury by weight). It is not unusual to find ratios as low as 1:1 now being employed. Such ratios are often referred to as minimal mercury technics or the Eames technic. Various types of proportioning devices are on the market, and most are satisfactory if adjusted properly.

Insufficient trituration and inadequate condensation pressure also contribute to excess mercury and to the resulting decrease in strength.

Trituration

As mentioned earlier, the purpose of trituration is to remove, by abrasion, the superficial coat of oxide left on each alloy particle. The clean metal is then readily attacked by the mercury. Of all the variables involved in the use of amalgam, none has a greater effect upon the physical properties than the length of trituration. Insufficient trituration results in a fast-setting amalgam from which less mercury can be expressed. The particles of the original alloy are not thoroughly bonded together, and a weaker framework is established. The final result is reduced strength and increased flow. Undertrituration must be avoided, not only because of the lowered strength but also because the finished surface will be rougher and more susceptible to tarnish and corrosion. There is ample evidence to demonstrate that underamalgamation results in an inferior restoration.

What is the appearance of the proper consistency of the mix? Fig. 15-9 gives examples of both undertrituration and a good mix. The length of time required to reach this consistency depends on many variables, such as the size of the mix, conditions of mortar, speed of trituration, type of alloy, and so on. Amalgamation, therefore, must be standardized according to the conditions present in each dental office. Certainly recognition of the proper appearance of amalgam when thoroughly triturated is imperative, and the mixing procedure then can be adjusted for the individual conditions that exist.

There is no evidence that mechanical devices, which are widely used for mixing amalgam, produce superior results to those obtained by a *careful* hand technic; however, mechanical trituration does tend to

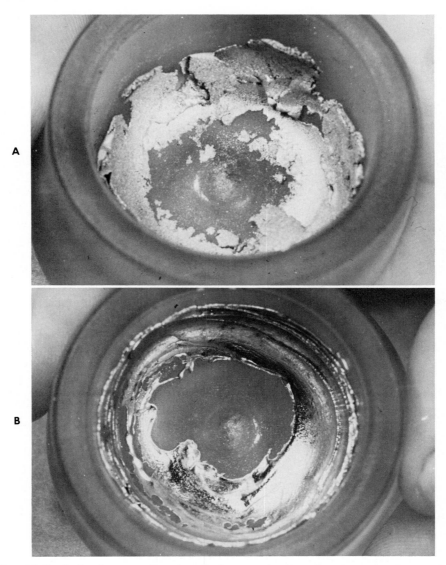

Fig. 15-9. A, Inadequate trituration. **B,** Proper mix. Use of such a granular consistency leads to low physical properties and clinical failure. (From Phillips, R. W.: J.A.D.A. **54:** 309, 1957.)

standardize the procedure. Herein, then, lies the real advantage of such devices. Individual types of amalgamators will vary in their efficiency and rate of amalgamation.

The degree of trituration does influence the dimensional change that occurs as the amalgam hardens; for example, the longer the mixing time, the less the setting expansion. There is, however, no evidence to indicate that the reduced expansion or possibly the few microns contraction that results from thorough trituration is clinically significant. Observations on clinical restorations made from thoroughly triturated amalgams, and even with a special

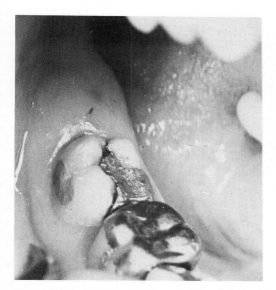

Fig. 15-10. Recurrent caries and the "ditched" appearance on this restoration are not caused by contraction of alloy but rather by certain other manipulative errors. (From Phillips, R. W.: J.A.D.A. **54:**309, 1957.)

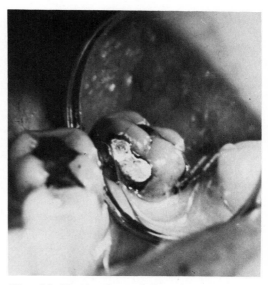

Fig. 15-11. Amalgam failure from severe expansion caused by moisture contamination of a zinc-containing alloy. (From Healey, H. J., and Phillips, R. W.: J. Dent. Res. **28:**439, 1949.)

alloy compounded to produce excessive contraction, have failed to reveal a single instance of open margins or recurrent caries. Restorations placed with thoroughly amalgamated mixes actually proved superior in surface condition and marginal adaptation. This seems to bear out the opinion of most investigators that it is better to err on the side of too much rather than too little trituration.

The "ditched" filling (Fig. 15-10), often attributed to contraction of the alloy, is more probably caused by poor condensation of the amalgam, which leaves this vital area weak and rich in mercury, or a thin feather ledge of amalgam left after carving. However, these remarks must not be construed as a recommendation for a contracting alloy or a haphazard technic. They merely emphasize that small-dimensional changes, as measured by present laboratory methods, may not be clinically significant and that the real danger in the trituration of amalgam lies in underamalgamation.

Effect of moisture

Excessive expansion of amalgam because of moisture contamination is a definite clinical problem. Such contamination may arise either from saliva being incorporated into the amalgam during condensation or from perspiration on the hands or fingers while the material is being handled. Approximately 16% of all failures can be attributed to this phenomenon. The zinc, present in most alloys, dissociates the water and liberates hydrogen gas. The trapped gas exerts a pressure within the restoration and results in an expansion, which may be as great as 500 μ (0.5 mm.) per centimeter, producing overhanging margins that invite recurrent caries, corrosion, and possible postoperative pain (Fig. 15-11). Likewise, the resulting voids that are formed reduce the strength of the restoration by approximately one fourth. Thus there is no alternative but to maintain a dry field during the operative procedure and to avoid handling the amalgam with the hands. Naturally this moisture contamination is a danger only during trituration or condensation. Saliva coming in contact with the packed surface immediately after condensation has no deleterious effect.

Because of this ever-present problem of moisture contamination, manufacturers have introduced zinc-free alloys, hoping to minimize this hazard. Since zinc is used to act as a scavenger for oxides, the manufacturer of a zinc-free alloy is probably a more delicate process and requires great care on the part of the manufacturer. Properly prepared, the alloy seems to have essentially the same physical properties as a zinc-containing alloy. The zinc-free alloys tend to be somewhat dirtier in handling than zinc alloys, but there is no sound correlation between this observation and clinical properties or behavior. The one characteristic that has not been evaluated adequately is the resistance to corrosion of the zinc-free alloys as compared to zinc-containing alloys. Short-term observations indicate that they could be more susceptible to corrosion.

Certainly, whenever the occasion arises when moisture contamination cannot be prevented, the zinc-free alloy should be used. It is to be hoped that the use of these new materials will not lead to a false sense of security on the part of the person using them. Moisture is always to be avoided, regardless of the composition of the alloy.

Tarnish and corrosion

Loss of esthetics because of tarnish or corrosion is a hazard with all metallic restorations and particularly with amalgam (Fig. 15-12). There is, of course, a difference between tarnish and corrosion. Tarnish is merely a surface deposit, while corrosion represents an actual chemical attack

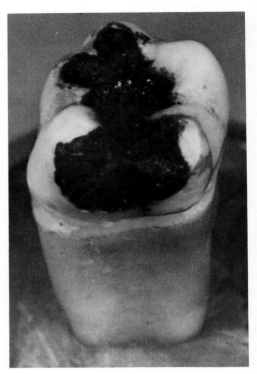

Fig. 15-12. Example of severe clinical corrosion. Oral environment and certain manipulative variables will influence its incidence and severity.

of the material. Tarnish, however, is often the forerunner of corrosion. The conditions in the oral cavity are extremely conducive to corrosion, since the environment is warm and moist, and conditions of variable acidity and alkalinity and food debris and plaque material are always present. Although the exact chemical nature of the tarnish layer is unknown, it is probably predominantly a sulfide with some lesser amounts of chlorides and oxides. As previously mentioned, it is the gamma-2 phase (Sn_8Hg) in the amalgam that is largely responsible for corrosion.

Certain variables not within the control of the dentist or hygienist certainly play a vital role in the frequency of tarnish. Factors such as mouth hygiene, diet, and pH and composition of saliva will unquestionably influence the susceptibility to tarnish. However, proper control of certain manipulative variables will contribute greatly to maintenance of esthetics. A smooth surface is less susceptible to accumulation of debris; thus surface irregularities in the restoration should be minimized. Small-grained alloys, thorough trituration, prevention of moisture contamination, and polishing the restoration will all aid in reducing discoloration.

The restoration is not completed until polished. During polishing the small scratches and pits left on the surface after carving the restoration are removed. If permitted to remain, debris will collect in the irregularities. The difference in pH of that debris, as compared to that of saliva, in conjunction with the metallic material creates a small electrical corrosion cell. This phenomenon is referred to as "concentration cell" corrosion and can produce a progressive deterioration through the body of the restoration. Care should be exercised at the time of polishing, and in all subsequent prophylaxis, to avoid generation of heat. Excessive heat will draw mercury to the surface and thus increase the possibility of both fracture and tarnish.

Galvanic action

The problem of galvanic shock in the oral cavity is one generally associated with the amalgam restoration. This phenomenon arises from the presence of dissimilar, or even similar, metallic restorations. When the restorations are in contact or when they are touched by another metal such as silverware, a sharp pain results. The incidence of such cases is relatively low, but it is frequent enough to be of concern. It is known that small currents in the magnitude of 0.5 μa do exist between dissimilar metal fillings. These currents persist indefinitely and normally do not cause discomfort. For the patient who is affected, the postoperative pain usually sub-

sides within several days, probably because of the reduced sensitivity of the pulp as it heals from the injury incurred during the operative procedure and from the caries process. Not much can be done to prevent this phenomenon except to coat the outside of the restoration with an insulating varnish, thereby insulating the metal from the saliva. If any corrosion is noted, the restoration should be repolished. This will often alter the potential of the cement enough to eliminate the sensitivity. There is no evidence that such currents contribute to any serious oral systemic dyscrasia.

The amalgam restoration still remains a fascinating and fertile area for research. Probably in no other material are the mistakes in manipulation so vividly exemplified under clinical conditions. Its success is dependent upon meticulous attention to detail during its manipulation, insertion, and polishing.

Mercury toxicity

Throughout the history of the amalgam restoration it has been speculated that the mercury could leach out in oral fluids, accumulate in body tissues, and thus produce local or systemic effects. The matter has been well studied and it is most unlikely that any danger can arise to the patient. Minor amounts of mercury diffuse out only during the period before the material has hardened. This mercury is present in the form of metallic mercury, not the toxic form such as the methyl mercury associated with fish food poisoning.

The dentist and his auxiliaries must be aware that mercury does vaporize rapidly when exposed to the office environment. Dental personnel are thus continually inhaling small amounts of mercury vapor when manipulating this material. While one should not be alarmed, normal hygienic procedures should be followed in handling the material in order to avoid excessive mercury contamination of the area.

Obviously the office should be well ven-tilated and all scrap amalgam should be stored immediately in a sealed container. Mercury suppressants are superior to vac-uum cleaners in cleaning carpeting if mercury is spilled.

IMPRESSION MATERIALS

There are two broad classifications of impression materials—elastic and inelastic. The inelastic type, such as plaster, com-pound, or wax, is the older. Although these materials are well suited for certain uses, such as impressions for complete dentures, their inelasticity and rigidity do not permit removal from undercuts or from around the crown of the tooth without rupture or distortion. In recent years various types of elastic impression materials have grad-ually replaced the inelastic ones in many dental technics. These flexible materials make impressions for partial dentures, in-lays, or bridges possible with greater ease, fewer steps, and little or no detectable per-manent deformation. In fact the advent of the reversible hydrocolloid technic revolu-tionized indirect technics for the construc-tion of inlays and fixed bridges. The fol-lowing discussion will be concerned with these elastic impression materials.

An explanation of indirect technics might be apropos at this place. With the direct technic for gold restorations, a wax pattern is formed in the actual tooth preparation in the oral cavity. The pattern is then re-moved and a gold casting made from it. In the indirect procedure an impression is taken of the tooth and cavity preparation. This impression is then poured in stone or metal to produce a working model. The wax pattern is now formed on this model. There are arguments for both technics; however, the indirect method saves chair time, secures better patterns in areas dif-ficult to see in the mouth, and provides easier finishing of the casting at the mar-gins.

Hydrocolloids

Hydrocolloids may be classified into two general types—reversible and irreversible. They are suspensions of aggregates of molecules in a dispersing medium of water, the water being held by capillary action. Dental reversible hydrocolloids are suspen-sions of molecules of agar, a seaweed. Al-though different chemically, they are com-parable in physical behavior to common gelatin. At elevated temperatures the agar forms a colloidal fluid *sol*, which may be safely injected into the cavity preparation. By means of water-cooled trays the sol material is then converted to a *gel*, which is firm, yet elastic; the agar forms a com-plete gel at approximately 102° F. This change from the sol state to a gel state is thermally reversible and is essentially phys-ical in nature rather than a true chemical reaction. In dentistry these materials are generally referred to merely as hydrocol-loids.

A proper armamentarium for boiling, storing, and tempering the hydrocolloid is essential (Figs. 15-13 and 15-14). Briefly, the material is handled as follows. It is first boiled for a minimum of 10 minutes to provide a fluid sol. There is no danger in overboiling, but insufficient boiling will lead to a granular, stiff mass of material. After boiling the hydrocolloid is stored at a temperature of approximately 150° F. until it is needed for injection into the cav-ity preparation or for filling the tray. Stor-age temperatures below 150° F. are too low and will permit some undesired gelation. Water-cooled trays with water at 60° to 70° F. are used to accelerate gelation. The tray must be held in position under passive pressure for a minimum of 5 minutes to assure adequate gel strength. Care must be exercised in removing the impression to avoid distortion. Contrary to common con-cept these materials are stronger and less apt to distort if subjected to a sudden load rather than a slow constant pressure. Thus they must be snapped out with a sharp

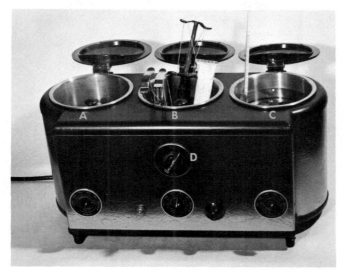

Fig. 15-13. A unit for preparation of a reversible hydrocolloid impression. A, Compartment liquifying material; B, storage compartment for solution; C, compartment for storage (tempering) tray impression material; D, timer.

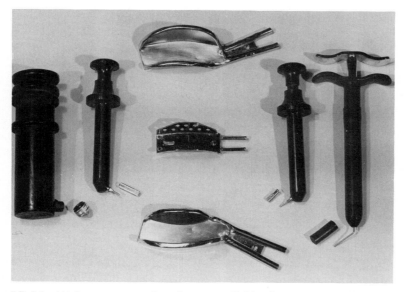

Fig. 15-14. Various trays and syringes available for reversible hydrocolloid technic. The trays are water cooled, and the small syringes are used for injecting the material into the cavity preparation. (From Hohlt, F. A.: Dent. Clin. N. Amer., pp. 139-155, March, 1957.)

thrust, as nearly as possible parallel to the long axis of the tooth, and must never be rocked or teased off of the teeth.

The irreversible hydrocolloids, commonly called alginates, gel by means of a definite chemical reaction, usually between sodium or potassium alginate and calcium sulfate. Other chemicals are present to regulate certain properties, for example, trisodium phosphate as a retarder to the set. The material is supplied in a powder and is mixed with the proper amount of water. The temperature of the water should be approximately 70° F. in order to provide ample working time. The warm oral temperature then promotes gelation. The tray is held in the mouth for approximately 2 minutes after obvious gelation.

The most common source of clinical error with either the reversible or irreversible hydrocolloids is failure to pour the impression immediately. Both reversible and irreversible hydrocolloids are approximately 75% to 85% water and tend to lose (syneresis) or gain (imbibition) water rapidly, depending on the storage environment. Likewise, all impressions contain a certain amount of internal stress from the manipulative procedures. This stress is relieved with time and results in distortion. Storage of the impression must not be prolonged for more than 15 minutes, for measured changes will invariably result (Figs. 15-15 and 15-16). There is no alternative but to pour the model as soon as possible after its removal from the mouth; if storage is necessary, the best environment is in approximately 100% relative humidity in a humidor type of arrangement. This does not prevent distortion but will minimize it.

Rubber base materials

More recently other elastic types of impression materials have been introduced. They are synthetic rubber materials that may be mixed with a suitable chemical to produce an elastic and accurate impression when carried into the oral cavity. One type

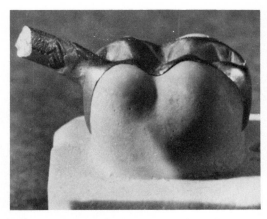

Fig. 15-15. Fit of a master casting tried on a stone die poured in a reversible hydrocolloid impression. The casting was actually fabricated on the original porcelain tooth and thus serves as a measure for the accuracy of the die. When the impression is poured at once, as shown here, no distortion is evident. (From Phillips, R. W., and Ito, B. Y.: J.A.D.A. **43**:1, 1951.)

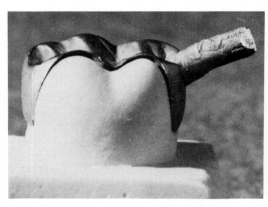

Fig. 15-16. Distortion resulting from impression that was stored for 1 hour in air before pouring. The same casting shown in Fig. 15-15 is used here. (From Phillips, R. W., and Ito, B. Y.: J.A.D.A. **43**:1, 1951.)

has as its principal ingredient a polysulfide compound and thus is classified as a polysulfide polymer, often more commonly referred to simply as a rubber base impression material. The other form of the dental

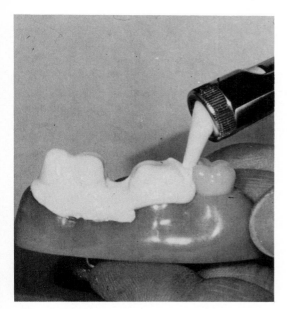

Fig. 15-17. An example of injection of a silicone impression material on a laboratory model. A similar technic is used with the reversible hydrocolloids.

rubber impression materials has a silicone rubber as its main component. The silicone type has a more pleasing color, odor, and handling characteristics, but both types are comparable to the reversible hydrocolloids in accuracy. They come in a paste form and are mixed with catalysts, in a paste or liquid, which produce "curing" in the mouth within a short time. They are available in both a thin-consistency as well as a heavy-consistency material so that they can be easily injected into the cavity preparation (Fig. 15-17). Their main advantages, as compared to hydrocolloid, lie in the simplicity of manipulation, lack of expensive armamentarium, and somewhat superior dimensional stability. However, it is still desirable to pour the impression immediately, since continued polymerization of the rubber will cause distortion.

Again, various manipulative variables will influence the accuracy of the result. The material must be held tenaciously by the tray or band, and this may be readily accomplished by painting the impression tray with a rubber cement. Mixing is not difficult, but care should be taken to incorporate the pastes thoroughly. The setting time is influenced by both temperature and humidity—the higher the temperature or greater the humidity, the more rapid the set. Contrary to the method using hydrocolloid, a minimum bulk of material between the tooth and the tray is desired. The impression must be held in the mouth for at least 8 minutes to allow ample curing, and as with hydrocolloid, it should be removed from the mouth with a sharp thrust.

CEMENTS

Several types of dental cements are used for widely different purposes—for actual restorations, for cementing gold restorations and orthodontic bands, as insulating bases for restorations, and for pulp capping. Generally speaking, as a class of dental materials they are the weakest. They have low strength, are readily soluble, and are easily stained. For maximal properties, even though they are less than desired, proper manipulation is imperative.

Zinc phosphate

The zinc phosphate cements, used primarily for cementation and as bases under metallic restorations, are made from a mixture of a powder and a liquid. The powder is primarily zinc oxide and magnesium oxide, while the liquid contains phosphoric acid, water, and certain buffering agents. Proper care of the powder and liquid is essential. The liquid contains a definite amount of water; if this balance is not maintained, the setting time is seriously altered, and the consistency of the mix will vary accordingly. More important is the effect on the physical properties of the cement. For example, if the water-acid ratio varies only 5% from that as supplied by the manufacturer, the solubility is doubled. Since this ratio will alter somewhat with time even when the liquid is properly cared for, the last one-fifth of the bottle should be discarded. The bottles of cement powder and liquid must be tightly stoppered at all times and the liquid discarded whenever any cloudiness or precipitate appears.

Such cements do not actually adhere, in a chemical sense, to the tooth surface. They cannot, therefore, be relied upon to hold an inlay or orthodontic band in place. They merely serve as a luting material to occupy the space between the restoration and the tooth. However, there is a close mechanical adaptation of the cement to irregularities in the cavity preparation and in the appliance. In order to maintain this adaptation, and thus prevent leakage, it is necessary to minimize solubility and to assure adequate strength to prevent fracture of these small projections. The manipulative factors that influence these properties will be discussed shortly.

Silicate

The silicate cements used in restorations have a powder consisting mainly of silica, alumina, and either calcium fluoride or cryolite (Na_3AlF_6). These fluoride compounds are used as a flux during the manufacture. The liquid is quite comparable to that of the zinc phosphate cements. Again proper care of both powder and liquid is essential.

Clinical surveys have shown that the incidence of recurrent caries around the silicate restoration is surprisingly less than around other types of restorative materials. This is probably because of the high concentration of fluoride present. During the setting of the cement, and possibly subsequently, the fluoride reacts with the adjoining tooth structure to reduce the acid solubility of the enamel. In essence it is comparable to a topical application of fluoride. The increased resistance of the tooth to organic acids accounts in part at least for the lowered incidence of caries. Many of the restorative materials are

believed to have some germicidal effect, especially the silver and copper ions present in amalgam. The exact effectiveness of each particular material in inhibiting bacterial action still remains controversial, however, and a great deal of research is being carried out to improve the germicidal characteristics. This is a particularly important area for research because, as has been discussed, no restorative material perfectly seals the cavity preparation, and microleakage is a real clinical problem.

Fluoride has been added to a variety of materials (for example, amalgam, resin, and zinc phosphate cement) in the hope of capturing the unique anticariogenic effect of silicate cement. Although a topical effect of the fluoride can often be demonstrated with such fluoride-containing materials, there is no documentation as yet that the benefits clinically will be comparable. The silicate restoration provides another fluoride mechanism that may not be present in these materials. It has been shown that the chemical composition of the plaque on the surface or at the margins of a silicate restoration is markedly different than the plaque associated with other types of restorative materials. Specifically the carbohydrate-nitrogen ratio is markedly higher. These data suggest that the fluoride may also be acting as an enzyme inhibitor to retard bacterial accumulations. Thus the anticariogenic effect of silicate cement may involve several different fluoride mechanisms that may be difficult to reproduce in other materials. Certainly for the moment the silicate restoration is often the material of choice, in spite of its other deficiencies. For example, in the mouth of a child patient with a high caries index, it is to be preferred because of its resistance to marginal caries, even though the restoration may not be as durable as those made of certain other types of materials.

• • •

As mentioned previously, solubility in dilute acids and in mouth fluids is the

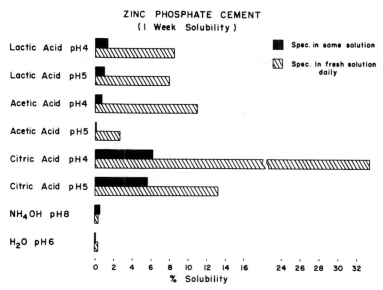

Fig. 15-18. Solubility of a typical commercial zinc phosphate cement in various media. Although distilled water (bottom of graph) is the conventional solution used to measure solubility, dissolution is much greater in dilute acids that may be present in the oral environment. Note that solubility also increases when the specimen is stored at lower pH's and in fresh solutions. (From Norman, R. D., Swartz, M. L., and Phillips, R. W.: J. Dent. Res. **36:** 977, 1957.)

primary weakness of dental cements (Fig. 15-18). Solubility certainly leads to recurrent caries around the cemented restoration, decalcification under orthodontic bands, stain, and loss of normal function of the restoration. The primary factor that controls the solubility, as well as the compressive strength, is the powder-liquid ratio. Solubility is directly related to the amount of powder that can be incorporated into the liquid. The soluble portion of the cement is the matrix, which forms around the original particles of powder. This matrix is crystalline for the zinc phosphate cements but is principally a gel for the silicates. The greater the amount of powder present, and thus the less of this matrix that is formed, the stronger and the less soluble will be the cement. The only way that the maximum powder can be incorporated for *any* desired consistency is by the use of a cool slab. The cooler the slab (although it never should be below the

dew point), the greater the amount of powder that may be incorporated and thus the greater the possibility for clinical success.

Because of the difference in the final chemical compound formed, zinc phosphate and silicate are mixed differently (Fig. 15-19). It is important that the silicate gel matrix not be disturbed as it forms because that would lower the physical properties. Therefore the mixing of silicate must be completed in approximately 1 minute. A large amount of powder is folded into the liquid immediately.

However, mixing time is not critical for the zinc phosphate cement. Small quantities are incorporated at a time, with the completion of the mix usually taking approximately 1½ minutes. The actual consistency will vary with the purpose for which the cement is to be used and for the individual operator.

Proper control of setting time is essen-

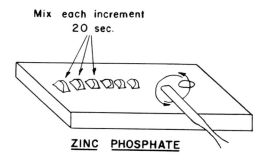

Mix each increment
20 sec.

ZINC PHOSPHATE

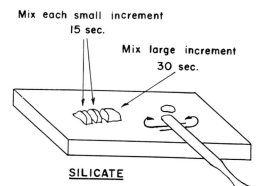

Mix each small increment
15 sec.

Mix large increment
30 sec.

SILICATE

Fig. 15-19. Diagram of mixing procedures for both zinc phosphate and silicate cements. Difference in mixing technic and time of spatulation is a result of the difference in chemical reactions that occur. In both cases, however, a maximum amount of powder must be incorporated.

tial to both of these materials, and one of the common difficulties encountered is gross deviation from the desired working time. When a cement sets too slowly, the cause is generally because the liquid has changed because of improper care, the mix is too thin, or spatulation was too long. If the set is too fast, it may be caused by mixing on a warm slab, insufficient spatulation, or too rapid addition of powder in the early stages of mixing.

Zinc oxide–eugenol

Another type of dental cement is prepared by mixing zinc oxide and eugenol. This mixture is particularly useful whenever maximum protection for the pulp is desired or where postoperative sensitivity may be likely. Zinc oxide–eugenol cements are considerably less irritating to the pulp than zinc phosphate cements, for example, since they have a pH of approximately 7.

Thus they are often preferred as a temporary restoration or as a base under permanent restorations. Their use as a permanent cementing agent has been limited because of the low strength of the set cement. As mentioned previously, a certain minimum strength is deemed desirable to assure mechanical retention of the casting to the prepared cavity. However, it has been found that certain additives, such as ortho-ethoxy benzoic acid, may be used to produce substantial increases in the compressive strength. Several such products have been introduced commercially and are now being subjected to critical clinical evaluation to determine their efficacy as permanent luting agents.

Polycarboxylate

Recently a new class of cements has become popular. Referred to as polycarboxylates, they are prepared by mixing a liquid of polyacrylic acid with essentially a zinc oxide powder. The cements are comparable to zinc oxide–eugenol in reducing sensitivity and in pulpal response. Furthermore, the cement apparently produces a chemical bond to tooth structure by a chelation reaction with the calcium present in the apatite structure of the tooth. The adhesive characteristics are so interesting that studies are now underway evaluating the efficacy of the cement in attaching orthodontic brackets to enamel without the use of bands. Certainly whenever past experience indicates that postoperative sensitivity is likely to be a major concern, these cements, or a zinc oxide–eugenol, are the materials of choice for the dentist for the cementation of a gold restoration.

Silicophosphate

The silicophosphate cements are essentially silicate cements that contain approximately 10% zinc oxide in the powder. They are often preferred over zinc phosphate cement for the cementation of porcelain jackets for esthetic reasons. Because of this somewhat high film thickness and inferior manipulative characteristics, their use in cementation of gold restorations has been limited. However, newer formulations seem to have overcome those shortcomings. As a class of cements, they offer the advantage of providing some anticariogenic protection at the margins since the fluoride mechanism is essentially comparable to that in a silicate cement.

RESINS

Plastics, referred to hereafter as resins, are ever increasing in their dental application. Originally confined to complete and partial dentures, they now are employed as filling materials, cements, artificial teeth, and prostheses of various types. The general field of plastics is one that is moving at an accelerated pace. There can be no doubt that the veritable avalanche of new resins eventually will result in revolutionary dental developments. It can be envisioned that some day resin materials will be available that will bond chemically to the tooth, that will possess physical and chemical properties that compare favorably to tooth structure, and that will have truly bacteriostatic or germicidal properties. Even more alluring would be the development of a durable adhesive resin film that could be applied to the intact tooth surface in order to serve as a barrier to caries or calculus formation, as was discussed previously. It is for this reason that the hygienist must have a keen interest and some basic knowledge of dental resins.

These materials, often referred to simply as acrylics, are usually derivatives of acrylic or methacrylic acid, although various other compounds, such as styrene, are employed to a limited extent in some of the newer types of materials. They are classed as thermoplastic resins as compared to the thermosetting resins that were previously used in dentistry, for example, vulcanite. The thermosetting resins differ from the thermoplastic resins in that they cannot be resoftened with the application of heat and their curing is a typical chemical reaction. On the other hand, the curing of the thermoplastic resins is more a combination of similar molecules. The appliance or restoration is generally formed by the curing of a mixture of a powder (the polymer) and a liquid (the monomer). Although the chemistry is somewhat complex, the process of curing this mixture into the finished hard denture or restoration is essentially one of changing the single molecules in the monomer into a long-chain molecule, similar to the molecule of the polymer itself. This process is referred to as polymerization. The physical properties of the final polymerized resin are dependent upon the degree of polymerization that takes place and the ultimate size of the molecule. The larger the molecule and the more complete the polymerization, the higher are the physical properties.

This polymerization may be accomplished by means of heat, light, or suitable catalysts. Although a catalyst, benzoyl peroxide, is incorporated in the powder of all types of dental resins to initiate the reaction, most appliances in the past have been cured primarily by the application of heat. For example, the denture is slowly heated from room temperature up to 212° F., generally in a water bath. Most of the polymerization occurs between 150° and 175° F. This reaction is strongly exothermic, with much heat liberated as the resin polymerizes. Therefore it is highly important that the curing progress slowly in order to prevent vaporization of the monomer. Any vaporization leaves bubbles and porosity.

Naturally it is impossible to use heat of this magnitude in the oral cavity. Thus polymerization of a resin cement, restorative material, or denture relining agent must be accomplished by chemical means. As will be explained later, with these self-cured resins an additional catalyst is added to the monomer in order to produce polymerization, even though the temperature is only 98° F.

For prosthetic appliances the acrylic type of resins generally have excellent esthetics, and certain of their physical and chemical properties are unusually high. They are insoluble in most oral fluids, generally have quite adequate resistance to fracture under biting stress, are easily fabricated or repaired, and have good color stability. Likewise the dimensional stability during usage is apparently satisfactory. The average change in contour of a full denture after 2 years of service is only approximately 0.2 mm. It is doubtful that the patient can detect fluctuations of this magnitude. Loss of fit of dentures with time is more likely to be associated with changes in the underlying tissues.

Proper care of the denture by the pa-

tient is essential if dimensional change is to be minimized and esthetics maintained. As yet the present resins do not have adequate resistance to abrasion; thus the patient must be warned against the use of harsh abrasives, such as household cleansers. The denture may be safely cleaned with soap and water or toothpaste. Hot water always should be avoided, since it will soften and distort the base. If the denture is stored for any period of time, it should be kept wet in order to prevent loss of the water that is normally present. Loss of this water is accompanied by contraction of the resin. The denture then will fit improperly until water from the saliva has been absorbed by the resin. Most cases of irritation under dentures can be attributed to improper fit or to poor oral hygiene. True allergy to acrylic resins seldom is seen in the dental office.

Restorative resins

The dental profession long has sought a material that would be less soluble than, and have superior esthetics to, the silicate restoration. One of the recent developments in that direction has been the use of the acrylic resins for this purpose. As mentioned previously, these materials are polymerized at mouth temperature by means of an additional catalyst in the monomer. This catalyst is usually dimethyl p-toluidine and is referred to as the activator. By proper adjustment of the concentration of this agent and the benzoyl peroxide in the polymer, polymerization can be reduced to a matter of a few minutes. This makes possible the use of the resin as a filling material or a cement or for the repair and relining of dentures.

Much of the early difficulty with the resins can be attributed to faulty materials, inadequate technics, and a lack of appreciation for their basic properties. These materials are excellent examples of the clinical difficulties that invariably arise when the basic physical properties of a

dental material are unknown or are ig-
nored. For example, because of low hardness and resistance to abrasion, their use
is generally contraindicated whenever they
are to be subjected to stress. They should
be confined basically to the Class V or
Class III restoration. Resin also may be
employed in the repair of the fractured
incisor (Class IV). In such cases a wire is
inserted into both the tooth and the resin
in order to provide the necessary retention
of the restoration.

The two main weaknesses with this material have been the lack of color stability
and the difficulty in securing adequate
adaptation to the cavity preparation. Rapid
discoloration of the early resins was common and could be attributed to deterioration of the activator. The oxidized by-prod-
ucts of the catalyst are usually colored
and lead to an overall darkening of the
restoration. Color stability has greatly improved, with better balance in compositions as well as use of different catalytic
systems (for example, *p*-toluene sulfinic
acid). Although the color stability is still
not perfect in some products, it is no
longer a real clinical problem.

As with any restorative material, it is
extremely important that the best possible
adaptation of the resin to the tooth surface
be secured. The resins contain no bacteriostatic or germicidal agents, and thus penetration of saliva and debris leads to unin-
hibited recurrent caries. As mentioned previously, the addition of fluoride to acrylic
resins may not be as effective as the addition of silicate cement. The high coefficient
of thermal expansion, 7 to 1 as compared
to that for tooth structure, may tend to
cause marginal seepage whenever hot or
cold food or beverages are taken into the
mouth. Table 15-1 indicates that the dimensional change, thermally, with resin
is considerably higher than with other common restorative materials. It is well to
emphasize, however, that the clinical significance of this characteristic is unknown.

Table 15-1. Coefficient of thermal expansion of
various restorative materials as compared to
that for tooth structure

Material	Factor*	$\left(\dfrac{\propto \text{ for material}}{\propto \text{ for tooth}}\right)$
Acrylic resin		7.1
Amalgam		2.2
Gold inlay		1.9
Gold foil		1.3
Silicate cement		0.8

*The higher the factor, the more dimensional change with
fluctuation in temperature.
$\propto$ = Linear coefficient of expansion.

For example, it is quite possible that the
temperatures to which the resin is actually subjected may not be severe because
of the buffering action of the mouth temperature and the location of the restoration. The low thermal conductivity of the
resin retards the diffusion of hot or cold
through the restoration. In other words,
the high coefficient of thermal expansion is
balanced somewhat by the fact that the
restoration does not tend to get hot or cold
rapidly, in contrast to metallic restorations. However, this property of the resin
is undesirable and emphasizes the need for
good adaptation to the cavity, which
would tend to prevent any dimensional
change.

Lack of adequate marginal seal is probably a major cause for subsequent pulpal
injury, but it is often blamed on the toxicity of the material itself. It is known that
the acrylic resins per se are no more toxic
than many other commonly used materials.
However, if gross leakage occurs, pulpal
injury must evolve irrespective of the filling material employed.

Adaptation of the resins has been greatly
enhanced by dentists who exert greater
care during insertion and who use improved
technics and auxiliary materials. The
use of brush-in technics for applying the
resin in increments rather than in one

large mass has definitely resulted in better adaptation. The use of special cavity lining agents, which are painted into the cavity before insertion of the resin, also results in superior adaptation. These lining agents should not be confused with cavity varnishes, which will be discussed subsequently. They are different in composition. A typical varnish prevents polymerization of an acrylic resin.

Another aid in improving adaptation is to swab the enamel surface within the cavity preparation with a 50% phosphoric acid solution. Such an "etching technic" cleans the tooth and thus increases the wettability of the resin. The resin penetrates into the small pits produced in the enamel by the acid and thereby increases the mechanical retention of the resin.

Resin systems other than acrylic now have become available in dentistry. One of these is used in the popular *composite* restorative resins preferred now by many dentists over the older acrylic resins. A composite material is one in which a filler has been added to a matrix material in such a way that the properties of the matrix substance is improved. The resin in these dental restoratives is a reaction product between an epoxy resin and methacrylic acid. To this resin, fillers such as glass beads or rods or particles of quartz are added in concentration as high as 78%. The combination of that particular resin and the high filler content produces a material with a lower coefficient of thermal expansion as compared to acrylic resins. The rapid polymerization, greater hardness and strength, and superior esthetics appeal to many dentists. Since their strength properties approach those of amalgam, they have been recommended for Class II restorations. However, their use in that type of restoration should be viewed with conservativism since wear during mastication may in time produce a change in anatomical contour. On the other hand, in those situations where esthetics are the predominate factor, such as in the bicuspid area, they may be the material of choice. Unquestionably the composite resins will increase in popularity and further improvements in their properties may be anticipated.

GOLD RESTORATIONS

The fabrication of a gold inlay, crown, or partial denture involves a series of steps making use of several different materials. The greatest single weakness of the cast restoration is, of course, the soluble layer of cement that is used as a luting material when the casting is seated. A thin margin of the cement is invariably exposed to oral fluids, and recurrent caries is directly related to the washing out of the cement. Naturally the better the fit of the casting, the smaller the amount of cement that will be exposed. One clinical investigation suggested that whenever the marginal discrepancy around a restoration exceeded 50 μ, secondary caries usually resulted. Thus all emphasis in the construction of the single gold restoration or the fixed bridge must center on securing finite accuracy in the casting. Although the perfect inlay never has been made, it is possible to produce, routinely, exacting restorations provided one has an appreciation and knowledge of the fundamentals involved. The essential components employed in the fabrication of the small dental casting are diagrammed in Fig. 15-20. The actual procedure will be outlined in the following discussion.

Wax pattern. The first step in the fabrication of an inlay is the preparation of the wax pattern. The wax pattern, which eventually forms the mold for the final casting, may be fabricated either directly on the tooth itself or on a die that is a replica of the prepared tooth. As mentioned previously, the former method is called the direct technic and the latter, the indirect technic.

The dental waxes contain paraffin as their main ingredient, with compounds

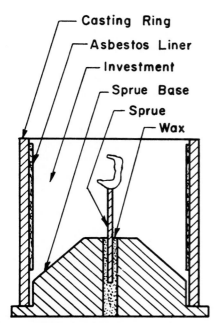

Casting Ring
Asbestos Liner
Investment
Sprue Base
Sprue
Wax

Fig. 15-20. Schematic drawing of components involved in the fabrication of gold casting.

such as a gum dammar and carnauba added to regulate the melting range and the working characteristics. For direct technics it is important that the flow of wax at mouth temperature be minimal in order to prevent distortion upon the removal of the pattern from the cavity preparation. However, when molding the plastic wax into the cavity, the flow must be high in order to secure maximum reproduction of the cavity. Thus the flow may be as much as 80% at a safe and comfortable oral working temperature of 115° or 120° F. This wide variation in flow at very little change in temperature is one of the specific and necessary requirements of a dental wax.

It must be remembered that the final casting can be no better than the original pattern. Therefore the wax must be well adapted at all margins, properly contoured, and carved to correct anatomy. One of the real hazards in the handling of wax is distortion, which may take place from the

time the pattern is removed from the preparation until it is invested. All wax patterns contain internal stress because of the natural tendency of the wax to contract on cooling, which changes the shape of the wax during molding and carving. The degree of stress will be dependent upon the amount and type of manipulation to which the pattern is subjected, but some stress is always present in any pattern. As soon as the pattern is no longer confined by the cavity preparation, the stress is relieved and distortion results. On a critical type of pattern this distortion can be readily detected within 30 minutes (Fig. 15-21). Thus a fundamental rule to be observed is to invest the pattern immediately. Even when the indirect technic is employed, wax distortion may occur on the die in the direction where the pattern is not confined by the die itself. Thus the margin always must be carefully checked before the pattern is removed from the die.

Investment. A sprue is attached to the pattern (Fig. 15-22). The sprue, either metal or wax, subsequently serves as the way for the molten metal to enter the mold. Care must be taken to avoid any overheating of the sprue, which will melt large areas of the pattern and cause distortion as the wax resolidifies. A small drop of wax is placed on the pattern at the point where the sprue is to be attached. After removing the pattern from the preparation and attaching the sprue, it is surrounded by a gypsum material called investment, placed in an oven, and the wax burned out. This leaves a mold of the original pattern into which the gold alloy is cast.

Dental gold alloys contract during solidification. The values given for this contraction range from 1.1% to 1.6%. An average value of approximately 1.4% seems to be acceptable. Unless this contraction is compensated for in some manner, the casting would be much too small. The compensation is accomplished in various

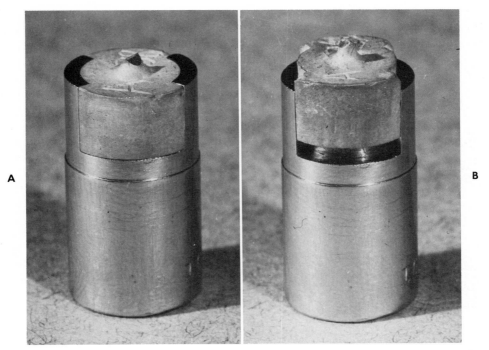

Fig. 15-21. Example of wax pattern distortion. **A,** Casting from a molded pattern invested immediately after removal from the model. **B,** Casting made from a pattern that had been allowed to stand 30 minutes off of the model before investing. (From Phillips, R. W., and Biggs, D. H.: J.A.D.A. **41**:28, 1950.)

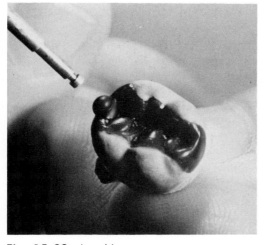

Fig. 15-22. Attaching sprue to a wax pattern.

ways, but all involve the expansion of the investment.

The investment is composed mainly of plaster or stone to provide strength and act as a binder and some form of silica to produce the thermal expansion. All investments have some setting expansion as the gypsum hardens, and all have varying degrees of thermal expansion when heated —investments containing the cristobalite form of silica expanding more than those that contain the quartz form. The third type of expansion possible in investments is hygroscopic in nature, produced by the sorption of water while the investment is hardening. Technics utilizing water baths or the additions of known amounts of water to the top of the setting investment make use of this type of expansion.

After burning out the wax, at temperatures varying between 900° and 1,300° F., depending on the technic and investment used, the gold alloy is melted and forced into the mold. This can be done by air pressure, centrifugal force, vacuum, or combinations of these.

Gold alloys. Various types of gold are used for different kinds of dental restorations. The requirements for a bridge abutment or partial denture clasp in terms of strength, resistance to abrasion, and attrition obviously will be more stringent than those for a simple one-surface inlay. As the casting becomes more complex or the demands upon it greater, the dentist usually makes use of harder and stronger alloys.

Pure gold, used in the gold-foil restoration, is referred to as 24 carat. The carat of all alloys is calculated on this basis; for example, an 18-carat gold alloy would consist of 18 parts of pure gold and 6 parts of other metals, and a 12-carat gold alloy would mean 50% pure gold. Dental alloys are complex, having six or more constituents. In addition to gold they usually contain varying amounts of platinum, palladium, silver, copper, and zinc. Each element is carefully balanced to give the desired color, hardness, melting range, and other physical properties. It is believed that the minimum precious metal content should be 75% to assure adequate resistance to tarnish and corrosion.

It is highly important that the casting have no porosity. Voids lead to corrosion in oral fluids and may drastically lower the required physical properties. The various types of porosity have been well studied. Briefly, density in castings may be assured by the following:

1. Using a sprue that has a diameter greater than the largest cross section of the casting
2. Locating the pattern within ¼ inch from the open end of the ring to permit rapid escape of the gases from the burned-out mold
3. Avoiding any overheating of the gold
4. Using adequate casting pressure
5. Giving the metal proper care during melting by keeping it in the reducing part of the melting flame and covering the surface of the metal with a flux to prevent oxidation of the metal

The fluxes used are powders, usually containing borax and charcoal. The finished casting is cleaned by "pickling" in warm acid. The casting failure is now the exception, and the ability to cast smooth, dense, and accurate restorations consistently (Fig. 15-23) is acquired early if attention is given to the fundamentals that have been discussed.

MISCELLANEOUS MATERIALS
Direct filling gold

Gold foil is one of the few pure metals used in the mouth. Gold foil is one of the oldest, and most satisfactory, of all restorations. The dentist uses small ropes, pellets, or a powder form of the foil to build the restoration, and the insertion does require special skill and proficiency. It is used primarily in the Class III and Class V restorations.

Impression compound

Compound, an inelastic type of impression material, long has been used in prosthetic dentistry for impressions of edentulous mouths or in operative dentistry to obtain impressions of single tooth cavity preparations. In the latter case the impression is secured by means of a proper-fitting copper band filled with the softened compound, forced on the tooth, cooled, and removed. Compound is composed of stearic acid, chalk, and synthetic resins.

Solders

Dental solders are used for joining individual units, such as in the construction of

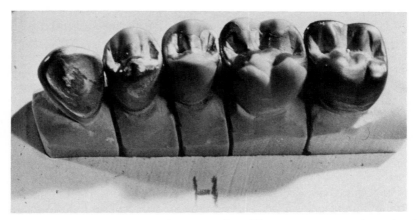

Fig. 15-23. Example of a series of castings for different type restorations showing fit on stone dies.

a fixed bridge. The soldering operation is a delicate one. If the appliance is not thoroughly cleaned or fluxed or the flame is improperly controlled, the resulting soldered joint will be weak and brittle. This loss in physical properties is probably caused by excessive crystal growth in the gold casting. A high percentage of the clinical failure of soldered appliances can be attributed to improper soldering procedures.

Chromium alloys

The base metal alloys have become popular as a substitute for gold alloys in partial denture construction. With trade names such as Vitallium or Ticonium, these materials are basically composed of chromium, cobalt, and nickel. Their properties differ greatly from those of the precious metal alloys. The chrome-cobalt alloys are much harder, are lighter, have greater tensile strength, and are more resistant to corrosion. On the other hand the gold alloys are less brittle and are easier to fabricate and repair.

Cavity varnishes and bases

Before placing the restoration the dentist may apply a varnish to the cavity prepara-

tion. This material is composed of a natural rosin or a synthetic resin dissolved in a solvent such as chloroform or ether. The varnish is applied in a thin layer, and the solvent evaporates to leave a film on the prepared cavity. This film is not thick enough to provide thermal insulation, one of the prime requisites of the base. The varnish does, however, reduce the marginal leakage around certain restorative materials such as amalgam. Likewise it tends to inhibit the penetration of acid when used under an acid-containing material such as a zinc phosphate or silicate cement. For these reasons the pulp reaction is reduced and postoperative sensitivity is less frequent.

The conventional base material is either a zinc oxide–eugenol or a calcium hydroxide–containing cement. Both are less irritating than zinc phosphate cement and tend to promote the formation of secondary dentin. The cement base is particularly important in the deep cavity preparation in order to provide thermal insulation under a metallic restoration and to form a strong foundation upon which the amalgam or gold foil restoration may be condensed.

SUGGESTED READINGS

Phillips, R. W.: Certain biological considerations in the use of restorative materials, New York Dent. J. 28:297, 1962.

Phillips, R. W.: The scientific bases of dentistry, Philadelphia, 1966, W. B. Saunders Co.

Phillips, R. W.: Advancements in adhesive restorative dental materials, J. Dent. Res. 45:1662-1667, 1966.

Phillips, R. W.: Elements of dental materials, ed. 2, Philadelphia, 1971, W. B. Saunders Co.

Phillips, R. W., editor: Symposium on dental materials, Dent. Clin. N. Amer., pp. 1-127, 1971.

Phillips, R. W., Swartz, M. L., and Norman, R. D.: Materials for the practicing dentist, St. Louis, 1969, The C. V. Mosby Co.

REVIEW QUESTIONS

1. List and justify the various physical and chemical properties essential to a dental restorative material.
2. Discuss the various manipulative factors that influence the clinical behavior of the amalgam restoration.
3. What is the element most likely involved in tarnish or corrosion of amalgam? Discuss the factors that influence tarnish of amalgam.
4. Discuss what is meant by galvanic action and its prevalence, clinical importance, and methods of prevention.
5. What types of amalgam failures are seen? What are the causes for such failures?
6. Discuss the influence of mercury on the physical properties of amalgam and the manipulative factors that influence the final mercury content of the restoration.
7. What are the causes and remedies for porosity in plaster or stone models?
8. What is the difference between the chemical formulas and properties of plaster and stone?
9. Describe the steps in fabricating a gold inlay.
10. How much do gold alloys contract when they solidify? How may this be compensated for?
11. Discuss causes for wax pattern distortion.
12. What is the difference in composition between the heat-cured acrylic resin and the self-cured ones?
13. How may the solubility of dental cement be minimized?
14. What is the difference in the chemical reactions of zinc phosphate cement and silicate cement? Are they mixed differently?
15. Explain the mechanisms for the anticariogenic behavior of silicate cement.
16. What is the difference in composition and mechanism of gelation of a reversible and irreversible hydrocolloid impression material?
17. What is meant by a composite material?
18. Discuss the problem of mercury toxicity from amalgam, both to the patient and to the dentist or his auxiliary.
19. What is meant by the microleakage phenomenon? Discuss its clinical significance.
20. Classify the various types of cements used by dentists.
21. Describe the final structure of silicate cement restoration.
22. What is the American Dental Association Specification Program for dental materials?
23. What is meant by the coefficient of thermal expansion? Compare this property for various restorative materials.
24. What functions are provided by a cavity varnish?

chapter 16

THE DENTAL HYGIENIST IN DENTAL PUBLIC HEALTH

Sidney L. Miller, B.S., D.D.S., M.P.H.

Ever since the practice of dental hygiene in this country was made permissible by amendment to Connecticut's State Dental Practice Act in 1907, the hygienist has served the dentist as a second pair of hands. Although this dental auxiliary was developed originally to perform oral prophylaxis on patients and to work as a health educator with children in schools and in the private dental office, the dental hygienist, by virtue of her specialized training, has a distinct role in public health programs. Indeed, early public programs in dental health employed a small number of dental hygienists—both in health departments and in school systems—for the purpose of fulfilling their fundamental role as provider of specialized care and health educator. Similarly, the earliest community programs for the prevention of dental caries utilized dental hygienists employed by the U.S. Public Health Service to apply topical fluorides to the teeth of selected groups of school children in order to evaluate the effectiveness of 2% sodium fluoride in reducing caries.

Thus were delineated the three primary functions of the dental hygienist in public health—namely, providing oral prophylaxis services, giving health education, and helping in the prevention of dental disease. Identification of the dental hygienist as a principal member of the public health team is readily understandable if one reviews the philosophy and purposes of public health as well as their application in community health programs.

WHAT IS PUBLIC HEALTH?

Public health is many things and is different things to different people, hence the need for a definition as the basis for a consideration of the scope of public health.

There have been many attempts at developing a working definition of public health. Undoubtedly, too, there will continue to be refinements, revisions, and modifications in any definition that is propounded, for change is one of the hallmarks of public health. Those definitions of public health that have been proposed in past years have ranged in length from one word—people—to scholarly dissertations covering as many as twenty-four pages of typewritten verbiage. The classic definition, finally adopted by the World Health Organization, is one that was developed by Dr. C. E. A. Winslow, which calls public health "the art and science of preventing and controlling disease, promoting health, and prolonging life through organized community effort."*

---

*Winslow, C. E. A.: The untilled fields of public health, Mod. Med. 2:183-191, 1920.

The concept of health is today regarded as "complete physical, social, and mental well-being, and not merely the absence of disease." Thus, within the definitions of public health and health are embraced many concepts and disciplines that touch upon not only the physical sciences but the social sciences as well.

Public health professionals find the key to a working definition of public health within a combination of the several definitions that have been proposed, because each one has some element of validity. The practice of public health may be said to encompass all community action to prevent and control disease, promote the public well-being, and prolong human life, and it includes input from all people in the community. *All* people must necessarily include not only professional full-time public health workers but also the community's health professionals, social scientists, and even the consumers of health care services themselves.

Public health is *all* people and everything that they do to improve the well-being of the community in a common endeavor to make man's existence safe and enjoyable at home, at work, and at play.

It should be kept in mind that the cardinal difference between public health practice and the private practice of medicine or dentistry lies in the fact that the patient in public health is the community, while that of the practitioner is the individual. The importance of individual health in this scheme of things extends usually only to the point where it constitutes part of the broader patient concept, the community. In the final analysis, the well-being of the community is the sum of the states of health of all individuals in the community.

DENTAL DISEASE: A PUBLIC HEALTH PROBLEM

Dental disease constitutes a legitimate public health problem because (1) it is widespread, (2) it poses a serious threat to the health and well-being of society, (3) there exists a body of knowledge for its control, and (4) that body of knowledge has not been applied. These four factors enter into a determination of when a disease merits the attention and concern of the public health authorities. Certainly, dental disease qualifies as a problem.[1]

Dental disease is universal in prevalence. By age 17 virtually 100% of all children who reside in a nonfluoridated area have experienced the discomfort of dental caries attack. Furthermore, the carious process is irreversible, progressive, and cumulative.

Perhaps of greater concern than the carious process to the profession and to society are the sequelae to caries attack—the ravages of dental caries. Up to age 34, dental caries is the principal cause for the loss of natural teeth in this country; after age 34, periodontal disease takes over as the chief cause for tooth loss. Alarmingly enough, approximately 13% of the nation's people are edentulous. Periodontal disease affects 100% of the population by age 60. Malocclusion and congenital and developmental defects are sufficiently prevalent among the population to pose serious threats to the well-being of society—not only physically, but economically as well. During the early years of World War II, more young men in this country were rejected for military duty because of dental disease than for any other single cause. Furthermore, dental care in the United States accounts for approximately 10% of the national expenditure for health care services.[2]

The private sector of the dental profession has, throughout the course of dentistry's evolution, attempted to control dental disease and to maintain the nation's dental health. The record is quite clear. Despite these efforts, dental disease occurs six times faster than it can be corrected; only 40% of the population visits a dental office each year, and there are many segments of society who cannot come to a dental office because of some physical shortcoming or because of the economic inability to purchase care, or who would not be welcome there even if they could come.[3]

It has become quite clear that the efforts of the profession at control of dental disease, which has followed the traditional pattern of remedial care, has not kept pace with the dental needs of the public. It is apparent that treatment services alone will never achieve the goal of control of dental disease in population groups. Especially is this true in light of the fact that the ratio of dentists to population has declined over the past several decades despite the fact that the demands for dental care have increased during this same period. In 1930 there was one dentist for every 1,700 people; today, the ratio approaches one dentist for every 2,100 people.[4] In point of fact, the resolution of the problem of dental disease calls for the mustering of all the health resources in the community and their concentration upon the total problem.

THE DENTAL PROGRAM IN PUBLIC HEALTH

The official agency entrusted with the community's health is usually the Department of Public Health, which exists at all levels of government. The maintenance of a Department of Public Health has become recognized as a major function of our modern society.

A modern Department of Health includes a combination of professional and supportive personnel who have been trained to utilize the health sciences in the public interest and for the common good. Through effective teamwork and community organization, the public health team engages in a unique set of services in a common effort and toward a common goal.

The several organizational units and their personnel within the Department of Health share in common the broad responsibilities of the Department. These responsibilities include participation in the planning and evaluation of the total program of the agency.

Since the organization of the first dental division within a state health department in 1921,[5] there have been great strides made in the development of effective programs in dental public health. Since then, there has been a new and increasing awareness of the essential role of dentistry in public health.[6] Today, after about 50 years, all but one state health department have a Dental Division within its organization. The Dental Division in public health functions as a specialized unit within the official health agency. Its responsibility is to motivate communities to utilize all valid preventive and control technics in the battle against dental disease.

For the past 35 years, since enactment of the Social Security Act of 1935, the people of the United States, as well as government at all levels, have been moving toward provision of better health care for all.[7] Dental health is today considered an essential health service that cannot be divorced from total health. The dental hygienist, an essential member of the dental health team, has a particular place in any program dealing with the dental health of the public.

Generally, a well-conceived program in dental public health today aims at achieving a reasonable and equitable balance between activities in health education, preventive dentistry, dental care services, and research. Fundamental to the direction and effectiveness of any public health program, however, is its administration.[8]

ADMINISTRATION OF A PUBLIC HEALTH PROGRAM

The training that a dentist undergoes in the handling of the individual patient serves as a guide to the management of a community as a patient. The procedure in public health administration follows the same steps that the dentist pursues every day in handling the individual patient who comes to him with a dental problem. The analogy is quite clear.[9]

In each case there is usually a chief complaint. The individual patient may have a toothache; in the case of the community, a school nurse may register with the authorities her alarm at observing a huge volume of decayed teeth in her students. Whatever the source or nature of the patient's chief complaint, the dentist in private practice will usually adhere to a specific routine in patient management. This routine follows an orderly pattern and proceeds step by step as follows:

1. Examination of the patient—clinical findings as well as radiographic examination, study models, and case history
2. Diagnosis—careful consideration of all the elements comprising the examination and noting a complete picture of the dental needs of the patient
3. Treatment plan—scientific correlation of all facets of the patient's needs as determined in the examination and diagnosis, with coordination of the logical sequence of treatment leading to restoration of the patient's dental health
4. Case presentation—presentation of the treatment plan to the patient, along with an explanation of purpose, justification, and goals in treatment
5. Fee and payment arrangements—fitting the treatment plan into the patient's budget and economic capability
6. Providing treatment—orderly procedures in accordance with the treatment plan presented by the dentist and approved by the patient
7. Assessment of treatment—a continuous determination by the dentist of

the elements of the treatment in reference to known standards, aspirations, and expectations

The foregoing steps, although not always followed in the suggested sequence, are exactly the same as those observed by the public health administrator in treating his patient, the community. However, he calls them by different names, as follows:

1. Survey—community examination to identify the problem in all its ramifications and the resources available for its solution
2. Analysis of the data—statistical analysis of the findings of the survey to serve as the basis for defining objectives or what needs to be accomplished. These objectives will serve as a basis for evaluating what will be accomplished.
3. Development of a program plan—a coordination of all resources that will be brought to bear against the problem in the attainment of the goals set forth as objectives
4. Selling the program plan—presentation to and preparation of the groups concerned in the program in order to gain acceptance and approval
5. Development of a budget—securing operational funds, within which the various program elements can be carried out
6. Operation of the program—who will be doing what, where, when, why, and how
7. Evaluation—periodic and continuous assessment of accomplishments to determine the feasibility of proceeding along the course outlined in the program plan

As is evident from a careful review of the foregoing series of administrative activities, good administrative procedure in dental public health requires skillful professional and personal relations, sound program planning and budgeting, practical organization of activities, judicious selection of staff, and continuing evaluation of the program elements.

All of these elements are interrelated. All need to be brought together equitably and judiciously if a program is to function smoothly and effectively.

In order to function effectively, the Dental Division in public health must receive the approval and support of the profession, of which the dental hygienist is a part. The dental hygienist who supports the public health program of the Dental Division can contribute to its success by interpreting its objectives and need to the public. Public acceptance and support will be reflected in the overt actions of its elected legislators whose support, moral as well as financial, is mandatory if the Dental Division is to function at all.[10]

ROLE OF THE DENTAL HYGIENIST IN PUBLIC HEALTH

In recent years the number of dental hygienists employed in public health programs has been increasing. Such progressive utilization of personnel is readily apparent if one reviews the definition and philosophy of public health, its program activities, and its administrative patterns, which have already been presented. As dental health programs continue to expand, more opportunities will present themselves for careers in public health for the dental hygienist.

Many of the early dental programs in public health were small, employing only one public health dentist or one administrator. As more funds became available, there was a resultant expansion of dental units in official health agencies. Additional positions were opened up for dental hygienists. With increased competency in preventive dentistry, such as the introduction of fluorides, new clinical functions that could be carried out by the dental hygienist have contributed to increased employment opportunities in public health for this dental auxiliary.

The dental hygienist has already demonstrated her value to public health dentists and, also, has seen the need for further training and education in public health for herself. The federal government has, in recent years, sponsored traineeship programs in public health for dental hygienists. Such government support has resulted in increasing the supply of dental hygienists who are properly educated in public health. However, the increase in the number of qualified public health dental hygienists has not kept up with an increased demand for their services.

Accurate data on the number of active dental hygienists in the country presently employed in an official or voluntary health agency are not available. However, they are estimated to comprise between 10% and 25% of the total number of practicing dental hygienists.[11, 12] A recent trend is their employment in Departments of Community or Social Dentistry in Schools of Dentistry and in Dental Public Health Units in Schools of Public Health.

The responsibilities and functions of the dental hygienist in public health are determined by and related to her educational background.[13] There exist today at least three levels of qualifications for the dental hygienist, with commensurate levels of service in public health.

The levels of service functions for the dental hygienist in public health are as follows:

1. Delivery of direct services as a clinician
   a. Oral prophylaxis
   b. Topical application of preventive agents
   c. Health education
2. Administration
   a. Supervision of clinical dental hygienists in a public program
   b. Administration of a program in dental public health
3. Faculty of a School of Dentistry or a School of Public Health

a. Teaching dental students and/or assistants the utilization of dental auxiliaries
b. Teaching expanded functions to dental auxiliary personnel
c. Evaluation of community dental programs

The particular role and function of the dental hygienist must necessarily be determined by her training and qualifications.

EDUCATION OF THE DENTAL HYGIENIST
Two-year certificate program

All formal schools of dental hygiene now offer the minimum 2-year course that meets the requirements for certification of the dental hygienist. Upon completing her education and receiving her certificate, the dental hygienist must take and pass a state board examination in order to acquire a license to practice clinical dental hygiene.

The clinical dental hygienist is qualified to perform oral prophylaxis, to conduct chairside patient education, to do topical applications of preventive agents, and to function as a resource person to teachers and to others. These services she may perform either in the private office of a dentist or in a public program operated by an official health agency or an institution of higher education.

Four-year degree program

Some schools offer a 4-year program leading to a bachelor's degree in dental hygiene. Usually, the 4-year program embraces the components of the standard 2-year certificate program plus an additional 2 years in the arts and sciences. The additional 2 years may be taken in courses designed specifically to develop skills of value in public dental programs. Most frequently, the additional 2 years of education precede the 2 years of clinical training.

The dental hygienist who earns a degree must also pass a state board examination. However, her advanced training qualifies her to perform functions that are above and beyond the capabilities of the 2-year dental hygienist. With her background she is capable of being a dental health consultant in a Dental Division of a public health agency. She is qualified to serve in a supervisory capacity to clinical dental hygienists in a state department of health, a school system, the U. S. Public Health Service, or the World Health Organization. She may be qualified to function as a faculty member in a School of Dentistry or in a School of Public Health.

Master's program in public health

The dental hygienist who has a bachelor's degree may continue her education and training toward a Master's degree in public health by attending a School of Public Health in a graduate program. This program may require 1 or 2 years of additional schooling. However, the dental hygienist who earns a Master of Public Health degree approaches in depth the training of the public health dentist.

Her Master's degree qualifies her to perform a number of specialized functions that ordinarily are outside the realm of competency of her less-trained counterparts. She will possess a generalized understanding of public health, including the administrative process, epidemiology, statistics, and health department organization. She will acquire an understanding of dental survey methodology and knowledge in depth of disease prevention and control on a community basis. She will acquire a background in the principles of education, which will improve her capabilities in one of her fundamental responsibilities as a dental hygienist, namely health education.

With such a background, she may qualify as a section head within an official dental division, a program supervisor, or an administrator. She will be qualified to participate in the planning and evaluation of the total program in public health.

DESIRABLE SPECIALIZED SKILLS
FOR THE PUBLIC HEALTH
DENTAL HYGIENIST

Interestingly enough, the restrictions imposed by state Dental Practice Acts on dental hygienists are not always carried over in the practice of public health. Although, in law, the dental hygienist is required to function under the direct supervision and control of a dentist, this is not always the case in public health.

The clinical distinction between the dentist and the dental hygienist as defined in the Dental Practice Acts does not always apply in the practice of dental public health. The determinant of authority and degree of freedom and individualized level of function, as stated earlier, is dependent upon the educational background, training, and experience of the individuals concerned. In the past, dental hygienists have functioned in top administrative positions in state and local dental public health programs. In short, the public health dental hygienist has some independence of action in her function as part of the public health team.[14]

Basic to service as a public health dental hygienist is the requirement that she be skilled in and have comprehensive knowledge of the practice of clinical dental hygiene. The hygienist in public health who functions as a consultant, supervisor, or administrator must, further, become knowledgeable about current developments and trends in all aspects of dental and dental hygiene practice. In order to maintain and improve her knowledge, she must scan many dental journals, be able to carefully evaluate pertinent articles, and attend refresher courses and dental meetings regularly.

If she is to function effectively as a consultant to clinical hygienists, other health workers, and school teachers, the public health dental hygienist must acquire skills in group dynamics. She should develop an understanding of those factors that condition and determine individual attitudes in her efforts to effect change in attitudes and social behavior. She should acquire skill in the technics of the education process in her efforts to motivate people to seek and adopt corrective and preventive service and to follow acceptable, effective health practices.

Her effectiveness in public health will depend to a considerable extent on her skill in public and individual communications. She must develop the ability to write effectively, with precision and clarity. She must be able to speak effectively. She should develop skills in the administrative process and the ability to think logically, prepare a written presentation of a program or report, and preside effectively at meetings and discussions.

One public health dental hygienist has stated quite succinctly that "dental hygienists, irrespective of their field of service, are primarily dental health educators and keenly interested in and concerned with the preventive aspects of dentistry."*

In summary, with this basic background and with additional training and education in public health, the dental hygienist will be able to:

1. Plan and conduct in-service training programs for other public health workers and teachers
2. Direct health education activities of staff dental hygienists
3. Obtain cooperation of local dental hygiene and dental associations
4. Present talks before lay audiences
5. Organize and participate in community health projects
6. Plan and participate in the preparation and dissemination of health educational materials

---

*Wisan, J. M.: Dental health education. In Pelton, W. J., and Wisan, J. M., editors: Dentistry in public health, ed. 2, Philadelphia, 1955, W. B. Saunders Co.

7. Help in developing a school health education program
8. Evaluate educational programs
9. Conduct dental surveys
10. Take an active and major role in planning and participating in programs for the prevention of dental disease[15]

REFERENCES

1. Council on Dental Health: Dental administration in the state health departments, J.A.D.A. **42**:61-75, 1951.
2. Health statistics, U. S. National Health Survey, Series B22, Washington, D. C., 1960, Department of Health, Education and Welfare.
3. Miller, S. L.: Dental care for the mentally retarded: a challenge to the profession, J. Pub. Health Dent. **25**:111-115, 1965.
4. Division of Dental Health, Public Health Service: Unpublished data.
5. Gerrie, N. F.: Dental public health, J.A.D.A. **40**:750, 1950.
6. Galagan, D. J.: The growing role of dentistry in public health, J. Missouri Dent. Assoc. **41**:12-19, 1961.
7. American Dental Association: The training and utilization of dental hygienists and dental assistants, Trans. Amer. Dent. Assoc. **108**:137-159, 1967.
8. Committee on Professional Education, American Public Health Association: Educational qualifications of public health dentists, Amer. J. Pub. Health **42**(1):188-191, 1952.
9. Young, W. O., and Striffler, D. F.: The dentist, his practice, and his community, ed. 2, Philadelphia, 1969, W. B. Saunders Co.
10. Young, W. O.: The program of the state health department's dental division, Chicago, 1957.
11. Kesel, R. G.: Dental practice. In American Council on Education: The survey of dentistry: final report, B. S. Hollinshead, Director, Washington, D. C., 1961, American Council on Education.
12. Blackerby, P. E.: Dental hygiene and dental specialties: public health and dental hygiene, J. Dent. Educ. **31**:484-487, 1967.
13. American Public Health Association: Educational qualifications of the public health dental hygienist, Amer. J. Pub. Health **46**:899-905, 1956.
14. World Health Organization: Expert committee on auxiliary dental personnel: report, Geneva, 1959, World Health Organization.
15. Collins, D. J.: A neglected resource: the dental hygienist, Chicago, 1969.

chapter 17

SHARPENING AND CONSERVING INSTRUMENTS*

James T. Andrews, B.A., D.D.S.

The dental hygienist must be thoroughly familiar with all the instruments and equipment she uses daily in performing her duties. Not only must she know how to use the instruments and equipment, but she also must have an understanding of the routine care and maintenance of them.

The dental hygienist, like the dentist, will come to value her time and the skill with which she performs her operatory procedures. She will soon discover that her efficiency is largely dependent upon the fine instruments and equipment with which she works. Some dentists and dental hygienists become almost fanatics, in the sense that they will refuse to tolerate the use of poor instruments or poorly sharpened instruments. Some will not even permit anyone but themselves to sharpen them; and they will always be sensitive concerning the kinds of instruments that they purchase and the care that is taken of them.

The very skills that the dental hygienist needs for sharpening and caring for her own instruments are those that are impor-

tant to the dentist in the additional instruments he uses. Because instrumentation is so dependent upon sharpening technics, this chapter will also acquaint the dental hygienist with some of the information that she ought to know about the care and the sharpening of the instruments that her dentist uses.

The objective of this chapter will be to describe the methods of sharpening the instruments used in performing a prophylaxis and the instruments used in cavity preparation by the dentist. Basic information will be included on the maintenance of handpieces, dental units, and their accessories.

One of the most important functions of the dental hygienist is the removal of deposits and stains from the teeth. In order that this may be accomplished most effectively, it is imperative that the hygienist use sharp instruments. Dull instruments not only require much more time on the part of the hygienist in scaling operations but they frequently do not remove all deposits from the teeth. These remaining deposits will act as a nidus for new calculus deposition. The use of dull instruments increases the discomfort to the patient by requiring more time in the chair, and it produces more trauma to tissue, since the hygienist must use more pressure in scaling operations.

---

*John Hembree, D.D.S., Associate Professor of Operative Dentistry, University of Tennessee College of Dentistry, prepared the illustrations for this chapter.

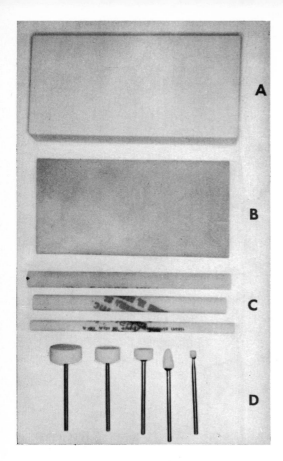

Fig. 17-1. Stones used for sharpening instruments. A, Flat Arkansas stone. B, Flat tapered Arkansas stone. C, Cylinder Arkansas stones. D, Composition handpiece stones. (Courtesy University of Tennessee College of Dentistry, Memphis, Tenn.)

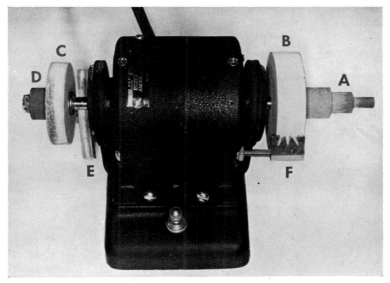

Fig. 17-2. Mechanical oscillating instrument sharpener. A, Stones for sharpening right-angled instruments with curved blades; B, large sharpening wheel; C, felt wheel to remove bur from instruments after sharpening; D, stone for sharpening left-angled instruments with curved blades; E, oscillating wheel; F, instrument guide. (Courtesy University of Tennessee College of Dentistry, Memphis, Tenn.)

EQUIPMENT

Hard Arkansas oilstones are preferred for the sharpening of cutting instruments, since they produce the finest edge. These stones should be lubricated with a fine grade light oil prior to sharpening instruments, and they should be wiped clean following the sharpening procedure. Hard Arkansas oilstones may be obtained in various sizes and shapes (Fig. 17-1) for use in sharpening by hand or by using the dental handpiece.

A mechanical instrument sharpener (Fig. 17-2) with oscillating sharpening stones is also available. This machine will perform most of the procedures that can be accomplished with the stones shown in Fig. 17-1. This sharpener is fairly simple to use because it has fixed guides for holding instruments as they are sharpened. The large sharpening stone should be thoroughly coated with black emery compound while the stone is rotating to prevent burning of the instruments and destroying the temper of the blade. Several types of mechanical instrument sharpeners are available. One model is like a miniature lathe that has an oscillating as well as rotary action.

METHODS OF SHARPENING

It must be remembered that whatever the method of sharpening employed, the objectives are to produce a sharp cutting edge on the instrument, to remove as little metal as possible from the instrument, and to retain the original bevels and shape of the instrument. Therefore it is necessary for the hygienist to know the dimensions, angulations, and shapes of the instruments she is sharpening so that they may be held in the proper relationship with the sharpening stone.

Instruments that are used routinely will not retain a sharp edge for very long; therefore, it is advisable to check all cutting instruments for sharpness after an operation and sharpen them if necessary prior

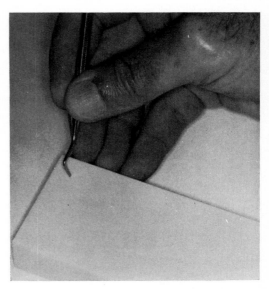

Fig. 17-3. Enamel hatchet sharpened on flat Arkansas stone. (Courtesy University of Tennessee College of Dentistry, Memphis, Tenn.)

to sterilization or disinfection. In the completion of difficult cases it may be necessary to have duplicate scalers available, since the instruments may become dull before the operation is complete. Sharpening of instruments may be accomplished at the chair in a few seconds with the flat, tapering Arkansas oilstone (Fig. 17-1, *B*) which can be sterilized by the dry heat method of sterilization.

Flat stones

Flat Arkansas oilstones (Fig. 17-1, *A*), at least 2 by 5 inches, may be used to sharpen most instruments. Instruments that have a cutting edge perpendicular to the long axis of the blade, such as enamel hatchets, chisels, and hoes, are the easiest to sharpen in this manner. The instrument is held with the thumb, index finger, and middle finger. The other two fingers are used for support on the side of the stone (Fig. 17-3). The bevel of the blade must approximate the stone completely, and it

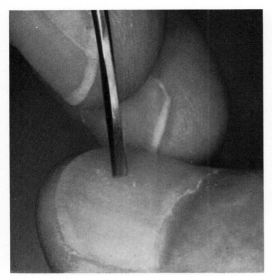

Fig. 17-4. Wedelstaedt chisel checked for sharpness by placing on thumbnail at an angle. If cutting edge does not slide, the instrument is sharp. (Courtesy University of Tennessee College of Dentistry, Memphis, Tenn.)

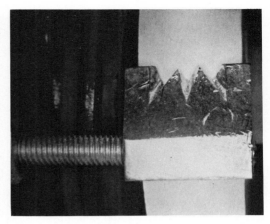

Fig. 17-5. Instrument guide on mechanical sharpener. (Courtesy University of Tennessee College of Dentistry, Memphis, Tenn.)

should retain this relationship to the stone as the hygienist draws the instrument toward her. This motion may be repeated several times if necessary. The instrument can be tested for sharpness against the thumbnail as shown in Fig. 17-4. Gingival margin trimmers and angle formers, which are instruments that do not have their cutting edges perpendicular to the long axis of the blade, may be sharpened in the same manner.

Flat tapered stones

Flat Arkansas oilstones that are thicker on one side and taper to a lesser thickness on the other side, with both the thick and thin sides rounded (Fig. 17-1, *B*), may be used in sharpening most sizes of curettes with whichever rounded edge best fits the curvature of the blade of the instrument. In addition the flat surface of the stone may be used in sharpening procedures.

Cylinder stones

Cylinder-shaped Arkansas oilstones (Fig. 17-1, *C*) of varying diameters may be used to sharpen prophylaxis and cutting instruments having a curved blade. A stone is selected that most nearly fits the curvature of the blade to be sharpened.

Straight handpiece stones

Straight handpiece stones are mounted composition stones. They are available in various diameters and are used in the same manner as the cylinder stones described previously (Fig. 17-1, *D*). Composition stones are not as hard as Arkansas stones; therefore, they will not produce as sharp an edge.

Mechanical sharpener

The mechanical oscillating sharpener is provided with an instrument guide, which holds the instrument stationary and allows a flat bevel to be placed on the instrument. This bevel may be increased or decreased by rotating the motor on its axis while the instrument is held parallel to the floor.

The instrument guide (Fig. 17-5) has three slots for the placement of instru-

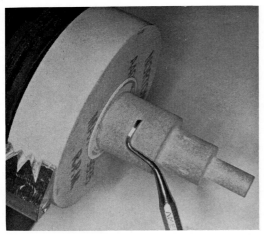

Fig. 17-6. Cleaning out concave surface of gingival margin trimmer with right-angled bevel. (Courtesy University of Tennessee College of Dentistry, Memphis, Tenn.)

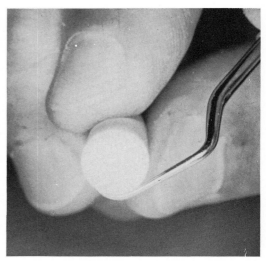

Fig. 17-7. Curette sharpened with cylinder Arkansas stone. (Courtesy University of Tennessee College of Dentistry, Memphis, Tenn.)

ments. The center slot is used for sharpening instruments in which the cutting edge is perpendicular to the long axis of the blade, such as enamel hatchets, chisels, and hoes; the other two slots are used when sharpening instruments in which the cutting edge is not perpendicular to the long axis of the blade, such as gingival margin trimmers and angle formers. Right-angle bevels are placed in the right slot and left-angle bevels are placed in the left slot.

Sharpening wheels of three smaller sizes are used for sharpening curved-blade instruments with a right-angle bevel, such as spoon excavators and scalers, and for cleaning out the concave surface of gingival margin trimmers with right-angle bevels (Fig. 17-6). The sharpening wheel (Fig. 17-2, *D*) is used for sharpening spoon excavators or cleaning out gingival margin trimmers with left-angle bevels.

To stop this instrument from oscillating, a wedge is placed between the oscillating wheel and the motor. The fixation of the large sharpening wheel is necessary so that the side cutting edges of the hatchets, chisels, and hoes may be sharpened.

PROPHYLAXIS INSTRUMENTS

As a rule, prophylaxis instruments such as sickle scalers, hoes, chisels, and curettes should be sharpened with hand stones because of the smallness of the blades. Mounted handpiece stones and the sharpening wheel of the mechanical sharpener will remove too much metal from the blade unless they are in the hands of experts.

Curettes may be sharpened with a cylinder Arkansas stone of appropriate size to fit the curvature of the blade by holding the instrument with the flat part of the blade parallel to the floor and moving the stone at right angles to the length of the blade while maintaining the stone in contact with the flat surface of the blade (Fig. 17-7). A flat, tapered Arkansas stone with rounded edges may be used to sharpen curettes in the same manner as the cylinder stones (Fig. 17-8).

Curettes also may be sharpened by using a flat stone and sharpening the outer surface of the blade. In this technic the blade is again held parallel with the floor, and

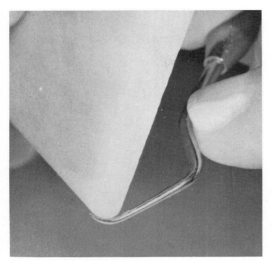

Fig. 17-8. Curette sharpened with rounded edge of flat tapered Arkansas stone. (Courtesy University of Tennessee College of Dentistry, Memphis, Tenn.)

Fig. 17-9. Flat tapered Arkansas stone used to sharpen the side of the curette. (Courtesy University of Tennessee College of Dentistry, Memphis, Tenn.)

the stone is moved downward following the curvature of the blade (Fig. 17-9).

Mounted handpiece Arkansas stones may be used to sharpen curettes. A stone fitting the curvature of the instrument is selected and positioned in the straight handpiece and then placed in contact with the concave portion of the blade (Fig. 17-10). The stone should be moved back and forward slightly to prevent grooving the blade.

The small stone on the mechanical sharpener can be used to sharpen curettes. This is accomplished by placing the concave surface in contact with the stone while using light pressure (Fig. 17-11). The bur produced in sharpening is removed by holding the convex surface of the blade against the felt wheel (Fig. 17-12).

Sickle scalers of large size can be sharpened by technics described for curettes, using cylinder Arkansas stones (Fig. 17-13), large cylindrical stones mounted in a straight handpiece (Fig. 17-14), or flat

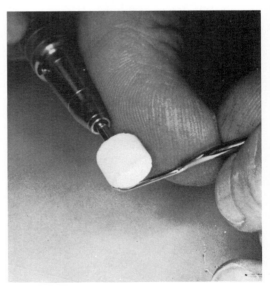

Fig. 17-10. Curette sharpened with composition handpiece stone. (Courtesy University of Tennessee College of Dentistry, Memphis, Tenn.)

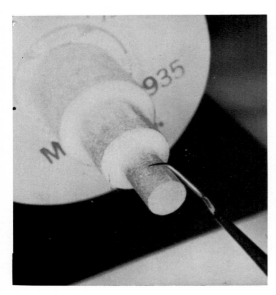

Fig. 17-11. Curette sharpened on mechanical sharpener. (Courtesy University of Tennessee College of Dentistry, Memphis, Tenn.)

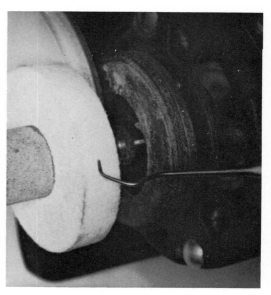

Fig. 17-12. Bur on cutting edge of curette removed by felt wheel of mechanical sharpener. (Courtesy University of Tennessee College of Dentistry, Memphis, Tenn.)

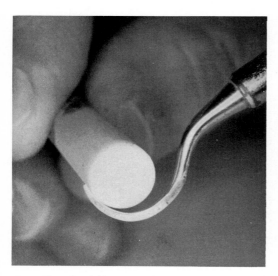

Fig. 17-13. Sickle type of scaler sharpened with cylinder Arkansas stone. (Courtesy University of Tennessee College of Dentistry, Memphis, Tenn.)

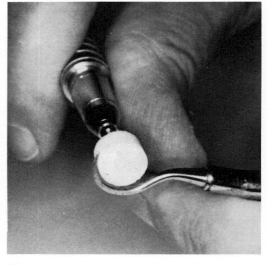

Fig. 17-14. Sickle type of scaler sharpened with composition handpiece stone. (Courtesy University of Tennessee College of Dentistry, Memphis, Tenn.)

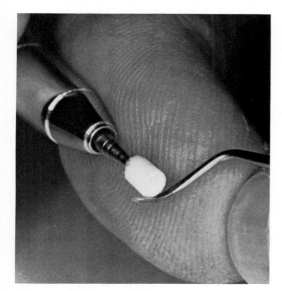

Fig. 17-15. Jaquette type of scaler sharpened with composition handpiece stone. (Courtesy University of Tennessee College of Dentistry, Memphis, Tenn.)

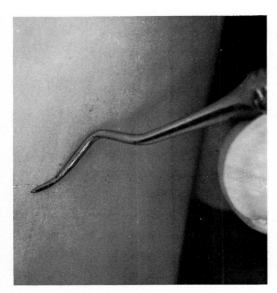

Fig. 17-16. Jaquette type of scaler sharpened with flat Arkansas stone. (Courtesy University of Tennessee College of Dentistry, Memphis, Tenn.)

tapered stones (Fig. 17-9). Scalers of the Jaquette type can be sharpened with a small stone in the straight handpiece (Fig. 17-15) or by use of the flat tapered stone (Fig. 17-16).

The *hoe* type of scalers are best sharpened with the large, flat Arkansas stone. The bevel of the blade is placed in apposition to the surface of the stone, and while using the remaining fingers to stabilize the instrument in this position, the instrument is drawn toward the hygienist (Fig. 17-17). The sharpening movement is from the shoulder, since the fingers, hand, wrist, and elbow should remain as fixed as possible while the instrument is moved across the stone in order to place one bevel on the blade instead of several bevels. This procedure may need to be repeated several times in order to produce a sharp edge.

The *chisel* type of scalers are sharpened in the same manner as that described for the hoe type of scalers (Fig. 17-18), or they may be sharpened with the mechanical sharpener (Fig. 17-19).

Files used in prophylaxis usually cannot be satisfactorily sharpened in the dental office, so they should be returned to the manufacturer for this procedure.

CAVITY PREPARATION INSTRUMENTS

Cavity preparation instruments may be sharpened with flat Arkansas stones, cylinder stones, and the mechanical sharpener. The flat Arkansas stones may be used in sharpening hatchets and other instruments of this type. The use of the mechanical sharpener is recommended for sharpening of cavity preparation instruments because of the ease of placing a single accurate bevel on the instruments and the facility with which the sharpening operation may be accomplished.

Hatchets, chisels, and *hoes* are all instruments that have the cutting edges of the blades perpendicular to the long axis of the blade. These blades are sharpened in the center slot (Fig. 17-20) of the instrument

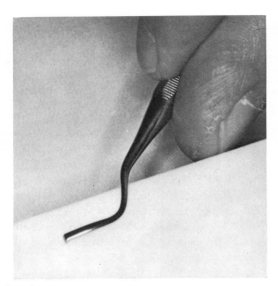

Fig. 17-17. Hoe type of scaler sharpened on flat Arkansas stone. (Courtesy University of Tennessee College of Dentistry, Memphis, Tenn.)

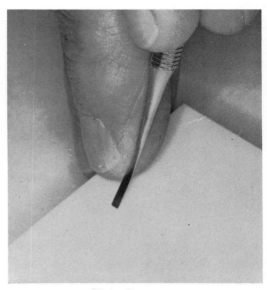

Fig. 17-18. Chisel type of scaler sharpened on flat Arkansas stone. (Courtesy University of Tennessee College of Dentistry, Memphis, Tenn.)

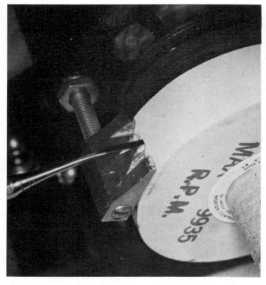

Fig. 17-19. Chisel type of scaler sharpened on mechanical sharpener. (Courtesy University of Tennessee College of Dentistry, Memphis, Tenn.)

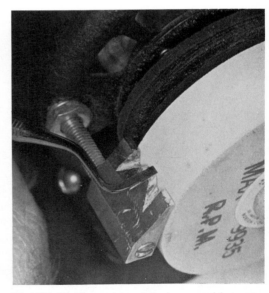

Fig. 17-20. Enamel hatchet sharpened in center slot of the instrument guide of mechanical sharpener. (Courtesy University of Tennessee College of Dentistry, Memphis, Tenn.)

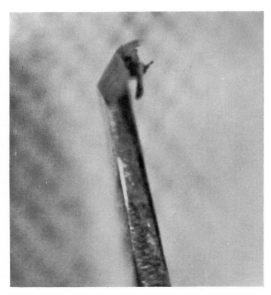

Fig. 17-21. Bur on cutting edge of instrument after sharpening on mechanical sharpener. (Courtesy University of Tennessee College of Dentistry, Memphis, Tenn.)

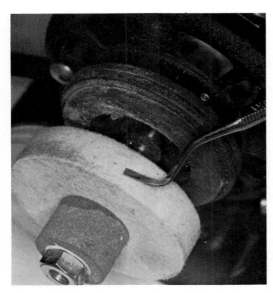

Fig. 17-22. Bur on cutting edge of enamel hatchet removed by holding the bur against the felt wheel. (Courtesy University of Tennessee College of Dentistry, Memphis, Tenn.)

guide of the oscillating mechanical sharpener. While holding the blade of the instrument parallel to the floor in the center slot of the instrument guide, the hygienist should rotate the motor either forward or backward until the bevel on the cutting edge of the instrument is duplicated when the instrument approximates the sharpening stone. She should apply gentle pressure until she can see the entire cutting edge in close approximation to the stone. A slight bur (Fig. 17-21) will be produced on the cutting edge of the instrument. This is removed by turning the blade over and holding it against the felt buffing wheel for a few seconds (Fig. 17-22). The blade is then removed and checked for sharpness as described in Fig. 17-4.

Instruments with cutting edges on the sides of the blades may be sharpened (Fig. 17-23) on the side of the large sharpening wheel after placing a wedge between the oscillating wheel and the motor, which will prevent the sharpening wheel from oscillating.

Gingival margin trimmers and *angle formers* are instruments with cutting edges that are not perpendicular to the long axis of the blade. These instruments are sharpened in the left and right slots of the instrument guide, with the left slot being used for left-angle bevels and the right slot being used for right-angle bevels. The instruments are approximated to the sharpening stone and sharpened, and the bur is removed as described for hatchets, chisels, and hoes (Figs. 17-24 and 17-25).

Spoon excavators are sharpened on the smaller stones (Fig. 17-26). If the spoons are not very dull, they can be sharpened by holding the convex side of the blade against the felt buffing wheel (Fig. 17-27). Small discoid spoon excavators are best sharpened by this method (Fig. 17-28).

Gold knives may be sharpened on the felt wheel (Fig. 17-29) or on a flat Arkansas stone.

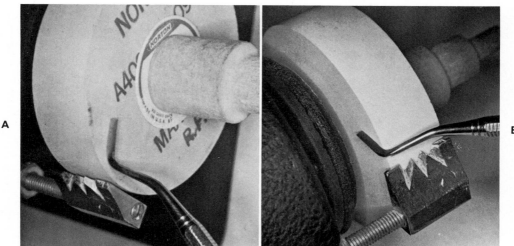

Fig. 17-23. A, Sharpening side bevel of enamel hatchet on mechanical sharpener. **B,** Sharpening side bevel of enamel hatchet on mechanical sharpener. (Courtesy University of Tennessee College of Dentistry, Memphis, Tenn.)

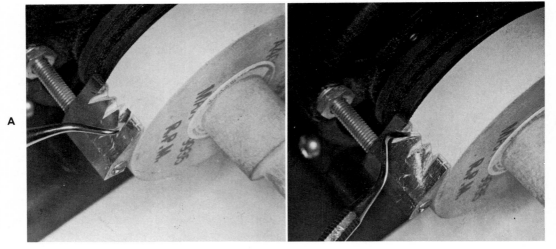

Fig. 17-24. A, Gingival margin trimmer with right-angled bevel sharpened in right slot of the instrument of mechanical instrument sharpener. **B,** Gingival margin trimmer with left-angled bevel sharpened in left slot of instrument guide of mechanical instrument sharpener. (Courtesy University of Tennessee College of Dentistry, Memphis, Tenn.)

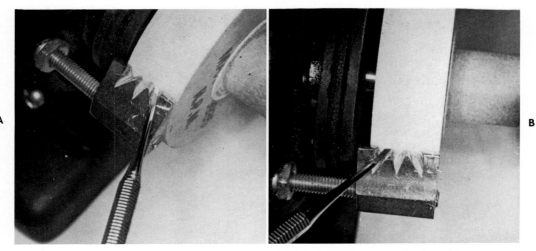

Fig. 17-25. A, Angle former with right-angled bevel sharpened in right slot of instrument guide of mechanical sharpener. **B,** Angle former with left-angled bevel sharpened in left slot of instrument guide of mechanical sharpener. (Courtesy University of Tennessee College of Dentistry, Memphis, Tenn.)

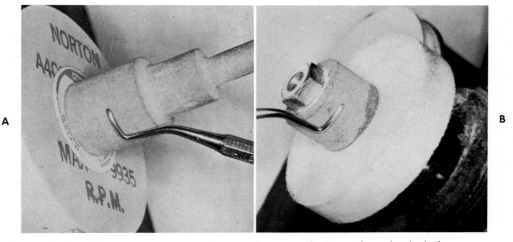

Fig. 17-26. A, Spoon excavator sharpened on small stone of mechanical sharpener— right-angled blade. **B,** Spoon excavator sharpened on small stone of mechanical sharpener—left-angled blade. (Courtesy University of Tennessee College of Dentistry, Memphis, Tenn.)

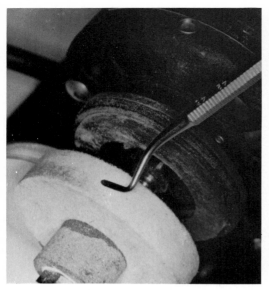

Fig. 17-27. Spoon excavator sharpened on felt wheel of mechanical sharpener. (Courtesy University of Tennessee College of Dentistry, Memphis, Tenn.)

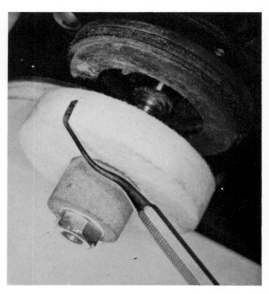

Fig. 17-29. Gold knife sharpened on felt wheel of mechanical sharpener. (Courtesy University of Tennessee College of Dentistry, Memphis, Tenn.)

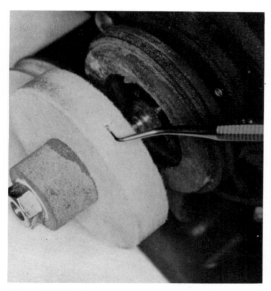

Fig. 17-28. Discoid spoon excavator sharpened on felt wheel of mechanical sharpener. (Courtesy University of Tennessee College of Dentistry, Memphis, Tenn.)

After the use of prophylaxis instruments at the chair the dental hygienist immediately should scrub all scaling instruments with soap, water, and a stiff brush to remove all blood and other debris, or they may be placed in an ultrasonic cleaner, which is a much more effective and efficient method of cleaning instruments.

After cleaning the instruments the dental hygienist should check them for sharpness, and those that are dull should be resharpened and cleaned again.

Most dental cutting instruments are manufactured of carbon steel, and they can be sharpened to a finer cutting edge than instruments made of stainless steel. Carbon steel instruments cannot be sterilized by the autoclave or boiling methods of sterilization, since these methods will dull the cutting edges of the instruments; therefore carbon steel instruments should be disinfected in a chemical solution to prevent damage to the cutting edges. Chapter 14 elaborates further on chemical disinfecting solutions. The dental hygienist never should forget to place antirust tablets in the disinfecting solution, if they need to be added to the particular solution being used, or else the instruments will be damaged.

Dry heat sterilization at a temperature of 160° C. for 1 hour is an effective method of sterilizing cutting instruments without damaging the cutting edges; however, if this method of sterilization is used, more duplicate sets of instruments will be necessary.

Stainless steel cutting instruments can be sterilized in the autoclave without damage to the cutting edges; however, one must sacrifice cutting efficiency when using instruments made of this material.

After sterilization or disinfection, instruments should be removed and dried with a sterile towel and placed in the instrument cabinet.

CARE AND MAINTENANCE OF EQUIPMENT

All equipment should receive routine preventive maintenance, and the equipment in the dental office is no exception. When one considers the cost of equipment in a dental office and also the fact that this expensive equipment will perform satisfactorily for many years if it is cared for, it is imperative to properly maintain it.

A good, safe procedure in the care and maintenance of all equipment is to follow the manufacturer's recommendation, since the equipment was operated and tested thoroughly before it was sold. Many hours of lost time can be saved by routine preventive maintenance as recommended by the manufacturer.

A schedule of periodic maintenance operations should be set up for all pieces of equipment in the dental office, and one or more of the auxiliary personnel should be assigned to perform these tasks. This may be accomplished by an index card file, typed schedule, calendar, or some other arrangement if it better fits a particular office.

One of the more important aspects in the care and maintenance of equipment is an appreciation of what can be done in the dental office with respect to the repair of equipment and when a dental repairman should be called in to care for the equipment. Most manufacturers provide a manual of instructions on the operation and maintenance of their equipment, together with some instructions on how to locate and correct malfunctions of equipment as they occur. Extra copies of these manuals may be obtained from local dental dealers. After following these suggestions, if the equipment malfunctions cannot be located and corrected, it is best to call the dental equipment repairman. Dental equipment has become highly specialized and complicated and requires special knowledge and training in its repair; therefore, most repairs will require the services of a trained repairman.

CONTRA-ANGLES
Prophylaxis angle

In the armamentarium of the dental hygienist the prophylaxis angle (Fig. 17-30) is the item of equipment requiring the most routine care and maintenance. Since this instrument is exposed to saliva, blood, debris, and pumice when used for cleaning and polishing operations in the oral cavity, it must be cleaned and greased after each prophylaxis to ensure a long period of use. A number of prophylaxis angles should be available in the dental office so that the hygienist does not have to pause between patients to clean the angle.

The cleaning of these instruments is best accomplished by running the complete angle on the straight handpiece in a cleaning solution. The gear barrel assembly (Fig. 17-30, A) should be removed and

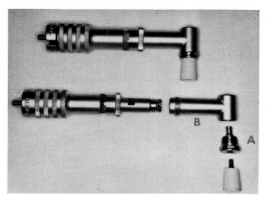

Fig. 17-30. Prophylaxis angle disassembled. *A,* Gear barrel assembly; *B,* head of angle. (Courtesy University of Tennessee College of Dentistry, Memphis, Tenn.)

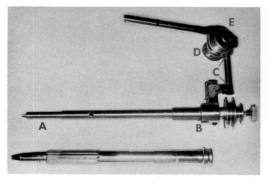

Fig. 17-31. Friction type of handpiece with sheath removed. (Courtesy University of Tennessee College of Dentistry, Memphis, Tenn.)

the remainder of the angle run in the cleaner to dissolve old grease. Old grease should be removed from the gear barrel assembly with cleaner and a brush, and the inside of the head of the angle should be blown dry with air. The head shell (Fig. 17-30, *B*) should be removed and the remainder of the angle again run in the cleaning solution to dissolve old grease. The gear barrel assembly should be replaced in the head shell and tightened. The head shell then is filled with grease and screwed back on the body of the instrument. These instructions for cleaning and greasing a prophylaxis angle are those recommended for the particular instrument in Fig. 17-30, but in all cases the dental hygienist should follow the instructions as recommended by the manufacturer for the instrument she uses.

In the event that these instruments are to be sterilized in oil, the instrument should be placed in the sterilizer with the head removed and greased after sterilization.

Friction angles

Friction angles are low-speed instruments primarily used for cavity preparation and finishing restorations. They will need lubrication after each use. They

should be cleaned and lubricated at the end of the day, following the manufacturer's recommendations for the type of angle used in the office.

Ball-bearing angles

Ball-bearing angles are precision-built, high-speed instruments requiring strict compliance with the manufacturer's recommendations for cleaning and lubrication. All ball-bearing angles, both long and short sheath, should be lubricated after each use. Cleaning of the instrument followed by lubrication should be done at the end of each day or more frequently if recommended by the manufacturer. Always use the type of oil specified in the instructions with the handpiece.

HANDPIECES
Friction handpiece

Most hygienists will be using a low-speed, friction-type straight handpiece. This instrument will be in routine use daily and will require constant cleaning, lubrication, and sterilization or disinfection.

The handpiece shown in Fig. 17-31 with the sheath removed should be oiled several times a day by placing a drop of oil at points *A* and *B*. At the end of the day the

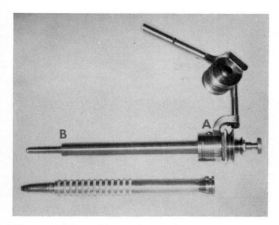

Fig. 17-32. Ball-bearing handpiece with sheath removed. *A,* Rear bearing; *B,* front bearing. (Courtesy University of Tennessee College of Dentistry, Memphis, Tenn.)

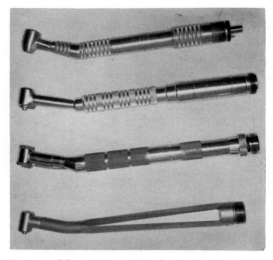

Fig. 17-33. Several types of airotor handpieces. (Courtesy University of Tennessee College of Dentistry, Memphis, Tenn.)

handpiece should be thoroughly cleaned and lubricated. The inside of the sheath should be cleaned with a bristle brush, dipped in cleaning solution, and dried off with air. The spindle should be cleaned with a piece of cloth and cleaning solution. The chuck is cleaned with a pipe cleaner dipped in cleaning solution. A drop of oil is placed at points *A, B, C, D,* and *E* in Fig. 17-31, and the handpiece is reassembled.

Ball-bearing handpiece

The handpiece shown in Fig. 17-32 is a high-speed, ball-bearing handpiece with sealed ball bearings that requires little lubrication. The rear bearing never requires lubrication, and the front bearing should be lubricated twice a month with 1 drop of oil. Since the spindle of the handpiece does not rotate against the sheath, no lubrication is necessary for the spindle. At the end of each day of use the sheath should be removed and cleaned with a brush and cleaning solution, and the spindle should be wiped clean with a small piece of clean cloth wet with cleaning solution. The chuck should be cleaned with a

pipe cleaner dipped in cleaning solution and 2 drops of oil placed down inside the bur hole.

Ball-bearing handpieces are precision instruments, and the manufacturer's recommendations should be rigidly followed, including the use of the type of lubricant recommended. The sheath may be sterilized by any means except immersion in a chemical disinfectant. The driving unit of the handpiece should not be placed in any type of sterilizer because the sealed bearings will be damaged.

Ultraspeed handpiece

Air turbine handpieces (Fig. 17-33) or airotors require little lubrication of the handpiece, since most of them have built-in lubricating systems; however, at the end of each day air only should be run through the handpiece for 30 seconds in order to remove any water in the head of the handpiece. The manufacturer's instructions for the particular type of ultraspeed instrument used in the office should be followed with respect to cleaning, lubrication, and routine maintenance.

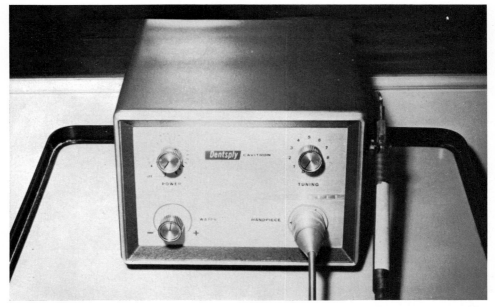

Fig. 17-34. Cavitron unit. (Courtesy University of Tennessee College of Dentistry, Memphis, Tenn.)

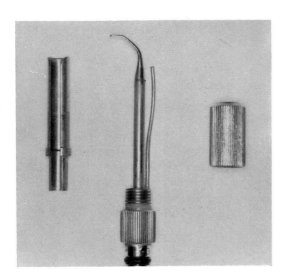

Fig. 17-35. Insert for Cavitron handpiece disassembled. (Courtesy University of Tennessee College of Dentistry, Memphis, Tenn.)

Most air turbine handpieces have a built-in lubricating system, with the oil reservoir located either in the dental unit or in an attached control box. It is imperative that the oil level be checked daily or even more frequently to ensure that a proper oil level is maintained in the oil reservoir to prevent damage to the handpiece. The type of oil recommended by the manufacturer always should be used, because an oil of a different viscosity will result in a different lubrication rate for the instrument and may damage the handpiece. The oil reservoir should be removed periodically and cleaned according to the manufacturer's recommendations.

The air supply to turbine handpieces contains an air filter to remove both moisture and minute particles of dust from the air before it reaches the bearings in the handpiece, because either moisture or dust will damage the bearings. The air filter should be purged daily by pressing a small, spring-loaded purging valve at the base of the air filter.

Cavitron unit

The Cavitron unit (Fig. 17-34) is an ultrasonic instrument designed for use in oral prophylaxis. It requires no preventive maintenance other than the removal of the insert from the handpiece after its use. Inserts may be dismantled (Fig. 17-35) for cleaning and sterilization and may be autoclaved, providing the temperature is not allowed to rise above 121° C. (250° F.).

GENERAL MAINTENANCE

Most pieces of equipment in the dental operatory will need maintenance regularly, either at short intervals or over longer periods of time. It will be the purpose of this section to state in general terms the maintenance procedures as they apply to equipment in the dental operatory, since there are so many different types of equipment on the market today.

Dental unit

The unit, including engine arm and pulleys, should be wiped clean with a dry cloth to remove dust and debris and should be cleaned and waxed periodically according to the manufacturer's recommendations.

The cuspidor bowl should be cleaned daily to prevent staining and the formation of odors. The cuspidor trap should be removed and cleaned at least twice a week.

Several cups of warm water should be flushed through the saliva ejector once a day and more frequently if a large number of metal restorations has been removed in daily operations. The metal strainer in the head of the saliva ejector should be removed and cleaned daily also.

Air, water, and multiplex syringes should be checked daily for leaks and proper function. If any irregularities are noted, they should be brought to the attention of the dentist.

The engine, engine arm, and engine arm pulleys require periodic oiling. The manufacturer's recommendations should be followed with respect to the time interval for lubrication and the type of oil used. When the engine cover is removed for oiling the engine, it is a good time to check the condition of the brushes in the engine and replace them if necessary.

The movable joints in the tray arm or bracket table arm and the operating light should be lubricated, if necessary, according to the manufacturer's recommendations.

The water supply strainer located in the unit should be removed and cleaned periodically, depending upon local conditions.

Foot rheostats should be checked and lubricated periodically. The manufacturer's instructions should be followed.

Oral evacuators

Oral evacuating units must be kept clean to prevent the formation of unpleasant odors in the operatory. Suction hoses should be rinsed with one or two cups of water following each use and when used in surgery; the hose should be rinsed before and after removing blood from the mouth. A germicide spray may be sprayed into the suction hoses once a day while the machine is operating, and at the end of the day the hoses should be rinsed with several cups of water.

If the evacuator has a collection tank that is not self-emptying, it should be drained twice a day, and the collection tank should be removed and cleaned twice a week following the manufacturer's instructions.

SUGGESTED READINGS

Blackwell, R. E.: G. V. Black's operative dentistry, ed. 9, South Milwaukee, 1955, Medico-Dental Publishing Co., vol. II.

McGehee, W. H. O., True, H. A., and Inskipp, E. F.: A textbook of operative dentistry, New York, 1956, McGraw-Hill Book Co.

Peterson, S.: The dentist and his assistant, ed. 3, St. Louis, 1972, The C. V. Mosby Co.

Schultz, L. C., and others: Operative dentistry, Philadelphia, 1966, Lea & Febiger.

chapter 18

DEVELOPING A DENTAL HYGIENE VOCABULARY

Kathryn S. Goller, C.D.A., R.D.H.
Shailer Peterson, B.A., M.A., Ph.D.

Everyone recognizes that people in different parts of the world speak different languages. Those who travel to foreign countries realize that it is difficult or even impossible to communicate with those persons who do not understand the same language. Language is an extremely important instrument in communications. Whether a person communicates with another person in conversation or in writing, it is important that they both understand the language that is being used. A Frenchman speaks and writes a different language than an Englishman or an American. However, this does not mean that all Americans can understand one another completely. First of all, there are regional differences in speech, so that an accent or a dialect in one part of the nation is so different from that spoken in another part of the country that sometimes the people from the two areas experience some difficulty in understanding one another. However, they are still speaking and using the same basic language, so that with a little care and perhaps by speaking and articulating slowly, each can understand the other person easily and accurately.

Just because two persons know the English language does not mean that they can converse and communicate on all subjects. The mother of a dental hygienist may be able to communicate with her daughter about the shopping tour that they have just completed and about the movie that they saw on television, but the mother may be completely lost in the conversation if her daughter started to talk about the work that went on at the dental office. Dentistry and dental hygiene have a vocabulary of their own. Similarly, this same mother who can talk to her son about the route that they should plan for their vacation may be completely lost when she hears him describing a football game or a basketball game. Every sport has its own rules and even its own vocabulary. Every business, every sport, and every profession have their own special vocabularies that are known best by the people who are involved closely with it.

A girl may have been a straight "A" student in English, French, and Latin in high school and yet fail half of the courses in the dental hygiene curriculum if she does not expand her vocabulary to understand what is required in courses in preventive dentistry, prophylaxis, dental materials, dental anatomy, microbiology, and all of the others that lead to her goal of being a registered and licensed dental hygienist.

It is fortunate that acquiring a dental hygiene vocabulary is not entirely a memo-

325

rization game. Most scientific words are put together like building blocks or tinker toys. If one knows the meaning of a single word part, she knows what a part of this word means whenever she sees this word part. If she knows that "sub" means "under," this automatically expands her vocabulary by dozens of words, for there are many that include that term. For example, there are such words as the following:

subagent	subcommittee
substation	subconscious
subphylum	subcontract
subsection	subtract
subsequent	subdominant
subepidermal	subindex
sublingual	submaxillary
submarine	submerge
subscribe	submit

Every word part, prefix, or suffix that one knows—just like "sub"—means that the dental hygienist has expanded her vocabulary by at least a half dozen words and possibly by a hundred or more.

New and special words are manufactured for the dentist or physician to save him time in saying what he wants to say. One should not be self-conscious about using these complicated words, for they are as much a part of the dental hygiene profession as are the words that the baseball fan expects everyone else to know when he describes something as a "double play" or when a football coach refers to his "T-formation" or his "balanced line" and so on. Words are not for the "show-off," but they are for the professional who finds that she needs special terms to describe accurately and quickly what it is that needs to be communicated.

One should never feel self-conscious or as if she were being a "show-off" by using the special words that have been developed for the dentist and his dental hygienist to use. Actually, she should feel self-conscious if she doesn't know the proper words to use and if she isn't able to use them at the right time and in the right way.

It is important to acquire an excellent vocabulary in dental hygiene for at least three reasons. First, the student who doesn't acquire this new vocabulary will not be able to pass the courses and be graduated as a dental hygienist. Second, it is important to acquire a good understanding of the terminology used by the dentist and his other office staff so that one can communicate with them and so that they can communicate with their new dental hygienist. Third, new patients who come to the office have their first opportunity to discuss their dental problems with the dental hygienist, who can then act as a teacher of all of the patients with whom she comes in contact. It is a challenging task to teach a new vocabulary to patients, for in teaching one proves to herself how much she really knows about the subject and the terminology.

The following material includes a large number of word parts that can be used in building new words with new meanings and a large number of words that the dental hygienist will confront in her textbook assignments and in her lecture courses. It would be *very unwise* to try to memorize all of the word parts and the words appearing in the following sections.

It is suggested that the reader scan over all of the word parts and check off those that she recalls seeing in previous reading. One should not try to scan the words in the glossary, for this is to be used much like one would use a dictionary, to find the meaning of unfamiliar words. As the reader covers the assigned reading in this or other books, she should practice using the glossary to be sure that she knows the correct meaning of new or strange words. Place a check beside every word that is searched for so that one can discover whether the same word or word part is continuing to give trouble. When one finds that she hunts up a word many times, then this is a word she must study. As one studies the glossary, it is a good plan also to scan through the pages and look at the various words that have been checked just to find out whether one does remember the meaning of these words that have appeared before as new and unknown words. The building of an excellent vocabulary is so very important that it is necessary that the student make a concerted effort to plan her method of building this vocabulary. Building an efficient vocabulary is just as important as getting a good grade in one of the required courses; this vocabulary will pay many dividends, for it will help one earn excellent grades in all of the courses that follow.

It was not too many years ago that both high school and college students were encouraged to study Latin and Greek because so many medical and dental terms were constructed from Latin and Greek words. It is no longer recommended that anyone study Latin and Greek for this purpose, even though a study of them can make one very appreciative of vocabulary rules and rules of composition.

Rather than having to take a course in Latin or Greek to help one know that "sub" means "under," any person who has been graduated from high school can recall a whole array of words that contain the word part "sub." Then by studying all of these known words, it is easy for this same person to come to the conclusion that there is one common meaning to all of these words, and this common meaning is "under."

Similarly, words that have "bi" in them all have reference to "two." All words with "cycle" have reference to wheel or circular. Therefore a "bicycle" is something with "two wheels."

The word part that is placed at the front of the word is called the *prefix*. This means that "leuko" (meaning "white") is the prefix in the word "leukocyte," which means "white cell." The word part "cyte,"

meaning "cell" is at the end of the word and is called the *suffix*.

One can also change words in order to change their words meaning. Singular words commonly can be made plural by adding an "s." Most present tense verbs can be made into past tense verbs by adding "ed."

There are many word endings that one uses everyday without thinking of the systematic manner in which they have become a part of the English language. Whenever one sees the ending "ology," it always refers to a "comprehensive scientific study," such as:

Biology	Archeology
Geology	Histology
Microbiology	Bacteriology

Similarly, the word endings of "ist" and "ian" always convert a word so that it means the person who is working in a particular field of endeavor, such as:

Hygienist	Physician
Chemist	Mathematician
Geologist	Optician
Oculist	Historian

In learning words or even word parts in a new vocabulary, the student will usually work out systems or procedures of her own to help her remember them. For example, when dealing with measurement in the scientific area, one is called upon to use the metric system instead of the old English system of pounds and ounces. The metric system uses a very systematic and meaningful method of combining word parts. A person can memorize these words endings and their meanings, but they can be memorized and recalled much more easily if the student studies them in a sequence that helps to reflect their meaning, such as the following:

*Kilo*meter	1,000 meters
*Hecto*meter	100 meters
*Deca*meter	10 meters
Meter	
*Deci*meter	1/10 of a meter or 0.1 meter
*Centi*meter	1/100 of a meter or 0.01 meter
*Milli*meter	1/1000 of a meter or 0.001 meter

Similar tables or charts can be made to show the meaning of milliliters, kiloliters, and liters. Also, weight measures to show the relationship between kilograms, grams, and milligrams can be written in a similar sequence.

WORD PARTS*

a-, an Negative, lack, without, as in asymptomatic

ab-, abs- Away, from, as in abnormal

ac-, acet- Sharp, sour, pointed, as in acetabulum, acetone

acou-, acu-, aco- Hear, as in acoustic

ad- Increase, motion toward, as in adherence

aden- Gland, as in adenitis, adenocarinoma

adip-, adep- Fat, as in adipose

-aemia Blood, as in anemia

aer-, ar- Air, breathe, as in aerobe

alb- White, as in albino, materia alba

-algia Pain, suffering, as in odontalgia, neuralgia

aliment- Food, as in alimentation

all- Other, foreign, as in allergy

ambi- Both, on both sides, as in ambidexterity

-ambl-, -ambul- Walk, as in ambulatory, somnambulation

ana-, an- Up, excessive, as in anaplasia

-ang-, angul- Sharp, bend, as in biangle

angi- Vessel, as in angiitis

angio- Relating to blood or lymph vessels, as in angioma

ante- Before, as in anterior, antecedent, anteroom

anti- Against, as in antibiotic, antidote, antiseptic

-apex, -apic Top or pointed extremity of any conical part, as in apicoectomy, apical

apo- From, opposed, as in apoplexy

aqu-, aqua- Water, as in aqueous

arth-, arthro- Joints, as in arthritis

-ase An enzyme, as in dextrinase

aud- Hear, as in audiometer, audiovisual

aut-, auto- Self, as in autotransplant

aux- Grow, increase, as in auxiliary

bacter- Stick or rod, as in bacteremia

bi-, bis- Two, twice, double, as in bicuspid, bifurcation, bicycle

bio-, bi-, be- Life, living, as in biology, biopsy

-blast- Germ, as in blastocyte; formative cell, as in osteoblast

brady- Slow, as in bradycardia, bradypnea

-bry- Grow, swell, as in embryo, embryology

bucc- Cheek, as in buccal, buccinator

burs- Pouch, as in bursa, bursitis

-cad-, cas-, -cay, -cid- Fall, as in casualty, decay, accident, deciduous

cal- Heat, as in calor, calorie

calc- Lime, calcium, as in calcification

carc- Cancer, as in carcinoma

card-, cardi- Heart, as in cardia, cardiovascular

cari- Rottenness, as in caries, carious

caust-, caus-, caum- Burn, as in caustic, cautery

-cav- Hollow, hole, or lesion, as in cavity, excavate

centi- One hundredth the size of the basic unit, as in centimeter

cephal-, cephalo- Relating to head, as in cephalometry

cerebr-, cereb- Brain, as in cerebral, cerebellum

-cern, -cret, cri- Separate, as in excrete, secrete

cervic-, cervix- Neck, as in cervical

cheil-, chil- Lip, as in cheilosis

chol- Bile, as in cholecyst, cholesterol

chrom-, chrom-, chromat- Color pigmentation, as in chromogenic, chromatism

-cid, -cis Cut, kill, as in suicide, incisal

-cidal Killing, as in bactericidal

cil- Lash, eyelash, as in ciliary

cing-, cinct- Encircle, gird, as in cingulum

cirrh- Orange-yellow, as in cirrhosis

-clast, -clas Broken, divided into parts, as in osteoclast

claus-, clos- Close, as in claustrophobia

co-, com-, con- Together, with, as in congenital

coag- Drive together, collect, as in coagulate

coll- Glue, as in colloid

contra- Against, opposite, as in contralateral

cosm- Order, beauty, as in cosmetic

cran- Skull, as in cranium, cranial

-cresc-, -crem-, cret- Grow, as in concrescence, increment

-cusp- Point, as in cuspid, bicuspid

cuti- Skin, as in cuticle

cyan- Blue, as in cyanosis

cyto-, -cyte Cell, as in cytology, leukocyte

de- From, not, separation, as in decalcification

deca- Ten times larger than the basic unit, as in decaliter

deci- One tenth the size of the basic unit, as in decimeter

den-, dent- Relating to teeth, as in dentist, dentin, dentition

-derm-, -derma- Relating to the skin, as in dermatitis, hypodermic

di- Double, apart from, as in diaphragm, diplococci

dia- Through, between, asunder, as in diaphragm

diastem- Space, interval, as in diastema

digit- Finger, as in digital

dis- Opposite, taking apart, as in disinfectant

---

*Hyphen before word part denotes prefix; hyphen after word part denotes suffix; hyphen before and after word part denotes root or stem.

dist-, disto- Remote, posterior, away from center, as in distal, distolingual

-drome Course, as in syndrome

-dur- Hard, as in durable, induration

dys- Difficult, bad, as in dystrophy

-ectomy Cutting out, as in gingivectomy, apicoectomy

edema- Swelling, as in edematous, edema

-emia Blood condition, as in bacteremia

endo- Within, into, as in endodontics, endoderm

epi- Upon, in addition, as in epidemic, epidermis

eryth-, erythro- Red, as in erythrocyte

-esthesia Sensation, as in anesthesia

eth- Air, as in ether, ethyl

etio- Cause, as in etiology

ex- Out, beyond, as in exodontics, excavate, exclude

extra- On the outside, beyond, as in extracellular

fac-, faci- Face, as in facial, maxillofacial

febr- Fever, as in febrile

fec- Excrement, dregs, as in feces, fecal

-flag-, -flam- Burn, flame, as in inflammation

fract-, frag- Break, as in fracture

gastr-, gastro- Stomach, as in gastritis

-gen- Beget, produce, as in genetics, glycogen

geni- Chin, as in genial

gero- Old age, as in gerodontics

geus-, gust- Taste, as in gustation

gingiv- Gum, as in gingivitis

gloss-, glot- Tongue, as in glossitis, epiglottis

gluc-, glyc- Sweet, as in glucose, hyperglycemia

-gnath- Jaw, as in gnathology, prognathia

-gno-, -gnos Know, knowledge, as in pathognomy, diagnosis, prognosis

-gram, -graph Tracing, mark, draw, as in radiograph

gyn-, gyne- Woman, as in gynecology

hecto- One hundred times larger than the basic unit, as in hectometer

-hem, hemo- Relating to blood, as in hemorrhage

hemi- Half, as in hemisection

hepa-, hepat- Liver, as in hepatitis

hist-, histo- Tissue, as in histology

homo-, homeo- Same, similar, as in homeostasis

hydra-, hydro- Relating to water, as in hydrated

hygie-, hygei-, hugi- Health, as in hygiene

hyper- Over, above, beyond, excessive, as in hypersensitive, hyperplasia

hypn- Sleep, as in hypnotic

hypo- Under, deficient, beneath, as in hypocytosis, hypofunction

-ia, -iasis Denotes a condition, pathological state, as in bacteremia

-ic, -ics Pertaining to, of, as in orthodontics, periodontics, pedodontics

idio- Peculiar to the individual or organ, distinct, as in idiopathic

in- Absent, without, not, as in inert, inactive

infer- Low, as in inferior

infra- Beneath, below, as in infraorbital

inter- Between, among, as in interproximal

intra-, intro- Within, inside, as in intraoral

-ist Person who practices, as in hygienist

-itis Inflammation, as in pulpitis, bronchitis, arthritis

kilo- One thousand times larger than the basic unit, as in kiloliter

labi- Lip, as in labial

lact-, lacto- Milk, as in lactation

lamin-, lamn- Flat plate, as in lamina dura

laryng-, laryngo- Larynx, as in laryngitis

-later-, -latero- Side, as in bilateral

leuco-, leuko- White, as in leukocyte

lig- Bind, as in ligate, ligament

lingu- Tongue, as in lingual

lip- Fat, as in lipid, lipoma

liqu- Pour, as in liquid

-logia, -logy Science or study of, as in pathology

-lysin, -lysis Setting free, disintegration, as in hemolysis

macro-, macr- Large, long, big, as in macrodontia

mal- Bad, poor, evil, as in malaria, malnutrition

marg- Edge, as in margin

med-, mes-, mid- Middle, as in median, mesial

met-, meta- Beyond, over, between, change, transposition, as in metabolism

meter-, metr- Measure, as in metric, diameter

micro- Small, as in microorganism

milli- One thousandth the size of the basic unit, as in millimeter

mio- Less, smaller, as in miosis

mono- Single, one, as in monosaccharide

muc-, muco- Mucus, slime, as in mucosa

myo-, my- Muscle, as in myocardium

narc- Stupor, as in narcosis, narcotic

nas-, nar- Nose, as in nasal, nasopalatine

necr- Death, as in necrosis

neo-, ne- New, as in neonatal

nephro-, nephr- Kidney, as in nephritis

non- Not, no, as in nonadhesive

nucleo-, nucle- Nucleus, as in nucleoprotein

ob- Against, toward, as in oblique, obliterate

ocul- Eye, as in oculist, oculomotor

odont-, odonto- Pertaining to teeth, as in odontoma, odontogenic

-oma Tumor, swelling, as in lipoma

op-, ops-, -opia Sight, eye, as in optics, myopia

or-, os- Mouth, as in oral

orific- Opening, as in orifice

ortho-, orth- Straight, normal, as in orthodontics

-osis Condition, disease, intensive, as in cyanosis

oss-, ost-, oste- Bone, as in osseous, ossification

oz- Smell, as in ozena, ozone

pan- All, entire, general, as in panacea

para- Alongside, beyond, as in parasite
path-, pathy- Disease, as in pathology
-penia Lack of, as in leukopenia
per- Excessive, through, as in percussion
peri- Around, near, as in periapical
phag-, phago- Eat, as in phagocyte
pharm- Medicine, as in pharmacy
-phobia Fear, as in carcinophobia
phon- Sound, voice, as in phonetics
-phylac-, -phylax-, -phylact- To guard, protect, as in prophylactic
-plas-, -plasm- To mold, shape, form, as in gingivoplasty
-plegia, -plexy Stroke, paralysis, as in hemiplegia
pneu- Relating to air or lungs, as in pneumonia
poly- Much, many, as in polysaccharide
pon-, pont- Bridge, as in pontic, pontoon
post- After, as in postoperative
pre- Before, as in preoperative
pro- Before, in behalf of, as in prognathic
prosop- Face, as in prosopalgia
prox- Next, next to, as in proximal
pseud-, pseudo- False, as in pseudomembrane
psych- Relating to the soul or mind, as in psychiatry
-pur-, pyo- Liquid inflammatory product as in pus, suppurate, purulent
pyr-, pyro- Fire, heat, as in pyrexia, pyrogenic
-ren, -renal Kidney, as in renal, adrenal
retro- Back, backward, as in retromolar
-rhage Profuse flow, breaking, as in hemorrhage
-rhea To flow, indicating discharge, as in pyorrhea
rube- Red, as in rubella
-rupt- Break, as in rupture, interrupt
sarco- Muscle, flesh, as in sarcoma
schiz- Divide, as in schizophrenia
-sclero- Hard, relating to sclera
-scope, -scopy To see, examine, as in microscope, microscopy
semi- Half, as in semipermeable
sen- Old, as in senile, senior
sept- Fence, wall, as in septum
-sial Saliva, as in sialogogue
-somn- Sleep, as in insomnia
stom-, stomat- Mouth, orifice, as in stomatology
sub- Under, below, as in subgingival
sulc- Groove, furrow, as in sulcus
super-, supra- Above, over, as in supernumerary, supragingival
sutur- Sewing together, as in sutural
syn- With, together, as in syndrome
syncop- Fainting, as in syncope
tachy- Swift, rapid, as in tachycardia
tact- Touch, as in tactile
therap- Treatment, as in therapeutic
therm- Heat, as in thermal
thromb- Lump, clot, as in thrombin

tox- Poison, as in toxicology
trans- Beyond, across, as in transplant
tropho- Relating to nutrition, as in hypertrophic
ultra- Beyond, excess, as in ultrasonic
-uria Relating to urine, as in dextrosuria
vacu- Empty, as in vacuole, vacuum
vas-, vaso- Vessel, as in vascular
vir- Poison, as in virulent
vit- Life, as in vital, vitamin
xer-, xero- Dry, as in xerostomia
zo- Animal life, as in zoology

GLOSSARY

abrasion The wearing away or wearing down of teeth because of mastication, that is, occlusal abrasion.

abscess Pus formation that is localized and limited in extent in any part of the body.

absorption Intake of fluids and other substances through the skin, mucous membranes, lymphatic system, and blood vessels.

abutment In the case of a bridge or other prosthodontic appliance, the tooth providing the point of anchorage and support.

acid A chemical substance that in aqueous solution undergoes dissociation with the formation of hydrogen ions; pH less than 7.0.

acidogenic Acid producing; for example, acidogenic bacteria cause decalcification through the action of the acid produced by the bacteria.

acidosis Condition caused by lack of components in blood that neutralize acid in blood.

acrylic resins Plastic materials used in the fabrication of dentures and crowns and as a restorative filling material.

acute Having severe and pronounced symptoms but of short course or duration; the opposite of chronic, which means of long duration.

A.D.A. Abbreviation for The American Dental Association.

A.D.A.A. Abbreviation for The American Dental Assistants Association

A.D.H.A. Abbreviation for The American Dental Hygienists' Association.

adhesive Sticky.

adsorption A surface phenomenon with material being attracted to the surface of a substance, as in meaning of the word *adhesive*.

aerobic Microorganisms that require oxygen to live.

A.H.A. Abbreviation for American Hospital Association.

alcohol An organic compound that is volatile, colorless, and nearly odorless and tasteless. In high concentrations it may be used as a disinfectant. It is nontoxic and readily evaporates without residue. It acts by a denaturation of protein and may precipitate a protective coat around bacteria contained in blood, pus, mucus, and the like; it should not be used on instruments unless they have been cleaned.

allergy The sensitiveness of a person to a specific substance, which in turn causes no reaction in a person who is not sensitive to this substance; protein incompatibility.

alloy The product (not a chemical compound) formed as a result of combining or fusing two or more metals; a mixture of two or more metals, mutually soluble when in a molten state. (*See also amalgam.*)

alopecia Loss of hair caused by roentgen rays, usually temporary.

alpha streptococci A group of microorganisms that produce a zone of green discoloration and partial hemolysis in the medium about the colony.

alveolar process The projection of the maxillary and mandibular bones that envelops the roots of the teeth and forms their alveoli. The alveolus is the cavity or socket in the maxillary and mandibular bones in which the root of the tooth is fixed.

alveolectomy (or alveoloplasty) The shaping of the alveolar ridge by surgical procedures for the removal of bony prominences, usually in preparation for the construction of a prosthetic appliance.

alveolus (alveoli) The tooth socket in the alveolar process.

amalgam An alloy composed of two or more metals, one of which is mercury. An amalgam composed of silver, tin, copper, zinc, and mercury is used extensively in dentistry for restorations.

ameloblast A dental enamel-forming cell; one of a group of cells from which the enamel on teeth is formed.

ammeter An electrical instrument, commonly found on x-ray machines and other equipment, that registers the flow of electrical current through a circuit. In the case of an x-ray machine it registers the current flowing through the x-ray tube; the greater this current, the greater the production of penetrating radiation. Therefore the high current permits exposures to be made in a shorter time because of the increased power of the rays.

amorphous Not having a definite crystalline structure. Some dental waxes are amorphous.

ampere A unit that describes the rate at which current is flowing through a circuit. One ampere is the rate at which current will be pushed through a circuit having 1 ohm of resistance if it is pushed through by a pressure of 1 volt. The current flowing through an x-ray tube

is usually measured in milliamperes; 1 milliampere is 1/1,000 of 1 ampere. (*See also ammeter.*)

ampul (ampule) A hermetically sealed container such as is used for storing measured doses of hypodermic solutions.

amylase An enzyme that converts starch into sugar.

anarobe
   facultative Microorganism that can exist under either aerobic or anaerobic conditions.
   obligative Microorganism that exists only in the complete absence of free oxygen.

analgesia Absence of sensibility to pain; loss of sensibility to pain without loss of consciousness; first stage of general anesthesia.

anatomical Pertaining to the anatomy; structural.

ancillary Little-used term that has been replaced by auxiliary to refer to personnel who assist the dentist by working under his direction and for whose work and service the dentist assumes the responsibility.

anemia A condition in which there is a significant reduction in the number of red blood cells, which, in turn, results in reduction in the oxygen-carrying capacity of the blood.

anesthesia A loss of sensation or feeling.

anesthetic A drug that produces anesthesia, or a loss of sensation. (*See also general anesthetic; local anesthetic.*)

Angström A unit of measure that describes the wavelength of certain very high-frequency radiations. The behavior and the penetrating power of radiations vary with their frequency, which is related to their wavelength. Broadcast radio stations have wavelengths of from 200 to 600 meters, and x-rays have a wavelength of less than 1 Å, or less than one billionth of a meter.

ankylosis Union or consolidation of two similar or dissimilar hard tissues previously adjacent but not atached, as a tooth and its surrounding bone.

anneal To temper glass or metal by alternate heating and cooling.

anode The positive terminal in an electrical circuit. In the case of an x-ray tube, the target is the anode, for it has a positive charge and is bombarded by electrons that are negatively charged.

anodontia Absence of teeth.

anodyne Any agent that neutralizes or relieves pain.

anomaly A deviation from a normal standard; may be a congenital structural defect.

anoxia Oxygen deficiency; a condition in which the cells of the body do not have or cannot utilize sufficient oxygen to perform normal function.

anterior Indicates a forward position or a position in the front part of the mouth; a term commonly used to denoted the incisor teeth.

anteroposterior From the front to the rear.

antibiotic The product of an organism that may be used to destroy other disease-producing organisms.

antidote An agent that counteracts or prevents the action of a poison.

antisepsis The destruction of germs that cause disease; fermentation or putrefaction.

antiseptic A substance that stops or inhibits the growth of bacteria but does not necessarily kill them.

antrum A cavity or chamber, especially one within cheek bones.

apex The point or extremity of a conical object, such as the end of the root of a tooth, which is called the apical end of the tooth.

A.P.H.A. Abbreviation for American Public Health Association.

aphasia Defect of loss of the power of expression by speech, writing, or signs, or of comprehending spoken or written language, as a result of injury or disease of the brain centers.

apical curettement Surgical removal of infectious material surrounding the apex of a tooth root, not involving removal of the root tip.

apical foramen The tiny opening of the pulp canal at the tip end of the root of the tooth. The vessels and nerves of the dental pulp pass through the apical foramen.

apicoectomy The surgical removal of the apex of the tooth root; most often done in conjunction with, or as an adjunct to, root canal therapy.

apoplexy Sudden loss of consciousness, voluntary motion, and sensation, caused by rupture or obstruction of an artery of the brain; commonly called a stroke.

appliance A device worn by a dental patient during a course of treatment.

aqueous Watery; prepared with water.

arch, dental The curved composite structure of the natural dentition, and the residual ridge or the remains thereof after the loss of some or all of the natural teeth.

armamentarium Technically, all the instruments, equipment, medicines, books, and journals needed by the dentist, dental hygienist, or physician in his or her profession. Practically, the term as used refers only to the instruments that are used.

articulate To unite or join the teeth of one arch in the proper position with the teeth of the opposing arch.

articulator An instrument for holding the casts of jaws or teeth in the proper relationship to one another.

artifact (artefact) A structure that is not natural, such as a shadow on an x-ray film that is caused by unnatural objects or by manipulation.

artificial stone A plaster-like substance used for making dental casts. The base of artificial stone is a gypsum material, hydrocal.

asepsis A method of treatment that creates an antiseptic condition by the exclusion of microorganisms.

asphyxia Suspension of breathing and animation because the body is deprived of oxygen, as in drowning or suffocation.

aspirator An apparatus employing suction.

asporogenic Not producing spores, such as the asporogenic bacteria.

astringent A substance that causes contraction or shrinkage and arrests discharges.

ataxia Failure of muscular coordination.

atrophy The wasting away of tissue or parts through lack of use or disease.

attenuation Reducing, thinning, or weakening; reduction of the virulence of a virus or pathogenic microorganism; in radiography, the process by which a beam of radiation is reduced in energy when passing through some material.

attrition Normal wearing away by friction. In dentistry, it refers to wearing down the surfaces of the teeth by mastication of food.

autoclave A sterilizer that performs its function by the generation of high temperatures that, in turn, are created by steam under pressure.

auxiliary personnel Persons such as the dental hygienist, dental assistant, and dental laboratory technician who work under the supervision or direction of the dentist.

axial The long or vertical dimension of the tooth, or the axis of the tooth.

bacillus A microorganism that is rod shaped.

bacteremia A condition characterized by bacteria in the blood.

bacteria Microscopic, typically unicellular plants whose undifferentiated rigid cells occur as spheres, rods, or spirals.

bacterial plaque A film-like covering on the teeth which is often very difficult to see in a well-kept mouth.

bacterial spore A resistant form of bacteria encapsulated by a thick cell wall that enables the cell to survive in environments unfavorable to immediate growth and division.

bactericide A substance or agent that destroys bacteria.

bacteriostatic Inhibiting the growth of bacteria.

base A chemical substance that in solution

yields hydroxyl ions and reacts with an acid to form a salt and water. A base turns red litmus paper blue and has a pH higher than 7.0.

baseplate A sheet of wax, metal, or other material used for making trial denture setups.

benign Not malignant.

Bennett movement The sliding of the rotational center of the condyle laterally while the mandible is in movement. The lateral movement of the mandible is the result of the movement of the heads of the condyle along the lateral inclines of the mandibular or glenoid fossa.

bevel The inclination one line or surface makes with another when they are not at right angles.

bicuspids Teeth with two cusps situated between the cuspids and molars. There are eight in the full complement of permanent teeth; also called "premolars."

bifurcation Division into two parts or branches, as in the case of two roots of a tooth.

biology The science of substances or organisms that either or have been alive.

biopsy Surgical removal of tissue for microscopic examination, primarily for the purpose of diagnosing the possibility of benign or malignant tumors.

bite-wing radiograph (or x-ray) A specific type of x-ray picture that shows, simultaneously, the crowns of upper and lower posterior teeth and a portion of their roots and supporting structures; generally used to diagnose the presence of dental decay in adjoining tooth surfaces.

boxing The construction of a retaining wall (usually in wax) around a dental impression, so as to hold modeling material until it sets.

bruxism The clenching or grinding of the teeth.

buccal Pertaining to the cheek. The buccal surface of a tooth is located toward the cheek.

buffer Any substance in a fluid that tends to lessen the change in hydrogen ion concentration (reaction) that otherwise would be produced by adding acids or alkalis.

bur A small rotary instrument of steel for cutting tooth structure, metal, and cement. Burs are operated by a dental engine or lathe.

burnishing Polishing by friction. Tinfoil is burnished for the purpose of adapting it to the cast.

calcareous Pertaining to a compound of calcium, such as calcium carbonate or calcium phosphate.

calcification The process by which organic tissue becomes hardened by a deposit of calcium and other inorganic salts within its substance.

calculus A hard, calcareous (calcium compound) material that is deposited on the surfaces of the crowns or roots of the teeth. Calculus may also be deposited in other parts of the body. The deposit of calculus on tooth structure is dependent upon an organic compound or matrix.

canine eminence A noticeable bulge over the cuspid tooth on the upper jaw just below and to the outside of the nose.

capsule A mucoid or gelatinous case that surrounds some bacteria and protects them from destruction.

carbohydrate Organic compound of carbon, hydrogen, and oxygen; includes starches, sugars, cellulose; formed by plants and used for growth and source of energy.

carborundum An extremely hard abrasive (harder than emery); registered trade name for silicon carbide. Carborundum stones and wheels are used in dentistry to polish restorations and teeth. They mount in the handpiece, and the unit motor makes them spin as a bur spins.

carcinoma A malignant tumor.

cardiac Pertaining to the heart.

cardiovascular Pertaining to the heart and the blood vessels.

caries Decay in tooth structure.

cariogenic Caries producing; conducive to caries.

carious Relating to decay in tooth structure.

carious lesion An area of tooth structure exhibiting caries, as identified by clinical or radiographic examination.

carrier. An infected person who harbors a specific infectious agent in the absence of discernible clinical disease and serves as a potential source of infection for man.

cartilage Firm, elastic, flexible connective tissue attached to articular bone surfaces and forming certain parts of the skeleton.

case history All the information the dentist is able to gather about a patient that will help in diagnosing and treating that patient. This information is strictly confidential.

cassette A rigid film holder in which are mounted two intensifying screens.

casting A process by which a reproduction is formed by forcing or pouring a liquid into a mold and permitting it to solidify, so that it will be of the desired shape when it has hardened.

catalyst A substance or agent that speeds up a chemical action but presumably does not enter into the chemical action itself. A so-called *negative catalyst* would slow down a chemical action.

cathode A negative terminal or electrode. In the x-ray tube, the filament is the cathode and emits the negative electrons that are attracted toward the target, which is the positive anode. (*See also anode.*)

caustic An agent that burns or corrodes and destroys living tissue; having a burning taste.

cauterize To burn, corrode, or destroy living tissue by means of a caustic substance, heated metal, or an electrical current.

cavities

one surface A carious lesion that involves a single surface of a tooth, either occlusal, buccal, labial, or lingual.

two surfaces A carious lesion that involve two adjacent tooth surfaces of an individual tooth, either the distal and occlusal surface (DO) or the mesial and occlusal surfaces (MO).

three surfaces A carious lesion that involves three tooth surfaces on an individual tooth, the mesial, occlusal, and distal surfaces (MOD).

cavity A hollow, hole, or lesion produced by dental caries.

cavity liner Material, usually a varnish, used to line the preparation in a tooth before the tooth is fitted or crowned or has an inlay placed.

c.c. Abbreviation for cubic centimeter.

C.D.A. Abbreviation for Certified Dental Assistant.

C.D.T. Abbreviation for Certified Dental (laboratory) Technician.

cementum A bone-like tissue that forms the outer surface of the roots of the tooth.

centigrade thermometer A thermometer on which there are 100 degrees between the freezing and boiling points of water; the freezing point of water is 0 degrees and the boiling point of water is 100 degrees. Temperatures are recorded in the centigrade scale for most scientific studies, whereas the Fahrenheit scale is commonly used in the United States for all non-scientific references to temperature. (*See also Fahrenheit thermometer.*)

centimeter A measurement of length. There are 100 cm. in 1 meter; 2.54 cm. equals 1 inch.

centric relation A relationship between the upper and lower jaws when the associated muscles are in balance, and one that must be considered when artificial teeth are positioned in the artificial denture.

Cephalometer A device for positioning the head for radiographic examination and measurement.

cephalometrics Scientific study of the measurements of the head.

cephalometry Measurement of the bony structure of the head using reproducible lateral and anteroposterior radiographs.

cervical Pertaining to the neck of a tooth or that portion near the junction of the crown and root of a tooth.

cervical line The line or landmark formed by the junction of the enamel and the cementum on a tooth.

cheilitis Inflammation of the lip.

chromosome One of the structures in ovum and sperm cells that are determiners of sex and other characteristics. (*See also gene.*)

chronic Of long duration; the opposite of acute, which means of short duration.

cingulum The lingual lobe of an incisor tooth.

clasp An integral part of a removable partial denture constructed of metal and used as a stabilizing and retaining device to keep both tooth and denture in passive apposition.

clinic, dental A physical facility to which patients are admitted for diagnosis, evaluation, and treatment of dental defects by two or more dentists practicing dentistry together.

coagulation Changing of a soluble into an insoluble protein; process of changing into a clot.

cocci Bacteria that are spherical in shape and appears in chains or clusters.

cold sterilization A process of sterilization through the use of chemical agents as a disinfectant. It is an unreliable procedure for destroying organisms and spores, and, when used for sterilization, it is necessary to follow a rigid regime. The use is usually limited to instruments that do not lend themselves to other methods of sterilization or to instruments that have sharp cutting surfaces that must be maintained.

colloid A mixture in which the dispersed particles are aggregates of molecules, which makes them larger than the particles or molecules that characterize the substance of a solution.

coma Prolonged loss of consciousness that does not reverse by itself.

complete denture A dental prosthesis that replaces the lost natural dentition and associated structures of the entire maxilla or mandible.

compound A chemical compound is one that has been formed as a result of a chemical reaction between two or more elements. The term *compound* is frequently employed in dental laboratories and clinics to refer to the wax-like substances that can be molded when heated.

congenital Existing at the time of birth.

contact point The area of a tooth's surface that touches a neighboring tooth.

contra-angle Attachment for straight handpiece that permits burs, stones, and disks to be used at a more effective angle in the mouth.

coronal Referring to the crown or visible portion of a tooth, as seen in the mouth.

corrode To wear away, as by the chemical action that occurs on the surface of a metal, as rusting and tarnishing.

C.P. An abbreviation used on labels for chemicals, which means that the substance meets the standards that permits it to be labeled as "chemically pure."

crown The portion of a tooth that is normally covered with enamel and that projects from the tissues in which the root is fixed. The portion that is visible under any normal or abnormal conditions is the *clinical crown*, but the portion that meets the basic definition is called the *anatomical crown*. An *artificial crown* is a cap of metal or plastic that acts as a restoration for the *natural crown*.

crown and bridge That branch of dental science primarily concerned with the replacement of missing or naturally destroyed teeth or tooth structures by use of permanent nonremovable dental prostheses or restorations.

curettage Scraping with surgical instruments.

curve of Spee An imaginary curve passing through the condyles and the cuspid teeth to the incisal edge of the lower centrals. A compensating curve; an imaginary line that contacts the tips of the buccal cusps of the bicuspids and molars extending to the condyles.

cusp A pronounced elevation, or point, on or near the masticating or occlusal surface of the tooth.

cuspid A tooth with one point or cusp. There are four cuspids in the permanent dentition, one on either side in each jaw situated at the corners of the mouth.

cutaneous Relating to the skin.

cuticle, primary A delicate membrane covering the crown of a newly erupted tooth; produced by the ameloblasts after they produce the enamel rods; also call Nasmyth's membrane.

cyanosis Blueness of the skin often caused by insufficient oxygenation of the blood.

cyst A sac-like structure containing liquid or other material, which may be normal or pathological.

cytology, oral exfoliative The microscopic diagnostic study of cells that have desquamated (fallen away) from the external or internal surfaces of the body. A diagnostic procedure used to asist in the detection of oral tumors.

D.D.S. An abbreviation to indicate Doctor of Dental Surgery, the academic degree given for the completion of the formal 4 years of study in an accredited dental school. The curriculum is essentially the same as that for the degree of D.M.D. (*See also* **D.M.D.**)

debilitant An agent for inducing weakness; a remedy that allays excitement.

decalcification Process by which calcium salts and other inorganic substances are removed.

deciduous That which will be shed, specifically the first dentition of man or animal; same as primary teeth.

DEF rate Similar to the DMF rate but used for primary dentition (baby teeth); the letter D, which stands for decayed primary teeth indicated for filling, and the letter F, which represents filled primary teeth, have the same meaning as in DMF. The letter E, however, represents only decayed teeth indicated for extraction. Missing teeth are not counted for this rate, since they often cannot be differentiated from teeth lost through natural exfoliation.

deglutition The act of swallowing.

dehydration Removal of water; the condition resulting from undue loss of water.

dental assistant A person employed by a dentist to perform chairside duties and any other duties assigned and supervised by the dentist.

   certified A dental assistant who has received formal training in dental assisting and who has met all requirements of the certification board of the American Dental Assistants Association.

   chairside Specifically, a dental assistant who assists the dentist in the rendering of dental treatment.

   coordinating A dental assistant who asists the dentist and the chairside assistant and in general coordinates the work procedures in the dental operating room.

   currently certified A dental assistant who has met the requirements of the certification board of the American Dental Assistants Association and has renewed her certificate annually.

dental health education A term commonly used in dentistry for instructing the patient in preventive and corrective methods.

dental health team A relatively new concept to the practice of dentistry, composed of the dentist, as the pivotal member, and a group of specially trained persons whom he employs and supervises in the performance of certain clearly defined duties. These persons are referred to as auxiliary personnel.

dental hygienist A person trained in and practicing the art of dental prophylaxis. Generally the only licensed person, other than a dentist, who receives specific training in dental health education and who is permitted to work directly within the oral cavity.

dental stone Materials that have essentially the same composition as plaster of Paris ($CaSO_4$)$_2$ · H_2O. However, the crystal differs physically and these materials are much stronger and harder. They are used to make dies and models from which inlays, crowns, and other dental appliances can be fabricated. Hydrocal is the proprietary name for dental stone.

dental technician A person self-employed or employed by a dentist or dental laboratory company who is essentially concerned with the fabrication of dental appliances or devices on the direct prescription or work order of the licensed practitioner.

dentifrice A substance, such as tooth powder or toothpaste, used with a toothbrush for the purpose of cleansing the accessible surfaces of the teeth.

dentin (dentine) The tissue that constitutes the chief substance of the tooth.

dentition A term that is used to designate the general character and arrangement of the teeth, taken as a whole.

dentoenamel junction The line of demarcation between enamel and dentin. Enamel can be deposited only on dentin.

dentofacial deformities Disabling abnormalities of the teeth, oral cavity, and face, usually congenital in origin; for example, oral clefts, severe malocclusion.

denture Artificial teeth that replace the natural dentition. A complete denture replaces all of the teeth in an arch, while a partial denture replaces only a portion of them. A denture also may replace tissues or structures adjacent to the teeth themselves.

fixed partial A restoration of one or more missing teeth that cannot readily be removed by the patient or dentist. It is permanently attached to natural teeth or roots that furnish the primary support to the appliance, generally referred to as a bridge.

immediate A dental prosthesis constructed for insertion immediately following the extraction of natural teeth.

partial An artificial replacement of one or more, but less than all, of the natural teeth and associated structures.

removable partial A prosthetic appliance that artificially replaces missing teeth and associated structures in a partially endentulous jaw and that can be removed from the mouth and replaced at will; it depends in part on the oral mucosa for its support.

desensitization Process of removing the reactivity or sensitivity.

desquamation Shedding or casting off, as of the superficial epithelium of mucous membrane or skin; a normal physiological process.

detergent A cleansing agent.

developmental grooves Fine, depressed lines in the enamel of a tooth that mark the junction of its lobes.

diabetes An inheritable, constitutional disease of unknown case, characterized by the failure of the body tissues to oxidize carbohydrate at a normal rate. It manifests itself in an excess of sugar in the blood, presence of sugar in the urine, and, in more advanced stages, acidosis and coma, with symptoms of intense thirst and hunger, weakness, and loss of weight.

diagnosis The procedures for the purpose of determining the nature or cause of a disease; also, the identification of the disease.

diagnostic services Procedures such as radiographs, clinical examinations, biopsies, blood tests, study models, and vitality tests that assist the dentist in determining the disease conditions present and the treatment required.

diastema A space or cleft; in dentistry, a space between teeth.

die An exact replica or model of an article or object, usually fabricated from metal or stone.

digital Pertaining to the fingers.

diplococci A pair of spherical cells adhering together, somewhat elongated; they are parasitic, growing best in the animal body.

direct flame sterilization A procedure using an open flame to sterilize needles and other metal materials.

direct technic A procedure for the preparation of casting of gold inlays or crowns. In this technic the wax pattern is formed and carved directly on the tooth that is being restored. (*See also indirect technic.*)

disease A deviation from a state of good health; a disturbance in the function of any organ of the body.

disinfectant An agent that effectively kills pathogenic microorganisms, including bacteria, viruses, and fungi.

distal Pertaining to a distant location or position. The distal surface of a tooth is the surface most distant from the median line.

D.M.D. Abbreviation for *Doctor of Dental Medicine.* (*See also* **D.D.S.**)

DMF rate For an individual, the number of permanent teeth (or for a group, the average number) that are decayed (D), missing (M) or indicated for extraction, and filled (F). The DMF rate is a measure of the cumulative effects of dental caries and a useful means for comparing the lifetime dental decay experience of groups of comparable age.

dram (drachm) A unit weight. One dram equals ⅛ apothecaries' ounce, or 60 grains.

dry heat sterilization A method of sterilization

that utilizes elevated temperature (about 160° C. or 320° F.) created in an oven.

ductile Describing the physical nature of a metal, indicating that it can be drawn into thin wires or hammered into thin sheets.

dysfunction A lack or impairment of function.

dysplasia An abnormality of development.

ectoderm The outermost of the three primitive germ layers of the embryo. From it are derived the epidermis and epidermic tissues, such as the nails, hair, and glands of the skin, the nervous system, the external sense organs (eye, ear, and the like), and the mucous membrane of mouth and anus.

edema Excessive accumulation of fluid in the tissues that causes swelling.

edentulous Without teeth.

electromagnetic spectrum Electromagnetic waves, including light waves, roentgen rays, radio waves, and many others whose characteristics depend upon their frequency or wavelength. The electromagnetic spectrum refers to the array of these rays, ranging from the shortest wavelength (highest frequency) to the longest wavelength (lowest frequency).

electron Negatively charged particle; unit of negative electricity; the arrangement and number of electrons when revolving about the nucleus of an atom determine many of the physical and chemical properties of the element.

embolus A clot or bit of foreign substance that obstructs the flow of blood in a vessel.

embrasure The opening with sloping sides formed by the adjacent surfaces of teeth.

embryo The fetus in its earlier stages of development, especially before the end of the second month.

emesis basin A basin, usually kidney shaped, used for receiving material expectorated or vomited.

emulsion A mixture of two liquids, neither of which is soluble in the other, as in the case of minute oil globules dispersed throughout water. *photographic* A gelatinous solution containing silver salts.

enamel The hard, calcified tissue that covers the dentin of the crown portion of a tooth.

endocrine glands Glands that secrete internally.

endodontics A branch of dentistry that deals with the treatment of pulpless teeth.

enzyme A complex chemical substance that acts to expedite and to catalyze the digestive process.

epidemiology The scientific study of diseases from the standpoint of their distribution and frequency of occurrence.

epithelium The covering of the skin and mucous membranes.

erosion In dentistry, the destruction of superficial layers of the tooth at the neck, beginning with the enamel and working inward. It is probably the result of a combination of chemical action and abrasion. The cavities have dense and polished surfaces.

eruption The process of a new tooth entering the mouth from its place of formation.

erythema Redness of the skin.

esthetic Appreciation of the beautiful in nature and art.

ethics The science of right conduct.

etiology The study or science related to the cause of any disease.

exfoliation The shedding of a horny layer or the shedding of a tooth, as in the case of a child losing his deciduous teeth.

exodontics A branch of dentistry that deals with the extraction of teeth. (*See also extraction.*)

exposure 1. An opening into the pulp chamber of a tooth, usually the result of injury or decay, whereby the pulp is brought into contact with the oral environment (including bacteria and saliva). 2. The time that ionization produced by an x-ray machine is permitted to come in contact with the object being radiographed. 3. A procedure whereby surgical removal of tissue permits an unerupted tooth to be visible within the oral cavity.

extraction The separation and surgical removal of a tooth from its natural state.

extraoral Outside the mouth.

exudate The material composed of serum, fibrin, and white blood cells in variable amounts that escapes from blood vessels into a superficial lesion of an area of inflammation.

F.A.C.D. Abbreviation for Fellow of American College of Dentists.

face bow An instrument or caliper-like device that is used to record the relationship of the maxillae to the temporomandibular joint.

facial surface Term used to designate the buccal and labial surfaces of the teeth collectively.

Fahrenheit thermometer A thermometer whose scale carries the name of its originator, G. D. Fahrenheit (1686-1736). On this thermometer the freezing point of water is 32° F.; the average normal body temperature is 98.6° F.; and the boiling point of water is 212° F. This temperature scale is used almost exclusively in the United States for everything except scientific experiments and research, for which the centigrade thermometer scale is used. (*See also Centigrade thermometer.*)

febrile Pertaining to fever; feverish.

fetus The unborn offspring in the uterus after the second month.

F.I.C.D. Abbreviation for Fellow of International College of Dentists.

film badge A pack containing a radiographic film or films to be used for the detection and measurement of radiation exposure in personnel monitoring.

filter

    added Objects placed within the x-ray beam for the specific purpose of absorbing some of the wavelengths. In dental x-ray machines the common filter material is aluminum.

    inherent Objects in the path of the x-ray beam that absorb some of the longer wavelengths, for example, the glass of the x-ray tube and the oil in which the tube is immersed.

    total In the case of filters used in the path of an x-ray beam this includes inherent filters plus added filters.

fissure A fault in the surface of a tooth caused by imperfect joining; a deep ditch or cleft; commonly the result of the imperfect fusion of the enamel of the adjoining dental lobes.

fistula A narrow passage or duct leading from one cavity to another, as from a periapical abscess to the oral cavity.

flora Bacteria living in various parts of the digestive tract.

    oral The microorganisms inhabiting the oral cavity of an individual, that live together in a symbiotic relationship.

flow The change in the shape of a material when placed under a stationary load. This generally may be considered a measure of plasticity. It is usually associated with noncrystalline substances, although there is an outstanding exception in amalgam.

fluorescence The property certain bodies manifest when irradiated; they emit light of a different wavelength from that of the light they absorb.

fluoridation The addition of fluoride to a community water supply as an aid in the control of dental caries, usually in quantities of 1 part per million (1 p.p.m.).

fluoride, topical application The direct application of solution of fluoride, usually sodium fluoride or stannous fluoride, to the crowns of the teeth as a measure for partially preventing the incidence of dental caries. Application is recommended on a routine basis through childhood and adolescence.

fluorosis The result of consuming excessive amounts of fluorine, as in the case of the enamel surface becoming mottled from drinking excessively fluoridated water.

focal infection A type of infection in which the bacteria are localized primarily in one place, such as in the tonsils or periodontal tissue, and sent into the blood supply from that focal point.

focal spot The area on the tungsten wafer in the anode that is bombarded by the electron stream and from which roentgen rays emanate.

foil, gold Small pellets of rolled gold foil that are malleted into a cavity preparation to restore the function and shape of a tooth; a type of dental restoration.

foramen A hole or perforation, such as the foramen in bone through which nerves or vessels pass.

formaldehyde solution A colorless, volatile fluid used as a surgical and general antiseptic and preservative.

fossa A round or angular depression in the surface of a tooth. Fossae occur mostly in the occlusal surfaces of the molars and in the lingual surfaces of the incisor.

four-handed dentistry The new concept in the practice of dentistry that utilizes the chairside assistant as the dentist's second pair of hands to perform dental treatment.

fracture The breaking of a cartilage or a bone.

frenectomy Surgical removal of the labial or lingual frenum (frena).

frenum

    labial The band of tissue that passes from the inside of the lip to a point midway between the central incisors.

    lingual The band of tissue that passes from under the tongue to the lingual aspect of the midpoint of the lower jaw.

fringe benefits Benefits, such as a health insurance, vacations, and disability income, provided either as a result of collective bargaining or unilaterally by the employer.

fulcrum The point of a lever system that is stationary. Being stationary, the "rest" finger position used in prophylactic technics acts as a fulcrum to provide security and surety of lever movement.

fumigation Exposure to the fumes of sulfur or to the action of a disinfectant gas. (This method of sanitation of premises is presently believed to be ineffective.)

fungicide An element or compound capable of inducing the destruction of fungi.

fusion The act of melting; uniting, as by melting together.

gamma streptococci Members of the streptococci family in which no change occurred in the medium surrounding the colonies.

gel A gelatin-like substance, generally containing large quantities of water or other liquid. Gels are actually solid forms of colloids and are extensively used as elastic impression materials, reversible hydrocolloid, alginates, and silica gels.

gene One of the hereditary germinal units in the chromosomes that carries a hereditarily transmissible character.

general anesthetic A drug, such as ether and nitrous oxide, that produces anesthesia throughout the entire body, as opposed to a local anesthetic, where the anesthesia is localized in one portion of the body or around one area of tissue.

germicide Any substance that kills germs.

gerodontics That branch of dentistry that treats all problems peculiar to the oral cavity in old age and aging including clinical problems of senescence and senility.

gingiva The portion of tissue enveloping the necks of the teeth crown-wise from the attachment at the gingival line.

gingivectomy The surgical removal of diseased gingiva with scaling and root planing of the tooth surfaces to eliminate periodontal pockets.

glossitis Inflammation of the tongue.

gram Unit of weight in metric system; 454 grams equals 1 pound.

grit The size of abrasive particles.

groove A long depression in the surface of a tooth.

guards The position assumed by the thumb and fingers of the left hand to steady the parts operated upon and protect them from injury in case of accidental slipping of the instrument.

gutta-percha A sticky, gum-like material obtained from the juice of various trees found in the Malayan peninsula (a temporary stopping).

halitosis Offensive or bad breath; may be related to systemic disease or uncleanliness of the oral cavity.

health State of complete physical, mental, and social well-being, not merely the absence of disease.

heavy metals Names given to those metals that have a relatively high molecular weight. Heavy metals such as silver, mercury, and copper inhibit bacterial growth in low concentrations and are bacteriostatic.

hematoma A blood clot formed from blood that has been released by trauma or pathology and that accumulates within a tissue.

hepatitis, infectious A disease of the liver whose incidence is related to close communal living. The virus is very resistant to heat, cold, chlorine, and alcohol. The incubation period is approximately 30 days. Prevention of the disease is dependent upon the maintenance of high levels of sanitation and personal hygiene. The only safe method for sterilizing instruments as far as this disease is concerned is boiling and autoclaving for 15 minutes.

histology The scientific study of the structure and composition of the tissues.

homogeneous Uniform, similar in makeup throughout.

hormone A chemical substance produced in an organ that, when carried to an associated organ by the bloodstream, influences its functional activity.

horn, pulpal A slender or blunt-pointed process of the pulp of a tooth extending toward the point of a cusp.

host Plant or animal in or on which a parasite lives.

hot water sterilization Most widely applicable agent for sterilization of inanimate objects; immersion of articles in boiling water (100° C., or 212° F.) for 10 to 20 minutes. This method is quick and economical, requires no special apparatus, leaves no toxic residue, has great penetrating power, and is harmless to a wide variety of materials, but it should not be used for cutting instruments.

hydrated Combined with water.

hydrocal See dental stone.

hypercementosis An excessive formation of cementum, usually at the apical portion of the root of a tooth, giving a bulbous appearance.

hyperpituitarism Excessive activity of the pituitary gland.

hyperplasia Abnormal increase in the number of cells.

hypersecretion Excessive secretion.

hypertrophy Abnormal increase in the size of the cells.

hypnotic Inducing sleep.

hypo A prefix meaning either a deficiency or beneath, as in "hypothyroidism," "hypodermic," and "hypogastric"; not to be confused with the chemical solution, sodium hyposulfite, which is often called a "hypo" solution.

hypochlorites A salt of hypochlorous acid; used as a disinfectant for *Brucella* species (undulant fever).

hypochlorous acid An acid used as a bleach or a disinfectant.

hypothyroidism Morbid state produced by deficient secretion by the thyroid gland.

idiopathic Self-originated; of unknown cause.

idiosyncrasy Any tendency, characteristic, or the like peculiar to an individual.

immunity The condition of an organism that permits it to resist disease.

impacted tooth Commonly, a tooth embedded in either the soft or bony tissues of the jaw in such a way that it has not erupted or has erupted only partially.

implantation The placement within body tissues of a foreign substance—for example, metal or plastic—for restoration by mechanical means.

impression A negative likeness of a form or model. Impressions are made of tissues in order to produce models of the original tissues.

in vitro Outside the living body; in a test tube or other artificial environment.

in vivo Refers to vital processes occurring in the living being.

incipient Beginning to exist, coming into existence.

incisal edge The surface of an incisor or a cuspid that is the cutting edge.

incisor A tooth with a cutting edge. There are four incisors in the upper jaw and four in the lower jaw, called the upper and lower right and left central incisors and the upper and lower right and left lateral incisors.

inclination

of a surface The deviation of a portion of the surface of a tooth from the general plane of that surface.

of a tooth The deviation of the long axis of a tooth from the perpendicular line, as the mesial inclination of the incisors.

incubation The keeping of a microbial or tissue culture in an incubator to facilitate development.

incubation period The time between exposure to a communicable disease and the appearance of clinical symptoms.

indirect technic A technic in which an impression is taken of the tooth or teeth after the cavity preparations have been made. Models, generally stone, are then made, and the wax patterns are fabricated on this die outside the mouth. (*See also* *direct technic*).

inert Without intrinsic active properties; no inherent power of action, motion, or resistance.

infectious disease An impairment of function that an organism suffers because of the activities of some other organism that lives within or upon it.

inflammation A reaction of living tissue to injury; a defense reaction of the body characterized by heat, redness, swelling, pain, and loss of function.

inlay, dental A dental inlay is generally a cast-gold restoration prepared by making a wax pattern to fit the cavity preparation, carved to restore the missing anatomy of the tooth. This pattern is reproduced in gold by casting and is then cemented in the tooth.

instrument exchange The passing and receiving of hand and rotary insrtuments between the dentist and the chairside assistant.

instrument exchange area The designated place where the dentist and chairside assistant exchange hand and rotary instruments. The exchange area is directly in front of the patient's chin, never more than 2 to 4 inches from the operating zone. In children or apprehensive patients, the exchange area may be directly behind the patient's head.

instrument grasps The manner of grasping and holding instruments to their work. The four fundamental instrument grasps are inverted pen, palm and thumb, palm-thrust, and pen grasps.

inverted pen Similar to the pen grasp, except that the position of the instrument is reversed, so that the working part points toward instead of away from the operator.

palm and thumb The handle of the instrument rests in the palm of the hand and is grasped by the four fingers, while the thumb usually rests on some adjoining surface.

palm-thrust The end of the large handle is grasped in the center of the palm, the shank being held between the balls of the thumb and first and second fingers.

pen The instrument is held like a pen, the shank being in contact with the thumb and first and second fingers.

interdental Situated between the teeth.

interdigitation Meshing of upper and lower cusps in occlusion.

interproximal space The v-shaped space bounded by the proximate surfaces of the adjoining teeth and the border of the septum of the alveolar process. Normally, this space is filled with gum tissue.

investing The utilization of a substance (investment material) for covering an object, such as a tooth, in order to produce the mold that will be used to fabricate artificial crowns, inlays, and so on.

investment A material for enveloping or embedding a cast or denture in a flask.

ion An atom or group of atoms having a charge of positive or negative electricity.

ionize To render a substance electrically conductive by the production in it of small electrified particles or ions. Ionization takes place when a substance (such as a compound) breaks up into its ions, which in turn have an electrical charge, thus rendering the material conductive.

jacket A specific type of crown, generally fabricated of porcelain or acrylic resin or a combination of precious metal and porcelain or acrylic resin; often called a cap.

jaundice A condition in which there are bile pigments in the blood and deposition of bile pigments in the skin and mucous membranes with resulting yellowish appearance.

keratinization The production of a horny or hard tissue.

kilo A prefix meaning one thousand, as in "kilogram," "kilovolt," and "kilometer."

kilovolt A unit of 1,000 volts.

labial Pertaining to the lips, as a position toward the lips. The labial surface of a tooth (incisor or cuspid) is that surface that is close to the lips.

laboratory stone See *dental stone*.

lacerations Breaks or cuts.

Lactobacillus A rod-shaped organism that has been isolated from the alimentary tract of man and animals, from carious teeth, and from milk that has undergone fermentation.

lamina dura Thin, hard bone lining the tooth socket.

lesion Any change in continuity of a tissue caused by disease or injury, or the loss of function of a part.

ligature A cord, thread, or wire used to tie off or bind. One type is used to hold rubber dam in place. Another type is used in an orthodontic appliance.

lingual Pertaining to the tongue, as a position toward the tongue. The lingual surface of a tooth is the surface that is close to the tongue. All teeth have lingual surfaces.

liter Unit of volume measurement in metric system; 1 liter equals 0.908 quarts dry and 1.057 quarts liquid.

lobe A part of a tooth formed by any one of the separate points of the beginning of calcification.

local anesthetic A drug that produces anesthesia in one portion of the body or around one area of tissue, as opposed to a general anesthetic, which produces anesthesia throughout the entire body.

macroglossia Enlargement of the tongue.

malaise The French word for *illness;* any indisposition, discomfort, or distress.

malar Referring to the cheek or cheekbone.

malignant Tending to go from bad to worse; the opposite of benign.

malocclusion Deviation from the normally accept-

able contact of the teeth in the opposing arches.

mammelons The three rounded prominences seen on the cutting edges of the incisors when they first erupt through the gums into the mouth.

mandible The lower jawbone.

mandibular Pertaining or referring to the mandible.

manikin Model of the human body or a part; used for teaching purposes.

marginal ridge A ridge or elevation of enamel, forming the margin of a surface of a tooth; specifically at the mesial and distal margins of the occlusal surfaces of premolars and molars and the mesial and distal margins of the lingual surfaces of incisors and canines.

mastication The act of chewing.

materia medica The division or branch of science that deals with the preparation of medicines.

maxilla The upper jawbone.

maxillary Pertaining or referring to the maxillae.

median line The periphery of the median plane; the vertical, central line dividing the body into right and left.

medication Administration of remedies; a medical agent.

membrane A thin layer of tissue that covers a surface or divides a space or organ.

mesial Toward or situated in the middle, as toward the median line of the dental arch. Those surfaces of the teeth that, as they stand in the arch and, following its curve, are toward the median line, are called mesial surfaces.

metabolism The total of chemical changes occurring in the body; chemical process of transforming foods into complex tissue elements and of transforming complex body substances into simple ones, along with the production of heat and energy.

metastasis The transfer of disease from one organ or body part to another, as in the case of a transfer of cells through blood vessels or lymph channels.

meter Unit of distance measurement in metric system; 1 meter equals 1.094 yards.

microorganisms Animal or vegetable organisms too small to be seen without a microscope.

microscope Instrument with a lens or combination of lenses for making small things look large.

milliampere One thousandth part of an ampere.

milliampere-second The product of the number of milliamperes of tube current, multiplied by the number of seconds of the exposure; used to designate the factors of a roentgenogram.

milliroentgen One thousandth part of a roentgen.

molar A grinding tooth.

morphology A branch of biology that deals with

the form and structure of animals or plants during any stage of their life.

mucin A glycoprotein found in the secretions of the mucous glands.

mucous membrane The moist, pink membrane that lines the mouth, nasal cavities, and alimentary canal.

mutation A change in form or quality. In biology a permanent, transmissible change in the characters of an offspring from those of its parents.

N.A.C.D.L. Abbreviation for National Association of Certified Dental Laboratory (Technicians).

narcotic A drug that relieves pain and tends to produce stupor or sleep at the same time, depending on the dosage.

nausea Sickness at the stomach, together with a tendency to vomit.

necrosis Deadness of a certain portion of tissue, not the entire body. Dental necrosis is decay of a tooth.

neoplasm A new growth, such as a tumor.

nitrous oxide A gas used in some general anesthetics; same as "laughing gas." Its first use in dentistry was by Dr. Horace Wells in 1844.

nomenclature Terminology; a system of names in a particular science, art, or field of knowledge.

obese Excessively fat.

oblique ridge A ridge running obliquely across the occlusal surface of the upper molars. It is formed by the union of the triangular ridge of the distobuccal cusp with the distal portion of the ridge forming the mesiolingual cusp.

obturator An artificial appliance that closes an opening in the palate, prescribed for patients with cleft palates.

occlude To shut, close. (*See also occlusion.*)

occlusal The chewing or grinding surface of a tooth.

occlusion The natural closure and fitting together of upper and lower teeth; the relation of the mandibular and maxillary teeth when closed or during those excursive movements of the mandible by which masticating efficiency is obtained.

odontology The science that deals with the teeth, their structure, and their development; used frequently as a synonym for dentistry.

onlay An inlay that is built upon the occlusal or incisal edges of the tooth; often used to restore lost tooth structure and to increase the height of the tooth.

operative dentistry The branch of dentistry primarily concerned with restoring carious, diseased, or damaged natural teeth to a satisfactory state of health, function, and esthetics.

oral examination Those procedures performed by a dentist that aid in making diagnostic conclusions about the oral health of an individual patient.

oral medicine The branch of dentistry that deals with the diagnosis and treatment of diseases of the oral cavity in the perspective of their relationship to diseases or conditions in other parts of the body.

oral pathology The branch of dentistry concerned with the study of disease processes of the hard and soft tissues of the oral cavity.

oral surgery The branch of dentistry concerned with operative procedures in and about the oral cavity and jaws.

organism A plant or animal having organs or an organized structure.

orthodontics The branch of dentistry that deals with the prevention and correction of irregularities of the teeth and malocclusion.

osmosis The passage of solvents or solutions through a semipermeable membrane that is selective in the substances it will permit to pass.

osteology The scientific study of bones and their structures.

oxidation The act of oxidizing or combining with oxygen.

oxidizing agent Anything which produces oxidation (such as the excess of oxygen in the flame of a blowtorch applied to casting gold).

oxygen A colorless, odorless, gaseous element that combines readily with most elements. It is necessary to all animal and vegetable life and for combustion. It makes up 20% by weight of the atmosphere and about 88% of water.

palate The roof of the mouth.

    cleft A palate with a fissure in the median line of the roof of the mouth, present at birth.

    hard The anterior part of the roof of the mouth, the bony palate.

    soft The posterior part of the palate near the uvula.

palliative Treatment of pain or discomfort affording relief from the primary concern of pain but not necessarily effecting cure.

palpation The act of applying fingers lightly to the surface of the body to determine the condition of the parts beneath in physical diagnosis.

palpitation Rapid beating of the heart.

papilla A small nipple-shaped elevation.

    incisive A rounded projection at the anterior end of the palate.

    interdental The triangular pad of gum that fills the space between the necks of the teeth.

lingual Any one of the papillae of the tongue.

paradental personnel Term coming into usage for reference to the auxiliary dental personnel such as dental hygienists, dental assistants, and dental laboratory technicians.

paramedical personnel Auxiliary medical personnel, such as nurses, medical technicians, and medical laboratory technicians.

pasteurization sterilization Process used in food sterilization. Fluid held at 143° F. for 30 minutes or 160° F. for 15 minutes is pasteurized. This process kills all vegetable cells of pathogenic bacteria; its purpose is to disinfect and to postpone spoilage.

pathogenic Disease-producing.

pathology The science that deals with the nature of disease and its causes and effects.

pedodontics The branch of dentistry that deals with dental conditions of children.

periapical Pertaining to that area of the tooth around the apex (tip) of the root.

pericoronitis Inflammation of the soft tissues surrounding the crown of an erupting tooth; frequently seen in association with erupting mandibular third molars and usually accompanied by infection.

periodontal Surrounding a tooth, as the periodontal membrane.

periodontics The branch of dentistry that deals with the prevention and treatment of diseases of the bone and soft tissues surrounding the teeth.

periodontium Surrounding a tooth, such as the periodontal membrane.

periphery The outward part or the surface or border; a term frequently used to describe the border of a denture or an impression.

permanent teeth The teeth of adult age, as distinguished from the deciduous (temporary or primary) teeth.

pH The symbol of a value that denotes the degree of acidity of a material. It is dependent upon the amount of ionizable hydrogen present. A pH of 7 is considered neutral; a value of less than 7 is acidic; a value greater than 7 is basic or alkaline, with a pH of 14 being the upper limit of alkalinity.

phagocyte White blood cell that usually engulfs bacteria or foreign bodies. Other tissue cells such as the giant cell also may destroy bacteria by this engulfing process.

pharmacology The scientific study of drugs.

phenol coefficient Germicidal power of a chemical; represents the strength of an antiseptic, relative to that of phenol; a measure of antibacterial activity that can be quantitated readily and expressed mathematically.

phonetics The study of the production and understanding of speech sounds, including variations by individuals and groups. Phonetics also includes the classification of the sounds produced.

pit A sharp, pointed depression in the enamel. Pits occur mostly where several developmental grooves join, as in the occlusal surfaces of the molars and at the endings of the buccal grooves on the buccal surfaces of the molars.

plaster of Paris See dental stone.

pneumatic Pertaining to gas or air. Some dental instruments are operated by air pressure, that is, by pneumatic pressure.

pocket A gingival sulcus pathologically deepened by periodontal disease.

point angles The meeting of three surfaces at a point, forming a corner. Those angles formed by the junction of three surfaces, as the mesiobuccoocclusal point angle.

pontic The portion of a dental bridge that replaces the missing tooth.

porte-polisher A hand instrument in which an orangewood point has been inserted. The point is dipped into a polishing agent and then placed on the tooth and moved up and down with a wrist movement to polish the teeth.

post-dam A raised ridge ⅛ inch wide at the posterior border of the denture, designed to seal the denture against the palate.

posterior teeth Those teeth of either jaw that are to the rear of the incisors and cuspids.

preprepared tray system A system whereby the armamentarium for a specific dental procedure is prepared in advance of usage and stored until needed.

preventive dentistry The branch of dentistry devoted primarily to averting oral diseases and inhibiting the progress of diseases already present. Some elements of prevention are inherent in all branches of dental practice.

primary dentition Specifically, the first dentition of man or animal.

prognosis The act of predicting the course or outcome, as of a disease.

prophylactic Given for the purpose of preventing disease.

prophylaxis The removal of calculus (tartar) and stains from the exposed and unexposed surfaces of the teeth by scaling and polishing.

prosthesis The replacement of an absent part of the body by one that is artificial.

prosthodontics The branch of dentistry that deals with the replacement of missing teeth and adjacent structures by artificial teeth and devices.

proximal Nearest, next, immediately preceding, or following; same as proximate.

psychosomatic Pertaining to the mind-body relationship; having body symptoms of a psychic, emotional, or mental origin.

ptyalin An enzyme found in the saliva of man and some of the lower animals, which changes starch into dextrin, maltose, and glucose.

public health dentistry That branch of dentistry concerned primarily with the prevention and control of dental diseases and the promotion of dental health through organized community efforts.

pulp The soft tissue that fills the pulp chambers and root canals of the teeth.

pulpectomy The complete surgical removal of the pulp of a tooth.

pulpotomy The partial removal of the pulp of a tooth, usually performed on children as a treatment after dental caries or a fracture has penetrated to the pulp.

pus A liquid made up of white blood cells (leukocytes) and a thin fluid called liquor puris. It is the product of inflammation.

pyogenic Refers to the production of pus.

radiation Divergence from a center; the emission of radiant energy; a structure made up of divergent elements; energy propagated through space, as in the case of radiation from x-rays or radiation of heat.

radiograph A roentgenogram; an image produced on a sensitized film by roentgen rays.

radiology The science of radiant energy and radiant substances, especially the branch of medical and dental science that deals with the use of radiant energy.

radiolucent A substance that, because of its lack of density, permits the passage of x-rays with only very light resistance. Radiolucent objects appear dark on radiographs.

radiopaque A substance that, because of its density, resists the passage of x-rays. Radiopaque objects appear light on radiographs.

ramus (ramus mandibuli) The ramus of the lower jaw—the bone back of the posterior teeth, which reaches upward to the head of the condyle.

R.D.H. Abbreviation for Registered Dental Hygienist.

rebase A process of refitting a denture by the replacement of the denture-base material without changing the occlusal relations of the teeth.

recall system Any method for periodically reminding patients to return for examination.

referral Sending a patient to another dentist or a member of another health profession, usually a specialist, for diagnosis or treatment.

rehabilitation, oral The complete reconstruction of the masticatory apparatus to as nearly a normal condition as possible; includes the replacement of lost teeth and tissue parts and the restoration of esthetics and function.

reline To resurface the tissue side of a denture with new base material to make it fit more accurately.

removable denture See denture, removable partial.

resin Certain plastic materials. Some types are used in dentistry for denture bases, artificial teeth, and filling materials.

resorption Gradual destruction of tooth root.

restoration Broad term referring to artificial structures that are constructed to replace missing structures.

restorative dentistry See operative dentistry.

rests A position of the third and fourth fingers to steady the right hand in order that the instrument may be held securely to its work without slipping.

resuscitation Restoration of life or consciousness; restoration of heartbeat and respiration.

retromolar pad Area behind the lower molar teeth.

ridge A long elevation on the surface of a tooth.

R.N. Abbreviation for Registered Nurse.

roentgen The international unit quantity of x-radiation or gamma radiation; the associated corpuscular emission per 0.001 gram of air produces, in air, ions carrying one electrostatic quantity of electricity of either sign.

roentgen ray Short-wave, high-energy radiation produced when electrons traveling at high speed impinge on various substances, especially the heavy metals.

roentgenogram See radiograph.

roentgenology The branch of radiology that deals with the diagnostic and therapeutic uses of roentgen rays.

root The portion of the tooth that is fixed in the bony walls of the alveolus, or socket, and is covered with cementum.

root canal The space within the root of a tooth containing pulp tissue and connecting the pulp chamber with the apex of the root.

R.Ph. Abbreviation for Registered Pharmacist.

ruga (rugae) Ridge, wrinkle, fold.

    palatal The irregular ridges in the mucous membrane covering the anterior part of the hard palate.

saddle Pertaining to the base. The part of the base of a denture that contacts and covers the soft tissue of the edentulous bony arch.

sarcoma Malignant neoplasm of connective tissue elements.

scaling A dental procedure performed to remove calculus (tartar) and necrotic tissue from around the necks and roots of the teeth; commonly performed in the "cleaning" of the teeth or in periodontal treatment.

screening of applicant Any examination of individuals or their records to ascertain their abilities or talents for a respective position.

sedative An agent that quiets activity and, hence, produces a state of sedation.

sepsis A poisoned state caused by the absorption into the bloodstream of pathogenic bacteria and their products from a region of infection.

septum A partition; the portion of the alveolar process that lies between the roots of the teeth, separating their alveoli.

serum The clear, liquid part of blood separated from its more solid elements after clotting; the blood plasma from which fibrinogen has been removed in the process of clotting.

silicate cement A type of dental restorative material used primarily to restore anterior teeth to their proper form, function, and esthetic coloring; occasionally referred to as "synthetic porcelain," a misnomer.

sloughing Peeling; loss of the outer tissue layer.

solubility The degree to which a substance (the solute) will dissolve in a given amount of another substance (the solvent).

solute The dissolved substance.

solution A homogenous mixture with no definite composition. The molecules of the dissolved substance (the solute) are dispersed among those of the dissolving medium (the solvent).

solvent The dissolving substance; a substance, usually a liquid, that can dissolve other substances.

space maintainer An appliance constructed for the purpose of preventing adjacent and opposing teeth from moving into the space left by teeth lost prematurely; a method of preventing malocclusion.

spasm A sudden, violent, involuntary muscular contraction.

spatulation The act of mixing or spreading with a spatula.

specialist One who has acquired special skill and knowledge beyond that acquired in either dental or medical school. In some cases, the dentist will announce to the public his area of special interest, and, in some cases, he may restrict his practice to this single area. The dental profession permits the use of the term *specialist* only in connection with those specialities that are officially recognized by the American Dental Association—oral surgery, orthodontics, prosthodontics, periodontics, pedodontics, oral pathology, and dental public health. Other groups are applying for similar recognition.

spirillum A cylindrical form of bacteria characterized by a number of bends or spirals along the long axis.

spirochete An elongated, flexible organism twisted spirally around its long axis and exhibiting motility without possessing flagella.

splint A rigid or flexible appliance for fixation of displaced or movable parts, such as broken jaws.

spore A single cell capable of growing into a new plant or animal.

sprue An attachment of metal or wax to the wax pattern that produces the funnel or channel for the molten metal after the wax pattern with sprue is invested.

staphylococci Normal body parasites; arranged in small groups or clusters.

sterilization Making incapable of reproduction; destruction or removal of all forms of life, with particular reference to organisms.

stomatology The branch of science that deals with the diseases of the mouth.

strain Used in connection with dental materials; the deformation that results when the external forces exerted become greater that the internal forces that resist them.

streptococci A group of spherical bacteria that multiply by dividing in only one direction, usually forming chains; often cause serious infections.

stress The internal resistance of a body, opposing deformation, when it is subjected to mechanical force.

study model A reproduction of an organ or part in plaster, clay, wax, stone, metal, or other material; used as an aid in diagnosis and in planning treatment of certain conditions.

subacute A transitional phase between acute and chronic.

sulcus, gingival The space between the free gingiva and the tooth.

supernumerary tooth A tooth in excess of the regular or normal number.

suppuration Formation of, conversion into, or act of discharging pus.

suture A surgical stitch; the line of junction of bones in the head; the material used to sew up a wound.

syncope The act of fainting. It is directly caused by an insufficient supply of blood to the brain.

syndrome A group of symptoms and signs that, when considered together, characterize a disease or lesion.

synthetic A substance prepared by artificial means, as opposed to a substance formed naturally.

tactile Pertaining to touch.

target In radiography, the tungsten button in the anode at which the electrons produced by the cathode are directed.

tarnish Surface discoloration on a metal, the result of oxidation.

temporomandibular joints The joints just ahead of each ear upon which the lower jaw swings open and shut and can slide forward.

terminology The complete system of scientific or technical words applying to a science, art, or subject.

therapeutic Pertaining to the treatment of disease.

therapy Treatment; specifically, the treatment of disease.

tic An involuntary purposeless movement of muscle that usually occurs under emotional stress; a twitching, especially of facial muscles.

tincture A solution in which alcohol is the solvent.

topical Pertaining to a specific location, as in the case of topical application of fluoride solutions on the teeth.

topography The detailed description and analysis of the features of an anatomical region or of a special part.

torus A bulging projection.

  mandibularis A bony prominence found in the region between the first and second bicuspids.

  palatinus A bony prominence often found in the center of the palate.

toxin Any poisonous product of animal or vegetable metabolism, especially one of those produced by bacteria and constituting the causative agents in certain diseases.

transformer An electrical instrument composed of coils that transforms or transfers electrical energy from one circuit to another, usually changing high voltage to low voltage or changing low voltage to high voltage.

traumatic Pertaining to that which has been caused by injury.

traumatic occlusion The injury to periodontal tissues caused by occlusal forces.

treatment plan A series of operations of procedures proposed to treat a specific dental disorder or disease or used for the attainment of a given state of oral health.

trituration The process of producing a powder from solid substances by rubbing.

tubercle bacillus A parasite that produces tuberculosis.

tuberosity, maxillary A broad, rough platform or eminence on the bone, located at the end of the maxillary ridge.

tumor A swelling or enlargement, especially one caused by morbid growth of a tissue not normal to the part.

typhoid bacillus A microorganism that causes typhoid fever.

ulceration A break in the continuity of overlying mucous membrane or skin.

ultrasonic Very high frequency, usually above the frequency of audible sound.

U.S.P. An abbreviation for *United States Pharmacopeia,* which is a volume of formulas that are recognized as standards.

vascular Pertaining to vessels, as blood vessels.

vasoconstrictor A substance or a nerve that causes the constriction of blood vessels.

virulence The relative infectiousness of a microorganism, or its ability to overcome the body defenses of the host.

virus One of several living agents or substances of submicroscopic size that causes certain diseases.

volt A unit of electricity that is the electrical force or pressure necessary to push electrical current at the rate of 1 ampere through a resistance of 1 ohm.

xerostomia Dryness of the mouth caused by functional or organic disturbances of the salivary glands.

x-ray See roentgen ray.

zoology The branch of biology concerned with the animal kingdom and its members as individuals as well as classes.

zygomatic arch An arch of bone commonly known as the "cheekbone." It begins just in front of the ear, arches slightly outward and forward, and then curves slightly inward to an area just below the outer corner of the eye. The "arch" portion of this bone is just above the ramus of the mandible; it is blocked by muscles.

INDEX

Boldface numerals indicate that term appears in an illustration or table. Proper names appearing in the text or in the caption of a figure are indexed; those in credit lines or in references are not indexed.